STABLE CONDITION

Stable Condition

ELITES' LIMITED INFLUENCE ON HEALTH CARE ATTITUDES

Daniel J. Hopkins

Russell Sage Foundation   NEW YORK

LIBRARY OF CONGRESS CATALOGING-IN-PUBLICATION DATA

Names: Hopkins, Daniel J., author.
Title: Stable condition : elites' limited influence on health care attitudes / Daniel J. Hopkins.
Description: New York : Russell Sage Foundation, [2023] | Includes bibliographical references and index. | Summary: "To what extent can political elites reshape public opinion through their words or policies? Stable Condition addresses that question through a detailed study of Americans' opinions about the Affordable Care Act (ACA) between 2009 and 2020. While researchers have produced a rich body of scholarship about the role of specific factors in shaping ACA attitudes, this book departs from prior research by providing a competitive assessment of several credible explanations for Americans' views on the ACA. These explanations range from personal experiences with the policy to messaging, partisanship, racial attitudes, and thermostatic responses to presidential policymaking in which the public gravitates toward the status quo. By considering varied explanations simultaneously, this book is positioned to advance this study's broader goal: the characterization of the potential for enduring elite influence on public opinion. A central tenet of representative democracy is that elected officials act with the consent of the governed, which has come to mean at least the periodic authorization of the citizenry via elections. But the prospect that political leaders can bend public opinion threatens to invert that relationship. The risk is that instead of acting on some vision of the public interest, leaders will manipulate public opinion so as to build support for their own ends. Even in a democracy, leaders may not enact the will of the people so much as reshape it to match theirs. Assessing elite influence in democracies requires us to consider its two main avenues together: messaging and policy"—Provided by publisher.
Identifiers: LCCN 2022037668 (print) | LCCN 2022037669 (ebook) | ISBN 9780871540287 (paperback) | ISBN 9781610449205 (ebook)
Subjects: LCSH: Public opinion—United States. | Health care reform—United States.
Classification: LCC HN57 .H57 2023 (print) | LCC HN57 (ebook) | DDC 362.1/04250973—dc23/eng/20220923
LC record available at https://lccn.loc.gov/2022037668
LC ebook record available at https://lccn.loc.gov/2022037669

Text design by Linda Secondari.

RUSSELL SAGE FOUNDATION
112 East 64th Street, New York, New York 10065
10 9 8 7 6 5 4 3 2 1

To my mom Alice Prince, my late father Smith Hopkins, my brother Benjamin Hopkins, and all my family members who have worked in medicine.

CONTENTS

LIST OF ILLUSTRATIONS *ix*

ABOUT THE AUTHOR *xv*

PREFACE *xvii*

Chapter 1: Introduction *1*

Chapter 2: The Elite-Level Politics and Policymaking of the ACA *22*

Chapter 3: The Stability of Public Opinion *43*

Chapter 4: Public Opinion and the Medicaid Expansion *64*

Chapter 5: The Offsetting Effects of the Exchanges *85*

Chapter 6: The Indirect Role of White Americans' Racial Attitudes *114*

Chapter 7: Framing's Limited Short-Term Impacts *145*

Chapter 8: Conclusion *177*

APPENDIX A (CHAPTER 3) *191*

APPENDIX B (CHAPTER 4) *199*

APPENDIX C (CHAPTER 5) *205*

APPENDIX D (CHAPTER 6) *219*

APPENDIX E (CHAPTER 7) *225*

NOTES *231*

REFERENCES *261*

INDEX *301*

ILLUSTRATIONS

Figures

Figure 3.1 Support for Repealing the ACA over Time, by 2008 Partisanship, 2012–2020 *48*

Figure 3.2 Favorable Attitudes toward the ACA over Time, 2010–2020 *50*

Figure 3.3 The Prevalence of Arguments in Favor of the ACA, 2009–2018 *53*

Figure 3.4 The Prevalence of Arguments against the ACA, 2009–2018 *54*

Figure 3.5 The Prevalence of Mentions of Personal Experience and References to Salient Social Groups in Public Opinion about the ACA, 2009–2018 *58*

Figure 3.6 Favorability toward ACA Repeal When the Program Is Presented as the Status Quo and When It Is Not, September 2017 *62*

Figure 4.1 Support for Medicaid Expansion in Maine as a Function of Share of Town with Public Assistance Income, 2017 *71*

Figure 4.2 Support for Medicaid Expansion in Oklahoma as a Function of Share of County with Public Assistance Income, 2020 *73*

Figure 4.3 Proportion of Medicaid Recipients and Favorability toward the ACA before and after Expansion *76*

Figure 4.4 Relationship between Medicaid Receipt and ACA Favorability over Time *81*

Figure 5.1 Distribution of HTP Respondents by Health Insurance Source before and after the ACA's January 2014 Implementation *95*

Figure 5.2 ACA Favorability by Health Insurance Status and Source, 2010–2018 *96*

Figure 5.3 ACA Attitudes among Respondents to the 2012–2018 ISCAP Panel Who Completed the November–December 2016 and October 2018 Waves *100*

Figure 5.4 Smoothed Favorability Ratings for Sixty-Four-Year-Olds and Sixty-Five-Year-Olds, 2010–2018 *106*

Figure 5.5 Change in HTP Respondents' ACA Attitudes Associated with Turning Sixty-Five Pre- and Post-ACA Implementation *108*

Figure 5.6 Average ACA Favorability among HTP Respondents by Age, 2011–2019 *110*

Figure 6.1 White Americans' Perceptions of the ACA's Beneficiaries, 2016 *123*

Figure 6.2 Regression Coefficients and Confidence Intervals for White Respondents' 2012–2013 Anti-Black Prejudice (–1 to 1) When Predicting Support for Repealing the ACA over Time (1 to 7) *127*

Figure 6.3 Variable Correlations for White Respondents, 2018 *132*

Figure 6.4 Variable Correlations for All Respondents, 2018 *133*

Figure 6.5 ACA Favorability among White Voters in Calhoun County, Alabama, by Experimental Racial Prime and Presidential Preference, 2017 *136*

Figure 6.6 ACA Favorability among White Voters in Online Patient Survey by Experimental Racial Prime, 2018 *138*

Figure 6.7 ACA Favorability among White Voters in SSI Survey by Experimental Racial Prime and Political Party Identification, 2018 *140*

Figure 6.8 Attitudes toward Expanding the ACA among White Activists by Experimental Racial Prime and Political Party Identification, 2016 *141*

Figure 6.9 Attitudes toward Expanding the ACA among White Voters by Experimental Racial Prime and Presidential Preference, 2017 *142*

Figure 7.1 Support for the ACA under Different Experimental Trust-Related Frames, 2011, 2017, and 2018 *156*

Figure 7.2 Number of U.S. Senators' Health Care–Related Press Releases by Month, Key Legislative Events, and Select Surveys, 2009–2010 *160*

Figure 7.3 Variation in Topics over Time in Senators' Press Releases, 2009–2010 *161*

Figure 7.4 Variation in Open-Ended Responses from Health Care Reform Supporters and Opponents over Time, 2009–2010 *166*

Figure 7.5 Difference in Citizens' Word Usage for ACA Supporters and Opponents as a Function of Each Word's Frequency on the Log Scale, 2009–2010 *169*

Figure 7.6 Distances or Correlations between Words Used in Senators' Press Releases and All Survey Respondents' Open-Ended Responses before and after the Issuance of Press Releases, 2009–2010 *171*

Figure 7.7 Respondents' Enrollment via the Exchanges after Receipt of Different Randomly Assigned Letters from the U.S. Government Encouraging Enrollment, 2015 *174*

Figure C.1 Personal Benefit or Harm Attributed to the ACA, 2010 *206*

Figure C.2 Coefficients for Being Uninsured in 2016 and 2018 (Included in the Same Model) When Predicting 2018 Support for ACA Repeal *213*

Figure D.1 Word Clouds of Open-Ended Responses by SSI Respondents *221*

Figure E.1 ACA Support across Different Experimental Trust-Related Frames among Low-Trust Respondents, 2011, 2017, and 2018 *226*

Figure E.2 Variation in Topics, April 2009 to February 2010, with Topic Probabilities Smoothed over the Prior Twenty-Eight Days *227*

Tables

Table 5.1 Multilevel Models Fit to KFF Respondents from 2015, 2016, and 2017, with Insurance Market Conditions (and Other Independent Variables) Predicting ACA Favorability, Measured on a 1–4 Scale *103*

Table 6.1 Relationships between Group Benefits and ACA Support or ACA Repeal, 2016 *124*

Table A.1 ISCAP Panel Waves and Sample Sizes *192*

Table A.2 Demographics of Respondents across Surveys *193*

Table B.1 OLS Models Predicting Town-Level Support for the Medicaid Expansion in Maine, 2017 *200*

Table B.2 OLS Models Predicting County-Level Support for the Medicaid Expansion in Oklahoma, 2020 *201*

Table B.3 OLS Regression Estimates from Models Predicting a 1–4 Measure of ACA Favorability among Respondents under Sixty-Five *202*

Table B.4 Multilevel Models Predicting ACA Favorability (1–4) Using the HTP for 2014–2016 and 2017–2019 *203*

Table C.1 Key Variables and Their Associations with Insurance Sources among Respondents to Surveys after December 2013 *205*

Table C.2 Open-Ended Keywords Used by Uninsured Respondents to Denote Harm by the ACA Pre- and Post-Implementation *208*

Table C.3 Open-Ended Keywords Used by Respondents with Self-Purchased Insurance to Denote Benefit from the ACA Based on Mutual Information, Pre- and Post-Implementation *209*

Table C.4 Select Coefficients from Fitted Models of Kentucky Respondents' Support for the ACA, Including Indicators for Those Who Received Subsidies and Used Kynect *210*

Table C.5 OLS Models of Anti-ACA Attitudes, Measured on a 1–7 Scale, as a Function of Various Variables, Fall 2018 *211*

Table C.6 Select Coefficients from a Change Score Model of the Change in Respondents' Support for Repealing the ACA, Measured on a 1–7 Scale, Fall 2016 to Fall 2018 *212*

Table C.7 OLS Model of Anti-ACA Attitudes, Measured on a 1–7 Scale, as a Function of Various Variables, Fall 2018 *214*

Table C.8 Full Multilevel Models with Insurance Market Conditions (and Other Independent Variables) Predicting ACA Favorability, Measured on a 1–4 Scale and Fit to KFF Respondents, 2015, 2016, and 2017 *215*

Table C.9 Regression Coefficients, Standard Errors, and *t*-values for Potentially Confounding Dependent Variables Predicted by Being Sixty-Five or Older *217*

Table C.10 RDD Models Fit to Respondents between Sixty-Two and Sixty-Eight before and after the ACA's Implementation *218*

Table D.1 Regression Results Predicting ACA Attitudes over Time *220*

Table E.1 Means and *t*-tests for the Listed Variables Comparing Those Randomly Assigned to the Trust Argument with the Control Group, 2011 *228*

Table E.2 Means and *t*-tests for the Listed Variables Comparing Those Randomly Assigned to the Trust Argument with the Control Group, 2017 *228*

Table E.3 Means and *t*-tests for the Listed Variables Comparing Those Randomly Assigned to the Trust Argument with the Control Group, 2018 *229*

Table E.4 Most Commonly Occurring Words in Each of the Six Clusters of Open-Ended Responses Identified through LDA, 2009–2012 *229*

ABOUT THE AUTHOR

DANIEL J. HOPKINS is professor of political science at the University of Pennsylvania.

IT'S A BEAUTIFUL Saturday morning in May 2013, and I'm standing on what has become my favorite place in the world, a T-ball field in South Baltimore. The field isn't much—it's tucked between a new parking lot and an old industrial building. If the ball gets hit to left field, there's a chance a gopher will find it in the uncut grass before any of the five-year-olds do. But seeing as I am a newly minted T-ball coach, there's nowhere I'd rather be.

There's just one problem. A few of the kids can really throw hard, but none of them can throw with any accuracy, and they let the balls loose at me without warning, sometimes from multiple parts of the field at once. Usually, I'm pretty good at catching a wild throw, or at least moving out of the way. But today there's a blurry streak in my vision, so I'm having real trouble seeing them.

I first noticed the problem four days earlier. When I left my house and stepped into the sun, I thought for a moment that there was a streak of fog, even though it was a cloudless day. My left eye was clouded. I felt no discomfort, but by Thursday I was closing one eye to read, and a college friend with an MD convinced me I needed to get checked out—despite what I kept telling myself, I didn't just need a new glasses prescription. Twenty minutes later, I was in the emergency room at Johns Hopkins (no relation, a fact which the cascade of residents, fellows, attendings, nurses, and administrative staff I'd meet in the coming days and weeks would invariably ask about).

The doctor who saw me in the emergency room didn't see much cause for alarm and sent me home with an unidentified "eye disorder." But during the follow-up appointment, things took a more worrying turn. I heard a phrase I had never heard before, optic neuritis, along with one that I certainly had—multiple sclerosis, or MS.

I'm a politics and stats geek, not a doctor, or at least not that kind of doctor. So when one doctor observed that I might have optic neuritis, I didn't know what that meant. When she explained that optic neuritis is often the first symptom of MS, though, I knew to be alarmed. In the moment, I could only really conjure up one thing about the disease. I knew that Mitt Romney's wife Ann has MS, and that was reassuring—Ann Romney has been able to play a prominent public role even decades after her diagnosis.

Anxious people seek out information in an (often self-defeating) attempt to relieve their anxiety, as research by political scientists Bethany Albertson and Shana Gadarian has taught me. So I dove into the medical literature, hoping that some PhD training in applied statistics would compensate for my lack of knowledge about medicine.

There's no sugarcoating it: MS is a scary disease. It is a neurodegenerative disease that takes different forms but often gets worse over time, sometimes leaving people unable to walk. But optic neuritis doesn't always lead to MS, so a diagnosis of optic neuritis begins a state of limbo. As an applied statistician, I channeled my anxieties into a quest to estimate my own probability of contracting MS as precisely as I could.

I became fixated on a panel study in which the researchers had followed a set of patients for years after being diagnosed with optic neuritis. As a researcher, I knew all too well the limits of the study: because the respondents weren't randomly sampled, but rather clustered at a small number of hospitals, it was unclear whether the results would apply to me.

An optic neuritis diagnosis inaugurates a waiting game to see if other symptoms of MS develop. I've been lucky: nine years (and about that many MRIs) after my optic neuritis diagnosis, they have not. MS is defined by two discrete events, so my risk of having MS is now pretty low. As the months passed and life eased back to normal, I quickly disabused myself of the Didion-style magical thinking that had briefly led me to believe I should re-create myself as a biomedical researcher and devote my life to studying MS.

And I have been lucky in another way—I have employer-provided health insurance. Even if I had been diagnosed with MS, I would have been positioned to see the doctors I needed without a major financial burden. In that period before the implementation of the main provisions of the Affordable Care Act (ACA) in 2014, that wasn't true for millions of my fellow Americans.

Like me, the law spent years in a kind of limbo. As the months passed and my own prognosis became clearer, I began to see another, potentially more productive direction in which to channel my anxiety: the fate of the 2010 law that promised to extend affordable health insurance. Again and again, the law faced unexpected threats, whether from the courts, Congress, or the very officials charged with implementing it. Just as I had wanted the foresight to know my prognosis, I wanted to understand what the future held in store for the ACA—and what that could tell us about how American politics works (or doesn't work). And again, I sought to bury my anxieties in data. But as a political scientist, I was much better positioned to contribute to an understanding of the politics of the ACA than I was to understand the pathophysiology of MS. This book is the product of that attempt.

Like a teaching hospital, this book is only possible because of the work of many people, most of whom contributed at different times and are unknown to each other. In particular, I am grateful to Adam Berinsky, Tom Clark, Jonathan Cohn, Robert Erikson, David Fleischer, Zoltan Hajnal, Tim McBridge, Chris Pope, Evan Saltzman, Robert Shapiro, Leah Stokes, and Rick Valelly for comments, advice, and/or data. Thanks, too, to friends and family, including Rona Gregory, Andrew Coburn, and Luke McLoughlin, who probably didn't realize that friendship included help on research. I'm likewise grateful to seminar participants at the University of Wisconsin, POLMETH 2019, APSA 2019, the Yale Law School, the Yale Department of Political Science, the Texas A&M Department of Political Science, and the Leonard Davis Institute's 2020 Health Policy Retreat.

Andrea L. Campbell deserves a special acknowledgment: she served on my PhD committee more than a decade ago, her work and ideas animate much of this research, and she encouraged me to write this book and then kindly provided detailed comments in the midst of the Covid-19 pandemic. The other members of my PhD committee—Claudine Gay, Gary King, and Bob Putnam—will find their ongoing influence scattered across many pages, and I am grateful for their continued mentorship and friendship.

Not only was Will Hobbs the co-PI on two separate Russell Sage Foundation grants that enabled this research, but he also coauthored elements of the book that would become chapter 5 and provided valuable feedback. Andrew Reeves has been graciously talking about this research for years (and about research in general for decades) as well as finding time to comment amid the Covid-19 pandemic. Josh Kalla read the entire manuscript in the twenty-four hours after I sent it to him. Jacob Hacker's comments were incisive and perfectly timed.

Colleagues at the University of Pennsylvania provided invaluable assistance and insights in ways big and small. Special thanks to Roberto Carlos, Ezekiel Emanuel, Meg Guliford, Atul Gupta, Michael Horowitz, Dorothy Kronick, Yph Lelkes, Matt Levendusky, Julie Lynch, Michele Margolis, Marc Meredith, and Omer Solodoch. Matt, Michele, and Marc in particular fielded a seemingly endless number of email and text queries at all hours of the day. Kalind Parish coauthored the *Public Opinion Quarterly* article that is a foundational element of chapter 4. The Leonard Davis Institute of Health Economics at the University of Pennsylvania fostered interdisciplinary collaborations and opportunities to present these ideas; I gratefully acknowledge Dan Polsky, Rachel Werner, and the entire LDI team.

I have also been lucky to work with an amazing team of students and researchers at Georgetown University and now Penn. Special thanks to Emma Arsekin, Tiger Brown, Sonali Deliwala, Jacob Denenberg, Benjamin Dorph, Henry Feinstein, Nicholas Fernandez, Isaiah Gaines, Matt Garber, Max Kaufman, Douglas Kovel, James Kuang, Debra Lederman, Sarem Leghari, Sydney Loh, Adelaide Lyall, Kat McKay, Shaan Mishra, Sam Mitchell, Owen O'Hare, Bhavana Penmetsa, Matthew Rabinowitz, Dylan Radley, Janelle Schneider, Jacob "Jack" Starobin, Daniel Sun, Leanna Tilitei, and Elena Zhou. Camilla Alarcon and Alesha Lewis, both of whom I met through the Society for Political Methodology, made valued contributions as well.

David Aziz's inspired research laid the groundwork for key analyses. Samantha Washington provided incisive comments on two chapters. Thomas Munson and Haley Suh merit special recognition for graciously volunteering with data analysis when Covid-19 locked down many parts of the United States. Tori Gorton made extensive contributions to this manuscript as it came to life; her insights and edits are found in every chapter and on every page. Will Halm provided key help with editing.

The panel data reported here were collected thanks to support from the Annenberg Public Policy Center, the Institute for the Study of Citizens and Politics, the University of Pennsylvania School of Arts and Sciences and

University Research Foundation, and the Russell Sage Foundation (awards 94-17-01 and 94-18-07 to Daniel J. Hopkins and William Hobbs and 87-11-01 to Seth Goldman and Diana Mutz). The Russell Sage Foundation deserves particular recognition: alongside the grant support, this book benefited markedly from my time at Russell Sage as a visiting scholar in the spring of 2022. I am especially grateful to Suzanne Nichols for her insightful, timely, and detail-oriented work.

To my kids, you did so much to make this book a reality, dealing with an occasionally distracted dad while at other times providing much-needed distractions—and always being a powerful motivation to work toward healing the world. I know you both have a passion for the environment, and while this book isn't about environmental attitudes, I hope that its insights can help those fighting climate change.

Emily, every aspect of this book bears the deep imprint of more than two decades of our conversations and the inspiration of your tireless commitment to your patients, to your research, to medicine, and to service. Through nightly conversations, I have learned so much from you about primary care, pediatrics, Medicaid, and poverty. I am continuously in awe of you, of the life we've built together, and of my luck.

Mom, the genesis of my interest in health care probably dates back to taking phone messages for you and telling random callers that they didn't need to talk to you because you were going to prescribe cefuroxime anyway. I have always tried to follow in your footsteps—not, admittedly, by going to medical school, but by re-creating the remarkable blend of research, teaching, and one-on-one service you managed to achieve as a professor of medicine. In so many ways personal and professional, you have taught and inspired me to always try to do more and to do it better. Maybe this book dedication can take the place of a surgical residency? To be discussed . . .

To my brother Ben, I'm so grateful for so much—that we've been able to watch our families grow together, and that your willingness to pursue the family business by researching cancer freed me up to study politics.

I also dedicate this book to the memory of my father, a surgeon who treated AIDS patients when many would not, and the only parent on the sidelines of suburban soccer games wearing an ACT-UP T-shirt. Also a sharp critic of our health care system, you would surely have had lots of reactions to the ACA had you lived to see it. I am sorry that cancer took that conversation, like so much else, away from us.

CHAPTER 1

Introduction

IN 1993, NEWLY elected Democratic president Bill Clinton was trying to push comprehensive health care reform through Congress, while another Bill—Bill Kristol—circulated a memo to his fellow Republicans. Kristol argued that Republicans needed to do everything in their power to kill Clinton's bill. He was alarmed about its potential political impacts. "Because the initiative's inevitably destructive effect on American medical services will not be practically apparent for several years," he wrote, "its passage in the short term will do nothing to hurt (and everything to help) Democratic electoral prospects."[1] A conservative and a former chief of staff to GOP vice president Dan Quayle, Kristol worried that voters would reward the Democrats for passing health care reform, making it harder for Republicans to retake the White House. In his view, the long-term impacts of the bill's passage were even more concerning: the legislation, he argued, would "relegitimize middle-class dependence for security on government spending and regulation."[2] Like the New Deal before it, comprehensive health care reform would become entrenched over time, transforming politics by permanently shifting the relationship between citizens and government.

Embedded in Kristol's advice was a theory of how public opinion works: if policies today can reconfigure public opinion tomorrow, those in power may be able to propagate their own worldview, possibly for decades to come.[3] In the period after Kristol's 1993 memo, a fast-growing body of political science research on policy feedback effects concluded that policies sometimes *can* reshape public opinion.[4]

Bill Clinton's efforts at comprehensive health care reform ended in failure, as Congress did not even seriously consider his plan.[5] But years later the political world would get to see if Kristol's prediction about public opinion and health care reform was right. In 2010, the Democrats managed to enact sweeping health insurance reform through the vehicle of the Patient Protection and Affordable Care Act (ACA), or "Obamacare." The widest-ranging social policy reform in a generation, and the signature legislative achievement of Barack Obama's 2009–2017 presidency, the ACA was a complex bundle of public spending, taxes, and regulatory policies that sought to increase access to comprehensive health insurance.[6]

In theory, the ACA seemed to be precisely the kind of law that should bolster the fortunes of the party and ideology behind it, just as Kristol had feared. It created substantial new benefits. Its Medicaid expansion alone provided health insurance to 14.8 million additional people in 2019.[7] Its separate insurance subsidies were also substantial—in 2016, for example, the federal government spent $46 billion via the law's Premium Tax Credit, meaning that the average policyholder's subsidy amounted to just over $4,000.[8] That's not to mention the other avenues through which the ACA provided sizable benefits, such as by prohibiting discrimination against customers with preexisting conditions, ending higher premiums for women, and removing caps on lifetime insurance payments. The ACA was an inherently redistributive policy that used taxes on high earners to extend health insurance primarily to Americans with low incomes.[9] Research on other policy areas has found that more modest government benefits can bolster the incumbent or enacting party.[10] Given the size of its outlays and their impacts on people's lives, the ACA appeared likely to do so as well.

Yet far from fulfilling Kristol's prediction, the ACA seemed to be a major political liability for the Democrats in the years after its enactment. In 2010 and 2014, Republican congressional candidates campaigned primarily on the basis of their *opposition* to the ACA, which they tagged as an unnecessary expansion of governmental authority—and they swept those years' most contested elections.[11] Researchers estimate that in 2010 Democratic members of Congress who voted for the ACA lost a whopping 8.5 percentage points when running for reelection relative to Democrats who did not.[12] Overall, in 2010 the Democrats dropped a historic sixty-three seats in the House of Representatives along with six Senate seats; in 2014 they gave up thirteen House seats and another nine Senate seats. Presidential scholar George Edwards titled his book on Obama's early years *Overreach*, and the politics of the ACA was a major reason why.[13]

One explanation for the ACA's unpopularity centers on a second pathway through which political elites are thought to influence public opinion: messaging.[14] The *New York Times* stated the conventional wisdom in reporting that "the Obama administration and Democrats . . . largely lost the health care message war in the raucous legislative process."[15] Scholars have joined commentators in contending that politicians' rhetorical choices influenced public views of health care reform, singling out former Alaska governor Sarah Palin's use of the phrase "death panels" in a 2009 Facebook post as especially memorable and effective anti-ACA rhetoric.[16]

Politicians and pundits commonly emphasize messaging as an explanation for a policy's popularity. The journalist Michael Hiltzik wrote that "the Democrats' problem wasn't Obamacare so much as faulty messaging. Think of how things might have been different if every time a Republican . . . trotted out a purported Obamacare 'victim' (most of which cases were bogus), a Democratic organization produced an Obamacare winner from among those 10 million new insurance holders."[17] Such arguments presume that politicians' choices about messaging play a key role in the success of their policy goals.

This belief in the impacts of messaging can be self-serving, since messaging is among the few things that politicians (and their consultants) can consistently control. But it's also a belief with considerable grounding in political science. In fact, political scientist Cindy Kam describes this elite leadership model of public opinion—and above all John Zaller's *The Nature and Origins of Mass Opinion*—as "arguably the dominant paradigm today of public opinion formation."[18] Framing, elite cues, and other forms of messaging have already generated extensive study, just as research on policy feedbacks has.[19] But these two research literatures have proceeded largely in isolation. From the vantage point of political figures like Bill Kristol and Barack Obama, however, messaging and policy feedbacks are the primary tools through which they and other political elites can reshape public opinion and so tilt the landscape for future policy battles. To politicians, they are thus complementary, meaning that studying messaging and policy feedbacks jointly is key if we are to provide an overall assessment of the capacity for elite influence on public opinion.

The Motivating Mystery: ACA Attitudes, 2009–2020

Still, an initial look at the evidence suggests that neither messaging nor policy feedbacks were all that influential. For years post-enactment, the public's overall response to the ACA was both stable and cool: between 2010 and 2016, surveys consistently found pluralities or majorities voicing opposition. (That was despite the fact that many of the law's provisions were quite popular on their own, with 67 percent of American adults backing the creation of the exchanges and 62 percent wanting to expand Medicaid in 2010.)[20] As we will see in chapters 3 and 7, shifts in messaging during the initial debate over the law left a shallow imprint on public opinion. Even the implementation of the law's main provisions in January 2014 did surprisingly little to move attitudes.[21] The Democrats still lost the 2014 midterms badly. And in January 2015, a year after the ACA's main provisions went into effect, the Kaiser Family Foundation's (KFF) Health Tracking Poll (HTP) found that just 40 percent of Americans held favorable opinions toward the ACA, while 46 percent held unfavorable opinions.[22]

The general stability and negativity of Americans' ACA attitudes for several years is a lingering puzzle: given the very real benefits it provided, why didn't the law's passage and subsequent implementation do more to shift public opinion or to generate political support for its Democratic architects and defenders?[23] Why did the public like many of the law's pieces but not the law itself? More starkly, what was wrong with Kristol's theory of elite influence through policy?

The 2016 election of Republican Donald Trump only deepened the mystery. After Trump's general election victory, a slew of pundits and scholars argued that the Democrats had lost partly because they had put too much emphasis on identity-based appeals related to race, ethnicity, and gender. In this view, key states like Michigan, Ohio, Pennsylvania, and Wisconsin backed Trump because the Democrats didn't focus their campaign on the economic interests of white voters without college degrees.[24] But such claims reflect a touch of political amnesia. The Democrats' chief policy accomplishment of the preceding administration had been the ACA, a redistributive economic policy of precisely the kind that should have played to the

Democrats' advantage.[25] In theory, the promise of health insurance not tied to employment might have been especially welcome in the hard-hit manufacturing towns of the Northeast and Midwest. By 2016, however, the Democrats saw themselves as having little reason to highlight their support of the ACA, while Republicans had little reason to conceal their strident opposition. In fact, Trump campaigned in 2016 partly on a commitment to repeal the law.

Still, the story does not end there. After Trump's election, GOP politicians moved quickly to fulfill their repeated promise to roll back the ACA. But after having been stable for years, public opinion swung in the ACA's favor as soon as its repeal became a real possibility. By November 2018, 53 percent of respondents to a KFF poll reported *favoring* the ACA, up thirteen percentage points from 2015—and in 2018's midterm elections, it was the Democrats trumpeting their ACA position.[26] Indeed, Republican House leader Kevin McCarthy blamed the GOP's 2018 loss of control of the House of Representatives "on the GOP's push to roll back health insurance protections for people with pre-existing conditions."[27] Enacting the ACA had proven unpopular, but repealing it was even more so. Far from influencing public opinion, political elites seemed to retreat in the face of it.

The Core Argument: The Limits of Elite Influence

How do we explain these paradoxical post-enactment trends? And more generally, to what extent can political elites reshape public opinion through their words or policies? This book addresses these questions through a detailed study of Americans' opinions about the ACA between 2009 and 2020. Researchers have produced a rich body of scholarship about the role of specific factors in shaping ACA attitudes, but this book departs from prior research by providing a competitive assessment of several credible explanations for Americans' views on the ACA.[28] These explanations range from personal experiences with the policy to messaging, partisanship, racial attitudes, status quo biases, and thermostatic responses to presidential policymaking.[29]

By considering varied explanations simultaneously, we are positioned to advance this study's broader goal: the characterization of the potential for enduring elite influence on public opinion.[30] A central tenet of representative democracy is that elected officials act with the consent of the governed, which has come to mean at least the periodic authorization of the citizenry via elections.[31] But the prospect of political leaders having the ability to bend public opinion threatens to invert that relationship. The risk is that instead of acting on some vision of the public interest, leaders will manipulate public opinion so as to build support for their own ends.[32] Even in a democracy, leaders may not enact the will of the people so much as reshape it to match their own.[33] Perennially important in democratic political systems, the question of elite influence is especially critical now given Donald Trump's 2017–2021 presidency and growing antidemocratic movements within American politics.[34] Assessing elite influence in democracies, in turn, requires that we consider its two main avenues together: messaging and policy.

Analyses that rely exclusively on closed-ended survey evidence often characterize public opinion in pessimistic ways,[35] with most voters seen as holding inconsistent or ephemeral preferences.[36] To avoid stacking the deck, this book relies on a wide base of evidence that incorporates hundreds of surveys—including extensive evidence from open-ended survey responses—alongside twelve survey experiments with varied populations, one field experiment, and analyses of elite-level rhetoric. At times we employ a panel that allows us to track the same respondents' attitudes over several years.

The book's core conclusion is that political elites were quite limited in their capacity to influence public opinion on the ACA, especially among those outside their party. The contours of public opinion prove coherent and stable in the face of the two major forms of elite influence, a conclusion broadly consistent with prior work focusing on aggregate trends.[37] Even using individual-level data, we find noteworthy coherence, structure, and some subtlety in how Americans thought about the ACA. In broad strokes, this capacity to resist elite influence holds true for short-term influence via messaging and for medium-term influence via policy feedbacks. Although both pathways hold out some possibility of longer-term influence, such influence is hard to trace to specific politicians—and it is also unlikely to translate into discernible electoral support on politicians' time frames, which are often no longer than the two-year congressional cycle. The extent of contemporary political polarization—in general and on the ACA specifically—adds to the already powerful constraints on the substantive magnitude of elite influence.[38]

Certainly, both messaging effects and policy feedback effects have already been thoroughly established by prior research, so why does this book's argument seem to depart so significantly? There is a straightforward, two-word answer: effect sizes. Prior research has often framed its core questions in binary ways, asking questions about the direction of effects such as "Are there positive policy feedbacks?" or "Can framing move attitudes?" Here we build on a generation of progress in statistical methodology to ask not just about the existence of effects but about their substantive magnitude and political import.[39] Thus, this book's aim is not to argue for or against framing effects or policy feedbacks, but to contextualize them by offering a holistic assessment of such effects relative to other explanations of public opinion.

In his 2012 reappraisal of *The Nature and Origins of Mass Opinion*, John Zaller acknowledges that "public opinion that has not been shaped by elites has played an important role in some of the most significant aspects of American history."[40] This book seeks to show that the same can be said of the ACA, and that public opinion was relatively impervious to elite influence, even in a likely case in which political elites deployed all the tools at their disposal. Although we do find some evidence of policy feedback effects, they were small in comparison with the amounts of money being spent, they were sometimes undercut by other elements of the law, and they were most pronounced among populations less likely to vote. Policy feedbacks cannot account for some of the main features of ACA attitudes, including the public's lingering doubts about the law, the stability of public opinion during the law's 2014 implementation, and the pro-ACA shift in attitudes that followed Trump's election. That shift was more consistent with models of public opinion in which the public shifts against the policy direction advanced by the president and Congress.

Through messaging, political elites can effectively polarize public opinion in the manner that extensive research has already demonstrated.[41] But in the case of the ACA, this power to cue some citizens via partisan heuristics was just one chapter in a much broader story. Messaging did polarize opinion in the law's early months, but there is much that messaging cannot explain, such as the high level of opposition to the law, the stability in public perceptions of the law, and the asymmetric strength of the opposition until late 2016.

In some respects, this book's depiction of elite influence through messaging is analogous to the limited but real power someone has when faced with a large boulder at the top of a hill. Sure, she can push the boulder down the incline. But once the boulder is in motion, she can neither control where it lands nor return it to its starting point. By taking salient, differing stances on an issue, political elites can trigger the polarizing dynamics that have been the focus of prior work in the tradition of *The Nature and Origins of Mass Opinion*; that is, they can set the boulder in motion.[42] They can only move some opinions, however, and they can do so much more easily when nudging those opinions into alignment with citizens' existing ideologies.[43] Neither words nor policies are likely to dramatically shift the balance of public opinion in favor of a policy in the face of cross-party elite disagreement. And given the pervasiveness of contemporary political polarization, cross-party disagreement is the norm on most salient issues—most certainly including the ACA.[44]

At the same time, using the ACA to outline the limits of elite influence sheds light on related questions about public opinion. From climate change and economic mobility to immigration and racial inequality, many of today's most pressing domestic issues raise questions similar to those raised by the ACA. How is the public likely to respond to complex legislation with disparate impacts on specific groups of Americans? As fights over policy unfold in today's polarized political landscape, does political partisanship crowd out everything else? Are public responses different when policy is delivered indirectly, perhaps through market-based mechanisms or low-visibility regulations? More broadly, in an age sometimes termed "post-truth," what is the role of the concrete realities of a policy's operation in shaping the public's views about it?[45] And what about the role of America's long-standing racial divisions and disparities? If we do not understand the drivers of attitudes toward the ACA, we will not be positioned to understand how Americans are likely to respond when similar questions surface elsewhere.

The actual impact of policy on public opinion is one important question; how policymakers *perceive* that impact is a separate but also important question. To the extent that politicians believe that citizens' personal experiences or other factors influence public opinion, they are likely to redesign key policies in the hopes of bending those factors to their advantage. ACA architect and economist Jonathan Gruber said something to this effect when he argued that "a lack of transparency is a huge political advantage."[46] In that way, policymakers' assumptions about what drives public opinion may find themselves inscribed into law.[47]

The Critical Case of Health Insurance Reform

There are key advantages to using the 2010 ACA and proposals to replace it as a vehicle to test varied accounts of public opinion. Even before the Covid-19 pandemic, health insurance reform was a major issue with clear-cut impacts on Americans' lives. In the United States, where health care accounts for 17.7 percent of GDP, any significant reform has tangible effects on the lives of millions.[48] The ACA certainly did. In 2019 alone, some 26 million Americans were insured through its Medicaid expansion or via its exchanges.[49] Health insurance, in turn, can have profound impacts on those who gain it or lose it; research demonstrates that people who gain insurance use more health care, have better mental health outcomes, and are less indebted.[50]

Behind the raw enrollment numbers are millions of Americans and their personal experiences with the health care system. Almost by definition, experiences with health insurance and health care can be life-changing.[51] In her 2014 book *Trapped in America's Safety Net*, political scientist Andrea L. Campbell tells a harrowing story about public health insurance in the aftermath of a car accident that paralyzed her sister-in-law Marcella.[52] To ensure that Marcella received vital medical care through Medicaid before the ACA's implementation, her family had to adapt to strict income and asset limits at precisely the time when it faced major unanticipated costs and challenges.

Few Americans are as entangled in America's complex system of paying for health care as people with major disabilities. Yet even more common encounters with the health care system can leave a lasting imprint. In the preface, I recounted some of my own experiences with these issues. Although the particulars differ, millions of Americans have had similar experiences. In an October 2020 KFF survey, 47 percent of respondents told pollsters that they had a preexisting health condition.[53]

Already dominating headlines, health care became still more salient in the wake of the Covid-19 pandemic and the associated economic turbulence from 2020 to 2022. Health care is not a niche issue. It affects virtually everyone in the country, often in powerful ways. So it is quite plausible that Americans' reactions to the ACA were shaped by what the law meant for them personally.[54] This argument was voiced by none other than 2012 Republican presidential nominee Mitt Romney, who told allies that year:

"You can imagine for somebody making $25,000 or $30,000 or $35,000 a year, being told you're now going to get free health care, particularly if you don't have it, getting free health care worth, what, $10,000 per family, in perpetuity—I mean, this is huge."[55] It wasn't just Bill Kristol. The belief that policies like the ACA could pay political dividends was widely held.

Another advantage of studying the ACA comes from its complexity. Although the ACA was a single law, the variety of policy levers it included enables us to separately assess the impacts of each. And the ACA wasn't all upside—the taxes and regulations associated with it were likely to leave a major footprint on public opinion as well. The law levied substantial new taxes on the top 5 percent of the nation's taxpayers.[56] And until it was modified via a December 2017 tax law, it also imposed a sizable fine on those without insurance. What's more, cancellation notices were sent to 4.7 million Americans in 2013 because their health plans didn't meet the ACA's standards.[57] These cancellations undercut Obama's oft-repeated promise that, "if you like your health care plan, you will be able to keep your health care plan."[58] It turned out that regulators had to like your health plan too. The ACA affords us the opportunity to study the effects of negative experiences alongside positive ones.[59]

The Sources of Opinion Stability

Assessing the relative influence of elites on public opinion is a deceptively challenging task. It requires us to consider the full set of explanations for public opinion on the ACA. Given that, we identify several broad types of explanations for public opinion that may be at work and then discuss them—and their implications for elite influence—in more detail.

For one, in explaining public opinion, researchers have long pointed to the connection between Americans' political attitudes and their views on key social groups.[60] That orientation has led one stream of research on ACA attitudes to emphasize racial attitudes while another points to political partisanship.[61] A third strain of research highlights the lack of trust in government.[62] Still other research focuses on personal experiences and self-interest.[63] These are all broad classes of explanations, and each encompasses mechanisms of elite influence as well as non-elite opinion formation.

Given this range of explanations, the ACA offers a critical test: In a polarized era, within a fragmented information environment, and on a prominent issue, is there still room for personal experiences to influence public opinion? Or is public opinion largely explained by more symbolic, group-oriented predispositions, whether stemming from political partisanship, racial attitudes, governmental distrust, or other factors? Studying attitudes toward the ACA provides a broad vista into the drivers of contemporary public opinion as surely as attitudes on taxes did four decades ago.[64] Such an analysis positions us to assess long-standing arguments about the public's political knowledge alongside those about elite influence.[65] Even so, the ACA is a single case at a single historical moment in a single country. This study focuses on a Democratic health policy initiative and may tell us less about responses to Republican-backed initiatives or to other policy domains.

Personal Experiences and Political Attitudes

To the extent that policy shapes public opinion, it may well do so through citizens' personal experiences, which are thus a useful starting place. Because the ACA left Medicare and employer-based insurance intact, the overwhelming majority of Americans neither gained nor lost insurance on account of the law.[66] In addition, several of the key policy levers were back-door regulations, which either rendered them invisible to customers or obscured their connection to government policy.[67] Even the effects of the Medicaid expansion, one of the most prominent and popular elements of the law, were muted by beneficiaries' relatively low levels of voter turnout.[68]

It's no surprise, then, that most of the public responded to the law as a partisan and political symbol; for a majority of the country, that was primarily what it was, even after enactment.[69] And for that majority, attitudes toward the ACA followed much the same pattern as other political attitudes. Grounded in partisanship and to some extent racial attitudes, ACA attitudes were generally quite stable, as we will see in later chapters. Their dynamics emerged from predictable public shifts against presidential initiatives—a cousin of a well-documented effect called "thermostatic response"—as well as commonly observed behaviors in political psychology such as status quo bias and loss aversion.[70]

Although I do not come to praise personal experience as a mechanism of opinion change, I do not come to bury it either. The United States is a country of more than 330 million people, and the ACA had concrete impacts on millions of them. For those who came into contact with its most tangible elements, self-interest did shape their reactions to some degree. Among low-income Americans in states that expanded Medicaid, the ACA subsequently became more popular: the effect was equivalent to moving about 3 percent of the distance from being "very unfavorable" to being "very favorable" toward the law. When assessing the political impact of a policy, however, it is not sufficient to show that it does or does not have a detectable effect. It is also crucial to identify the size of the impact, the size of the affected population, and that population's level of political engagement.[71] So, while such effects among low-income Americans are detectable, they apply to only a small subset of the population and are not especially large even for that subset. Medicaid recipients' relatively low levels of voter turnout further dampen the electoral implications of their shifting attitudes.[72]

Thus, the mere existence of positive personal experiences with the ACA has not translated into a significant political dividend for its authors. Detectable effects are one thing. Effects that can induce politically meaningful shifts on election outcomes are quite another. From the vantage point of public opinion, the key facts about the ACA were not the size of its benefits but rather the law's complexity and the small fraction of Americans who were unambiguous beneficiaries. Complex policies can produce complex feedback effects. The limits on elite influence through policy design are pronounced.

To an important extent, the ACA's impacts on citizens' attitudes arising from their personal experiences were also self-canceling. Personal experiences fostered pro-ACA attitudes among some but anti-ACA attitudes among others, muting their overall impacts. Experiences are especially impactful when people lose something they already have.[73] Accordingly, among those Americans who were most likely to be uninsured and thus compelled to pay a fine after the ACA's implementation, opinions moved *against* the law. In these respects, the findings reported here are in keeping with recent research showing that when the event or issue in question is sufficiently powerful, and when its impacts are sufficiently well measured, personal experiences and self-interest can move attitudes.[74]

To illuminate the key factors driving public opinion toward the ACA, it's critical to also consider alternative theoretical accounts. As we will see, although most Americans' ACA attitudes were not grounded in personal experience, neither were they malleable or easily influenced by elite messaging.[75] In line with prior research grounded in in-depth interviews or letters to public officials, we show that Americans' ACA attitudes had more content, coherence, and consistency than some accounts (or late-night TV hosts) would lead us to expect.[76] This consistency provides another brake on mechanisms of elite influence.

Certainly, the initial choice by prominent Republicans to stridently oppose the ACA solidified opposition to the law, to the point that opposing the ACA became virtually synonymous with being a Republican.[77] That surely counts as a form of elite influence. And yes, partisans quickly came to adopt their side's arguments for and against the ACA. But this shift largely followed a predictable pattern of polarization. From there, the specific rhetoric employed by both sides did little to move public opinion among those who did not already agree with one of the parties' stances on the ACA. Put differently, models of elite influence do little to explain the post-enactment dynamics of ACA attitudes. For activists, political organizers, politicians, and citizens alike, this is one of the book's main takeaways: the influence of politicians' rhetoric on public opinion was quite limited.

Racial Attitudes as an Illustrative Case

Probing the sources of that consistency leads us to the role of not just partisanship but also of attitudes related to other salient social groups, most notably racial groups. In the United States, both political divisions in general and social policy attitudes in particular are grounded in racial divisions.[78] Put more starkly, to ask white Americans about redistributive programs like welfare and Medicaid is, to an important degree, to ask them about the deservingness of black Americans and other marginalized groups.[79]

There is particular reason to think that racial attitudes could prove influential in white Americans' assessments of the ACA.[80] The law was the signature achievement of the nation's first black president, and it was explicitly designed to reduce racial disparities in health care.[81] In 2015, the second year after the ACA's main provisions went into effect, black and Latino Americans accounted for 50 percent of all Medicaid enrollees while representing just 30 percent of the population.[82] What's more, as of 2022, eight of the twelve states that continued to reject the ACA's Medicaid expansion were members of the former Confederacy, signaling a blunt connection between the law, federalism, and the nation's legacy of profound racial inequality.[83] Given these observations, no study could aspire to provide a comprehensive account of Americans' ACA attitudes *without* considering racial attitudes and prejudices.

There are multiple mechanisms through which racial divisions could shape ACA attitudes, so racial divisions provide a critical test of claims about the stability of public opinion—and its unresponsiveness to elite influence. For centuries, politicians have commonly "played the race card," seeking political advantage by deepening the racial divides in public opinion.[84] Can such elite rhetoric foregrounding race shift views of the ACA?

The evidence uncovered here on the relationship between whites' racial attitudes and their ACA views is nuanced but cuts against claims of elite influence, particularly in the short term. On the one hand, we extend prior research by finding sizable correlations between whites' racial attitudes and their views of the ACA.[85] Many white Americans use long-standing narratives about beneficiaries' deservingness, work ethic, and government waste in justifying their ACA views—narratives that are given force by racial prejudice.[86] However, across seven separate survey experiments conducted in different times and places, we find very limited evidence that white survey respondents' ACA attitudes are affected by questions that prime them to think specifically about the law's black and Hispanic beneficiaries. Given the totality of the evidence, racial attitudes appear to be an upstream influence on ACA attitudes that shape those views primarily through their relationship with broad predispositions like partisanship and ideology.[87] That means that racial attitudes are better positioned to help explain the overall stability and partisan division of Americans' ACA attitudes than to account for those occasional moments when ACA attitudes shift. They are more of a brake on elite influence than a mechanism of it.

A comprehensive assessment of these varied explanations for ACA attitudes also positions us to characterize public opinion more broadly. With some frequency, prior research has examined the question of who influences whom: Does public opinion shape subsequent positions taken by politicians, or do politicians influence public opinion?[88] In assessing political representation, that question is undeniably essential. But it also presumes significant interaction between the two, as if they were dancers and the goal is to identify who's leading. The perspective advanced here instead emphasizes the extent to which public opinion and politicians' positions are divorced, each proceeding on its own logic and time frame.

Why Study Public Opinion on the ACA?

To understand how Americans respond to sweeping policy reforms, this book focuses on reactions to the ACA between 2009 and 2020. Throughout that period, the health reform law was a central vehicle for arguments between Republicans and Democrats. Those fights moved across many venues at a dizzying pace, from town hall meetings and the halls of Congress to the executive branch, the judicial system, state capitals, and political campaigns. Already those elite-level battles have given rise to numerous books and articles.[89] Although this book covers elements of those battles, especially in chapter 2, it differs in that it concentrates on citizens' reactions to the law rather than on the elite-level machinations.

Scholars of public policy have long known that politics doesn't end with the enactment of legislation and that interest groups, elected officials, bureaucrats, judges, and other actors continue to shape a policy long after the ink on federal laws has dried.[90] Still, the ACA stands out amid federal policymaking of the last century for the extent to which it was the center of an ongoing, highly salient political debate that lasted for years post-enactment.[91] The passage of the ACA was not the end of the political battle, but rather the end of its beginning. The law shaped the contours of every federal election between 2008 and 2020. It animated and reoriented many state and local elections as well.[92] Simply put, we cannot understand American public opinion during the consequential decade between 2010 and 2020—or fully understand the Obama and Trump presidencies—without understanding how citizens were thinking about the ACA. By the same token, if we understand the trajectory of Americans' ACA attitudes, we know a lot about their political views generally during a tumultuous period.

Even for those interested primarily in health care, a study of public attitudes toward the ACA is of more than historical interest. As of the Biden presidency, health care and the ACA continue to be some of America's central political battlegrounds more than a decade after the law's enactment. For one thing, debates about single-payer health care versus more incremental approaches were a salient feature of the 2020 Democratic primary debates, prompted in part by Senator Bernie Sanders's "Medicare for All" proposal.[93] Some of the 2020 Democratic presidential contenders' proposals would have ended private health insurance altogether, a change that would have induced massive, systemwide shocks to the health care system. The experience of the ACA is nothing short of a billboard-size warning sign to those who argue that abolishing private insurance would initially be popular.

The lessons of this study are by no means confined to the ACA or even health care. Even before the passage of the climate-oriented Inflation Reduction Act (IRA) in the summer of 2022, debates about climate change legislation had come to echo debates over the ACA in important respects.[94] Both reforms needed to survive the same policymaking gauntlet and face possible vetoes or dilution from institutions that include Congress, the presidency, executive agencies, the courts, and state-level officials.[95] Like health care, climate change is a complex issue, and legislation to address it is likely to have concrete but varying impacts on millions of Americans. As with the ACA, backers of climate change legislation have to decide how much to rely on complex, market-based mechanisms such as "cap-and-trade" policies versus policies involving direct government provision or subsidies. In a 2019 *New York Times* column, David Leonhardt cited the political vulnerability of the ACA's exchanges in arguing that "Democrats would be foolish to push for complicated market-based policies when Republicans are hostile and voters are skeptical."[96] For those who would expand the government's role in fighting climate change or on other issues, the ACA is a lesson in the political fragility of complex policies that employ penalties.

It's a lesson that the Democrats who developed the IRA appear to have internalized, as they eschewed a carbon tax or other punitive regulations in favor of straightforward, extensive subsidies for clean energy production.[97] The IRA relies on carrots, not sticks, to shift the U.S. away from a reliance on fossil fuels. It may thus avoid some of the backlash provoked by the ACA. But the ACA is also a reminder that in a nation as large as the United States, personal experiences do not typically account for more than a fraction of shifts in overall public opinion, especially positive ones. On a polarized issue, messaging does even less.

The IRA is unlikely to be the last word on climate policy, so this book will also help identify instructive differences between the politics of legislating on health insurance and on climate change. The ACA's chief benefits were targeted at specific individuals in the near term, as millions of people became able to purchase affordable, comprehensive insurance. The law's costs were targeted as well, falling principally on high earners (who paid increased taxes), the uninsured (who paid the individual mandate), those whose pre-ACA plans did not meet the law's standards, and those whose post-ACA premiums rose rapidly. Some of the primary benefits of climate change legislation, by contrast, are more diffuse, with many accruing over decades to people in countries around the world.[98] Depending on its breadth, future climate change legislation may well disrupt the status quo more than the ACA, as it may affect the cost of everything from heating a home to driving to work. For these reasons, some of the dynamics that limited the ACA's popularity may be even more pronounced in post-IRA climate change legislation.

Causal Inference and Multiple Explanations

This book differs from much contemporary political science research in a key respect. Encouraged by the growing emphasis on causal inference, contemporary political science research often emphasizes the effects of a single causal factor.[99] This research strategy has the tremendous advantage of fitting within the potential outcomes framework, the dominant approach for inferring causal effects.[100] But while the potential outcomes framework has fostered rapid progress on varied questions, its dominance has led research literatures to foreground some questions over others.[101] One particular risk is that bodies of research develop with a variety of individually credible but collectively unintegrated causal effects. On their own, such bodies of research may not be well situated to compare rival explanations or to examine which of several factors is especially influential. Imagine a doctor considering which cancer treatment to prescribe. She certainly needs to know the impact of a specific treatment regimen, but it's also important that she know how various treatments compare to each other and the order in which to administer them. Likewise, social scientists, policymakers, strategists, and advocates sometimes need to go beyond assessments of one specific treatment to identify which of a variety of actions are especially likely to be impactful and where in the causal chain they act.

In this book, I draw heavily from recent work on causal inference and operate squarely within the potential outcomes framework. But my goal is not simply to test policy feedbacks, messaging, or any single explanation for ACA attitudes. Instead, it is to compile a series of experiments and observational analyses that jointly provide estimates precise enough to allow us to compare prominent explanations to one another—and to test claims of elite influence broadly understood. Doing so also affords us leverage on where in the causal process different factors operate. Rather than concluding that elite influence does or does not matter in some binary way, I seek to identify the conditions under which it is more or less likely to matter and to characterize the magnitude of those impacts relative to other prominent accounts of the public's ACA views. I also consider causes that operate well upstream from the outcomes they affect. The effects of personal experiences with the ACA are discernible. But they are also substantively small and cross-cutting, especially when compared with key changes in national politics and policymaking. Political scientists can reach such conclusions only by studying multiple explanations simultaneously and competitively.

Chapter Outline

To understand public opinion, it is critical to understand the policy that the public itself is evaluating. The basic design of policies such as Social Security and the GI Bill can be described straightforwardly. But not so with the ACA: it cannot be understood without first understanding the patchwork system of public and private health insurance that preceded it. Chapter 2 thus begins by sketching the pre-ACA insurance system and the key levers through which the ACA was originally designed to work. Chapter 2 also summarizes the law's short but highly dramatic political history. Those already well versed in the ACA and the ongoing battles over its implementation can skip this chapter—although since they know how riveting the tale is, they may not want to.

Chapter 3 seeks to characterize public opinion toward the ACA between 2009 and 2020, relying on the KFF's rolling cross-sectional HTP as well as the 2007–2020 panel of the Institute for the Study of Citizens and Politics (ISCAP) and surveys by the Pew Research Center. As we will see, the dramatic shifts in the law's political and legal fortunes left little imprint on public opinion. Instead, public opinion toward the ACA was surprisingly stable from before the law's passage until at least 2016, when Donald Trump's election led to a substantial pro-ACA shift.[102] This chapter thus provides evidence of a profound and enduring disconnect between the ever-changing elite-level battles over the law and the consistency of public opinion surrounding it. At the same time, chapter 3 underscores that public views of the ACA displayed an unappreciated level of nuance. While some accounts of public opinion conceive of opinions primarily as partisan rationalizations, our analyses of open-ended survey data show considerable understanding and evolution on the part of the public.[103] To borrow a term from the political scientist Philip Converse, non-attitudes these are not.

In the subsequent two chapters, I turn to evaluating claims about elite influence through policy design. The Medicaid expansion, the subject of chapter 4, involved the direct provision of government-backed insurance, raising two key questions about the political impacts of self-interest.[104] First, was support for the Medicaid expansion driven by those most likely to benefit from it? The early sections of chapter 4 consider which groups of voters supported the Medicaid expansion when it was put to a statewide vote, focusing on Maine's 2017 initiative and Oklahoma's 2020 initiative. They show that the dynamics of initiatives on Medicaid expansion were overwhelmingly partisan, with only hints that communities that stood to benefit more were especially supportive. To answer the second question, this chapter next uses KFF survey data to show that the Medicaid expansion had a clear, positive effect on lower-income Americans in expansion states—precisely the people most likely to benefit from the expansion. Even so, the impacts were limited by varied factors, from its partial implementation to the fact that it targeted lower-engagement citizens. The politics of the Medicaid expansion is not principally the politics of self-interest.

The ACA's insurance exchanges were a somewhat different story, as chapter 5 explains. The architects of the ACA originally conceived of the exchanges as the law's centerpiece. From 2014 until 2018, the exchanges were also backed by an individual mandate, enforced by a fine for those without insurance. Chapter 5 employs various data sets to examine the attitudes of those most likely to be affected by the subsidies, exchanges, and individual mandate. As it shows, this complex combination of features meant that on balance the ACA's exchanges produced offsetting feedback effects that did little to move public opinion overall.

Chapter 6 turns to the influence of racial attitudes and views of the ACA and so focuses on the white American majority. Do racial attitudes provide an opportunity for elite influence, or are they instead a source of attitudinal stability? What we conclude about the white American majority's racial attitudes hinges on the evidence that we focus on. The ISCAP panel shows the clear imprint of racial attitudes. What white Americans think about the ACA is closely connected to their adherence to anti-black stereotypes. Yet other evidence cuts in the opposite direction. Across seven experiments conducted at different times and in different places using different survey modes, we find little evidence that calling attention to the black and Latino beneficiaries of the law reduces its popularity. One way to make sense of these results—and to fit them with prior work on this topic—is to recognize that racial attitudes are an upstream causal influence.[105] They operate primarily by shaping political divisions, sorting partisans, and lending force to narratives about social policy generally. Thus, elite attempts to shape attitudes in the short term through racial priming are likely to have limited success.

Many pundits and politicians alike are convinced that messaging is a vital ingredient in a policy's success. In chapter 7, we take up those claims, focusing on 2009 and 2010, when the ACA was being developed and ACA attitudes were likely to be more malleable. We first use survey experiments invoking distrust to benchmark the potential for framing effects. Next we analyze U.S. senators' press releases and politicians' appearances on major television shows to characterize politicians' rhetoric on the ACA. We then use a combination of data from the HTP and open-ended survey responses to explore the influence and limits of elite-level rhetoric on citizens. Public views of the ACA show none of the volatility of elite-level rhetoric. We do find evidence that the public adopts the language used by political elites in describing the policy to some degree. But overall, messaging does not prove to be a decisive influence on ACA attitudes, a finding reinforced through a large-scale field experiment. The broad narratives that the public employs to make sense of a policy can matter, but those narratives don't seem to be susceptible to elite influence, at least not in the short term.

The ACA was arguably the central vehicle for battles between Republicans and Democrats between its introduction in 2009 and the 2021 end of the Trump presidency. Its passage was Democrats' top legislative priority when they held unified control in 2009–2010, and its repeal was Republicans' top legislative priority when they were in the same position in 2017. It remained the target of high-profile legal challenges even after the 2020 election. And the Covid-19 pandemic put new strains on the law, as it did on the health care system generally. So any endpoint for an analysis of ACA attitudes is going to seem arbitrary and will leave the story incomplete. In chapter 8, however, we try to bring the story to a conclusion.

At a time of consistently close federal elections, parties understandably look for every electoral advantage.[106] But the evidence here shows that messaging and even policymaking are not likely to translate into short-term electoral gains—and that policymakers would do well to focus on designing policies that accomplish their policy goals while avoiding a sustained political backlash. In today's polarized environment, the expectation that piecemeal policies will build meaningful political support within a few electoral cycles does not seem realistic.

CHAPTER 2

The Elite-Level Politics and Policymaking of the ACA

EARLY IN THE morning of Friday, July 28, 2017, the U.S. Senate found itself voting on what some called a "skinny repeal" of the ACA. The legislation in question would have ended its individual mandate and delayed its employer mandate while leaving some key parts of the law untouched.[1] Ironically, the bill's Republican backers did not actually want that particular legislation to become law. In fact, GOP Senator Lindsey Graham had announced the prior afternoon that he was supporting the bill precisely because he had received assurances from the GOP Senate leadership that it would *not* become law.[2] But after months of failed attempts to find a proposal to repeal the ACA that could win the needed fifty U.S. senators, the Republicans had settled on a placeholder bill.[3] If it passed, the Senate would then be able to appoint members to a conference committee with the Republican-controlled House of Representatives to iron out a final bill that was likely to repeal key elements of the ACA. Senate Republicans were punting.

Republican senator John McCain, who was receiving cancer treatments in his home state of Arizona, had returned to Washington, D.C., earlier that week specifically for the vote. At the time, the Republicans held a two-seat majority in the Senate. But with Republicans Susan Collins of Maine and Lisa Murkowski of Alaska likely to oppose the measure, the bill needed support from every other GOP senator to produce a 50–50 tie that could be broken by the Republican vice president. As the GOP's 2008 presidential candidate, McCain seemed like an unlikely person to torpedo his party's top legislative priority. That was especially true given that the ACA was the principal legislative accomplishment of Barack Obama, McCain's 2008 opponent. But during the roll call vote early that morning, McCain strode into the Senate chamber, extended his arm, and then, turning his thumb decisively down, cast a "no" vote on the "skinny repeal."

We don't typically think of health policy legislation as dramatic, and yet, at that moment, the fate of the ACA—as well as the health insurance and taxes of millions of Americans and the related laws governing their lives— hung in the balance. Nor was that the first time that the ACA had hinged on a single person's choice.

In this chapter, we provide the background needed to understand the battles over the ACA in the decade following its enactment. We first narrate an abbreviated history of the attempts at comprehensive health insurance reform in the United States that led up to the ACA before explaining the law's key features. We then consider the brief, tumultuous political life of the ACA post-enactment.

The chapter has three core goals. The first is to provide a sketch of the ACA's path dependence—that is, the ways in which decisions made about health insurance decades ago have shaped the policy choices available to recent generations of reformers. In doing so, we can better understand why the ACA took the shape that it did, and we can think about what plausible counterfactual health care reforms might have looked like. Second, the chapter recaps the drama surrounding the ACA—in contrast to the stability of public views of the law, as we will see in the next chapter. Our portrait of all the elite-level shifts in the law's fortunes will put the public's lack of a strong reaction in sharp relief. Finally, to understand the ACA's elements that are more or less salient to the public, the chapter aims to illuminate what the ACA actually does. We cannot assess claims about how the law did or did not shape public opinion until we understand the complex ways in which it has touched Americans' lives.

A Brief History of Health Insurance Reform

Among developed countries, the United States has a system of health insurance that is an outlier in critical respects. For one, American health care is quite expensive. The United States spends 16.8 percent of total GDP on health care, a figure higher than in any other large developed country.[4] At the same time, the United States stands out for its system of health insurance: whereas many other developed countries have strictly public systems of health insurance, the United States has long had a complex hybrid system in which a majority of people get insurance privately through their employer.[5] This hybrid system is one cause of Americans' high levels of personal health care debt, a problem unknown in many other developed countries.[6] Still, key populations in the United States are insured directly through the government: those who are over sixty-five and eligible for Medicare (18 percent) and those with incomes low enough to qualify for Medicaid (20 percent). The U.S. military insures 9 million people via TRICARE. Through Veterans Affairs (VA), the government also directly provides health care to 7 million veterans.[7]

This patchwork system of insurance is the product of political evolution over many decades.[8] Wage controls and labor shortages during the Second World War encouraged employers to compete for employees through benefits rather than pay, and federal tax deductions for employers helped lock in a system of employer-sponsored insurance. But of course, not all Americans were employed, and not all employers provided health insurance.

Addressing clear gaps in health insurance provision, President Lyndon Johnson and Congress established systems in the mid-1960s to provide insurance for the elderly (Medicare) and the poor alongside some people with disabilities (Medicaid). Despite being established at roughly the same time, Medicare and Medicaid differ in critical respects. Medicaid was designed as a federal-state partnership that, along with other features, limited the benefits it provided to poor Americans.[9] By requiring states to pay substantial shares of the cost of Medicaid, the program created powerful incentives for state officials to keep health care spending low; no such incentives were built into Medicare. One of Medicaid's architects, Representative Wilbur Mills of Arkansas, even thought of it as "build[ing] a fence around Medicare" so as to prevent the more generous program's expansion.[10] Decades before Bernie Sanders advocated for expanding Medicare to all Americans, members of Congress were designing policies to preempt that very possibility.

The Clinton Push for Health Reform

From Harry Truman's presidency onward, Democrats proposed sweeping reforms that would move the United States toward a system of universal health insurance more like those in other developed countries. In 1992, Democrat Bill Clinton won the presidency after a campaign in which he had emphasized health care. With unified Democratic control of Congress and the presidency for the first time since the Carter administration in the late 1970s, the Democrats were poised to make another push for systemic health insurance reform.

After his election, Clinton tasked First Lady Hillary Clinton and aide Ira Magaziner with developing a health care plan. The resulting plan, dubbed "managed competition," relied on "regional purchasing cooperatives that would contract with private health plans and monitor the competition among them."[11] Unlike Medicare, Clinton's health care plan didn't call for a direct, government-run insurance program; instead, it "sought to achieve liberal ends of universal coverage through the conservative means of managed competition among private health plans, with a backup cap on the rate of growth in average insurance premiums."[12] In the words of the researcher Theda Skocpol, it was "a compromise between market-oriented and government-centered reform ideas," one that "substitute[d] regulations for revenue."[13]

Despite Bill Clinton's prime-time address to a joint session of Congress in September 1993, the bill met strident opposition after its release. As we saw in the introduction, some on the political right worried that a new middle-class entitlement would represent a critical setback in their effort to reduce the size and scope of government. But the opposition to Clinton's health reform came from moderate Democrats too. A year after Clinton's address, the plan's failure in Congress was clear.[14] Scholarly debates over the reasons for its failures presaged debates about the limitations of the ACA. Skocpol, for example, contends that Clinton's approach accepted too readily the fiscal constraints of deficit-cutting that it had inherited from the Reagan era. The proposal "assiduously avoided the 'tax and spend' modalities of traditional New Deal liberalism," she writes, "only to fall victim instead to the political pitfalls of substituting regulations for spending."[15] The sociologist Paul Starr, by contrast, contends that there was no pathway to pass more expansive legislation and that Clinton should have pursued a more limited plan more quickly.[16] For Sven Steinmo and Jon Watts, the nature of American political institutions, as they had evolved by the 1990s, gave interest groups such power as to render national health insurance "impossible."[17]

The Lead-up to the ACA

Even after the failure of comprehensive health reform in the first two years of the Clinton presidency, health insurance continued to be a central issue in federal politics. In 1997, the federal government enacted the Children's Health Insurance Program (CHIP) as part of a bipartisan agreement between the Democratic president and congressional Republicans. CHIP provided grants to states to insure children whose families were above Medicaid thresholds but below 200 percent of the federal poverty line.[18] In 2003, the Republicans sought to add a prescription drug benefit to Medicare, a move that they thought would help George W. Bush win reelection in the following year. As part of the Medicare Modernization Act (MMA), they enacted a prescription drug benefit for seniors known as "Medicare Part D," with the bill passing the House of Representatives by a single vote.[19] Votes on the House floor commonly last ten minutes, but that early-morning vote was held open for hours to give the GOP leadership additional time to wrangle votes from members of their own caucus who were hesitant about expanding government benefits. Politically, it was noteworthy that Democrats were largely opposed to the MMA, in part because the MMA provided a voluntary prescription drug benefit that came, not directly from the government, but through private insurers.[20]

Policy changes at the state level were key, too. In 2006, with the signature of Republican governor Mitt Romney, Massachusetts enacted legislation that significantly increased the state's fraction of residents with health insurance by mandating that residents have health insurance and that many employers provide it, while also authorizing subsidies for lower-income residents. Politically, some of Romney's advisers thought that the state's health insurance reform would position him well to run for president in 2008, as he could tout having accomplished a reform that had bedeviled Hillary Clinton, his would-be Democratic rival.[21] Notice that in the Massachusetts case as well as with CHIP and the MMA, the efforts to expand health insurance were bipartisan or even Republican-led. As of 2006, there was certainly reason to think that some form of health insurance reform could be passed through Congress with at least some Republican support.

The white whale of the Democratic Party—comprehensive health insurance—continued to be an animating issue in the lead-up to the 2008 presidential election. Hillary Clinton had emerged as the front-runner for the Democratic nomination, and true to form, she emphasized comprehensive health insurance reform as a central plank of her candidacy. Like the Massachusetts law, Clinton's health care plan included a mandate that all Americans have health insurance—and she was actually criticized for that mandate by one of her Democratic rivals, Illinois Senator Barack Obama.[22] But Obama, too, campaigned on a significant expansion of health insurance. And when Obama was elected in November 2008 with a sizable Democratic majority in the House of Representatives and a sixty-vote supermajority in the U.S. Senate within reach, the Democrats embarked on yet another attempt to extend health insurance to the millions of people who lacked it.

Barack Obama took office during the sharpest economic downturn in decades, and his immediate work was focused on passing an economic stimulus. His administration and fellow Democrats in Congress quickly pivoted, however, to tackle the issue of health insurance. To some, that represented a major political error, since the Democrats could well be perceived by voters as shifting away from the economic woes faced by much of the country.[23] But to some Democratic officials and White House aides, the economy and health care were closely connected: surging unemployment was causing millions of Americans to lose their health insurance, and millions more may have been locked in their jobs by the fear of losing insurance.

During the spring and summer of 2009, efforts to lay the groundwork for what would ultimately be the ACA continued, with bipartisan talks between a group of Democratic and Republican senators as well as feverish policy discussions in different parts of Washington, D.C.[24] Political actors are often keen to avoid what they perceive as their predecessors' key mistakes, and health care reform was no exception. Some Obama aides who saw the choice by the Clinton White House to draft the legislation itself as a political mistake plotted a course in which Congress would take the lead in writing the bill.

During the August recess in 2009, members of Congress were famously confronted at many of their town hall meetings by activists who would come to identify with the Tea Party.[25] Former GOP vice presidential nominee Sarah Palin also fanned false concerns about health care reform, writing on Facebook, "Who will suffer the most when they ration care? The sick, the elderly, and the disabled, of course. The America I know and love is not one in which my parents or my baby with Down Syndrome will have to stand in front of Obama's 'death panel' so his bureaucrats can decide, based on a subjective judgment of their 'level of productivity in society,' whether they are worthy of health care. Such a system is downright evil."[26] That the law included no such panels was beside the point.

That September, like Bill Clinton before him, Barack Obama delivered a prime-time address on health insurance reform whose aim was in part to recapture the initiative and prod Congress into action. But there, the stories of the Clinton and Obama pushes for health insurance reform diverged. The Clinton reform effort stalled after facing bipartisan opposition in Congress. After fifteen years of polarization, the Democrats in 2009 were more unified. Even Tennessee representative Jim Cooper, a centrist Democrat who had opposed Clinton's bill in 1993–1994, was on board with Obama's efforts.[27] By November 7, the House of Representatives had narrowly passed a health insurance bill whose contours were roughly similar to what would ultimately be the Affordable Care Act, although it did include a public option as well as a single nationwide health insurance exchange. In a signal of the partisan divisions to come, the House's health care bill received just one GOP vote, and that was from a freshman lawmaker representing a strongly Democratic district in New Orleans.

The Anatomy of the ACA

It's worth pausing the political narrative here to understand the key features of the ACA. As we have seen, the pre-ACA system of health insurance provision was a patchwork of public and private insurance, with private insurance typically tax-subsidized and provided primarily through employers.[28] Although there was a separate insurance market for individuals, it was small and had highly variable products, and insurers could reject applicants with preexisting conditions.[29] On the public side, Medicare was the federal program that insured a majority of those sixty-five and over, and Medicaid was a means-tested federal-state partnership that targeted households with children and varied markedly across states.[30] Others were insured publicly through CHIP or TRICARE. This hybrid system left 50 million Americans without health insurance, many of whom were middle-class and working age.[31] That fact had motivated the periodic efforts to enact comprehensive health care reform.

Rather than develop or expand a single program, the ACA sought to fill in gaps in the existing system. The law's centerpiece was arguably the establishment of exchanges or marketplaces through which individuals could purchase private insurance, which was subsidized for those making less than 400 percent of the federal poverty line. These exchanges are regulated markets in which customers can shop for health insurance products that are ranked according to their coverage; customers can access them online, enlist the help of a broker, or contact insurers directly. Insurers were allowed to charge older customers only three times as much as younger customers, and they could no longer deny coverage due to an individual's health history. Initial projections indicated that by 2019, 24 million more Americans would be insured through the exchanges and a further 16 million through the ACA's expansion of Medicaid.[32] The original expectation was that states would operate their own exchanges, but only a minority of states chose to do so. Moreover, the quality and pricing of the insurance offerings varied markedly by geography. Depending on where customers lived, they might have found themselves with various affordable insurance options—or with only a few.[33]

The law also expanded Medicaid eligibility to 138 percent of the federal poverty line and allowed able-bodied adults to participate irrespective of family status; prior to the ACA, income thresholds were lower but varied by state, while adults without children were typically ineligible.[34] Separate elements ended lifetime and annual caps on insurance company payouts, defined what essential health benefits plans must include, and enabled children to remain on their parents' insurance until age twenty-six.[35] Politically, the exchanges were also a potential keystone of ACA support overall, as they targeted a more middle-class constituency than did the Medicaid expansion.[36]

The exchanges themselves had various policy levers. As enacted, the exchanges were bolstered by a new tax penalty, or "individual mandate," for Americans who did not have qualifying health insurance, a mandate that had been featured in the Massachusetts plan and would limit adverse selection. (Simply put, adverse selection is a problem in insurance markets in which people who anticipate needing extensive coverage are more likely to buy insurance policies. Adverse selection thus risks driving prices up as insurers confront the costs of these claims.) In 2016, 5 million tax returns included such penalties, with a mean payment of $727.[37] The federal exchanges also had a notoriously rocky rollout. The healthcare.gov website was plagued by long waiting times and other technical difficulties during its fall 2013 opening.[38]

By contrast, Americans making below 400 percent of the poverty line were provided by the federal government with subsidies in the form of the Advance Premium Tax Credit (APTC). In 2016, 6.1 million American households received this credit, with a mean subsidy of approximately $4,000.[39] Notably, those with access to qualifying health insurance through employers were ineligible for subsidies on the exchanges. Separately, people whose incomes proved higher than expected were required to repay the excess subsidy.

The ACA gave states the authority to run their own exchanges, but to the surprise of the ACA's architects, a majority chose to have the federal government administer their exchanges instead.[40] Prices and the insurance products available on the exchanges varied markedly from state to state and market to market. States also varied in the extent to which they encouraged residents to use the exchanges.[41] In short, even those most likely to consider using the exchanges were likely to have very different experiences depending on their specific medical conditions and place of residence.[42]

One of Obama's stated goals in enacting health care reform was to make the law deficit-neutral, so the ACA also included taxes to fund the law. Some of those taxes fell on consumers via the health care industry, including taxes on pharmaceuticals, health insurers, medical devices (later repealed), and tanning salons. But two of the primary revenue sources were taxes on high-income taxpayers: a 0.9 percent payroll tax as well as a 3.8 percent tax on net investment income, both taxes being levied on those earning more than $200,000 per year.[43] The geography of American taxation led to these taxes being paid disproportionately by Democratic-leaning states.[44]

This brief synopsis has omitted a range of other ACA provisions, from the creation of the Center for Medicare and Medicaid Innovation to new limits on insurance companies' spending on administration.[45] While impactful, those provisions were invisible to most citizens. Chapter 5 considers yet another feature of the ACA—the provision that insurers covering dependents had to continue coverage until age twenty-six. But even with the selective discussion here, the ACA's complexity should be clear.

The Political Saga of the ACA

In J.R.R. Tolkien's *The Lord of the Rings*, one of the characters notes that "the quest stands upon the edge of a knife. Stray but a little, and it will fail."[46] While *The Lord of the Rings* is pure fantasy, complete with elves and wizards, the very real efforts to pass and then preserve the ACA could be similarly described. As in Frodo's fictional quest, the history of the ACA is replete with moments when a single individual or a subtle twist in fate would have ended the reform. We opened this chapter with one such moment—Senator John McCain stopping his fellow Republicans' legislative march toward repealing the law. But that moment was just one of many.

When Democratic senators negotiated over the ACA late in 2009, the Democrats had exactly the sixty votes in the U.S. Senate that they needed to pass legislation over the threat of a filibuster. In the absence of GOP support, a single defection from wavering Democratic senators, like Connecticut's Joe Lieberman or Nebraska's Ben Nelson, could doom the effort. Having a sixty-vote supermajority was a double-edged sword: because the Democrats had been so successful in Senate elections in 2006 and 2008, several of the more moderate Republicans who might have backed health care reform had lost their seats. When Pennsylvania's Arlen Specter switched to the Democratic Party, the Democrats gained a key vote, but the list of would-be bipartisan fig leaves also grew shorter. Maine Republican Olympia Snowe had voted for a version of health care reform in committee, but when she subsequently came to oppose the effort, the Democrats were forced to rely entirely on their own votes. So any Democratic senator could derail the train.

In December 2009, with the effort to pass health care reform on the line, Senate majority leader Harry Reid cut deals with senators who were on the fence to win their support. The deal that Reid made with Ben Nelson was so lucrative for Nelson's home state of Nebraska that it was widely derided as the "Cornhusker Kickback." But with all sixty Senate Democrats on board, Reid then proceeded to pass the sweeping health care reform bill that had been advanced by Finance chair Max Baucus, kickback and all.

However, the Democrats' elation at having passed the bill through the Senate was short-lived. On January 19, 2010, Republican Scott Brown shocked political observers by winning a Massachusetts special election to fill the Senate seat opened by the death of Ted Kennedy. The irony was obvious: Kennedy, one of the Senate's most outspoken supporters of comprehensive health insurance, was being replaced by a senator who had pledged to oppose the ACA. Given Brown's opposition and that of every other Senate Republican, even with the support of all fifty-nine of their remaining senators, the Democrats would be unable to pass any subsequent health care legislation that was subject to the filibuster in the Senate. The original plan to merge the Senate and House versions through a conference committee was dead. In response, some Democrats, including Obama's chief of staff Rahm Emanuel, argued for a less ambitious bill.[47]

However, there was still a narrow pathway to enactment, and Obama chose to take it. The Senate had already passed a health insurance bill, after all, so no conference committee would be needed if the House of Representatives passed the Senate's bill word for word despite its limitations—and despite the infamous "Cornhusker Kickback." On March 21, the House narrowly voted to pass the Senate bill. But it did so only after Obama issued an executive order to mollify the concerns of pro-life Democratic representative Bart Stupak. So Bart Stupak and House Speaker Nancy Pelosi joined Ben Nelson, Joe Lieberman, and Scott Brown as individuals whose decisions helped shape the course of the ACA. Shortly thereafter, the House and Senate used the budget reconciliation process to remove the Nebraska provision and make other fiscal changes without needing sixty Senate votes.

But the House passing a Senate bill word for word is not the typical road for major legislation, and that unusual birth made the ACA more susceptible to legal and policy implementation challenges in the years to come.[48] It's something akin to a student accidentally turning in a draft on a crucial assignment and being stuck with its typos and errors for years. As we discuss later, the ACA as enacted included drafting errors and omissions that made it an accessible target for legal challenges. For instance, it did not include a severability clause, which would have helped the bulk of the law to stand if a specific element were ruled unconstitutional.

A few of the ACA's elements came into force soon after its passage, including its ban on lifetime caps on insurance payments and its provision enabling children to stay on their parents' insurance until age twenty-six.

But the ACA was deliberately backloaded: almost four years passed between its enactment in March 2010 and the implementation in 2014 of key provisions like the main Medicaid expansion and the insurance exchanges. As a consequence, the ACA remained largely in limbo for years and faced existential political and legal challenges before its main provisions were even enacted.

Helen Levy and her coauthors estimate that several years after its enactment 83 percent of the ACA's provisions had been implemented as written.[49] Their research also highlights that Republican opposition was not the sole explanation for the elements that were not implemented. In 2011, the Obama administration itself declared an entire title of the law, the Community Living Assistance Services and Supports (CLASS) Plan, infeasible.[50] The ACA's so-called Cadillac Tax, a tax on high-end health plans, was repealed in 2019 with overwhelming bipartisan support.[51]

Many laws continue to be contested after passage.[52] But the ACA was an entirely different experience: soon after passage, it gave rise to lawsuits as well as implacable opposition from Republicans, opposition that grew notably stronger after the 2010 wave election shifted control of many statehouses to the GOP. The ACA's reliance on states to implement key elements like the exchanges had helped it win passage through the Senate. But that reliance also meant that key elements of the ACA were to be implemented by state officials who were committed to the law's repeal.[53]

One of the existential threats to the ACA came from a series of lawsuits that were heard by the Supreme Court in 2012. The suits challenged the constitutionality of the law, and in particular the mandate that all Americans receive health insurance; they also challenged the expansion of Medicaid under the law. Some legal scholars initially dismissed the suits' likelihood of success, but during extensive oral arguments in March of that year the justices' questioning led a prominent legal commentator to pronounce that the ACA was in serious legal jeopardy.[54] One critical legal question was about the constitutionality of the ACA's individual mandate: Did the federal government have the authority to mandate that Americans purchase a product from a private actor? That conundrum sparked further questions about the law's severability. The absence of a severability clause left open the question of whether parts could be unconstitutional without imperiling the entire law and potentially raised the stakes for any court decision.

When the Court's decision in *National Federation of Independent Business v. Sebelius* was announced in June 2012, *Fox News* initially reported that the law had been struck down.[55] But in fact, it had been upheld on a 5–4 vote. Subsequent reporting has made it clear that the decision could easily have gone the other way. In an internal conference among the Supreme Court justices in late March 2012, Chief Justice John Roberts reportedly voted that the ACA's individual mandate was unconstitutional while also voting that the Medicaid expansion could stand as written—as a nationwide policy, from which states could opt out only by forfeiting their existing Medicaid funding. But the other four conservative justices on the Court believed that striking down the individual mandate required voiding the ACA in its entirety, a step that Roberts did not want to take. To avoid overturning the entire law, Roberts needed to build a coalition of five justices; he ultimately did so by upholding the ACA's mandate as a tax while also concluding that the Medicaid expansion must be optional for states.[56]

This act surely adds John Roberts—and the four liberal justices who sided with him—to the list of individuals whose decisions powerfully shaped the course of the ACA. The law had been just one vote away from being invalidated by the Supreme Court. At the same time, two of those liberal justices wound up voting with the conservatives that the Medicaid expansion constituted a sufficiently different program from traditional Medicaid that states had to be given the ability to opt out of participation without jeopardizing their existing Medicaid funds.[57] The move to make the Medicaid expansion optional was a surprise: Justice Elena Kagan had commented during oral arguments that the expansion offered states "a boatload of money."[58] Moreover, the Medicaid expansion's constitutionality had not been central to the legal challenges against the law.[59] Together, those facts suggest that making the Medicaid expansion optional was the price of winning Roberts's vote to uphold the individual mandate as a tax.[60] But it proved to be a hefty price to pay: even nine years later, in 2021, twelve states had not expanded Medicaid, leaving 2 million Americans without access to the program.[61]

As a political scientist, I am far more comfortable summarizing the political views of millions than speculating about the views of a single person I haven't surveyed or interviewed. But the *NFIB v. Sebelius* decision—and its unexpected move against the Medicaid expansion—does encourage us to consider what John Roberts's motives may have been. Did making the

Medicaid expansion optional bring the ACA closer to his conservative policy preferences? Or was there a political calculation involved? Did Roberts think that making the expansion optional might prevent the law from becoming entrenched? To the extent that Roberts was motivated by the latter possibility, that reinforces the point that political actors' *expectations* of policy feedbacks are themselves influential.

Implementing the ACA, 2013–2014

This account of the ACA emphasizes the profound influence of individual decisions, whether those of Barack Obama, Bart Stupak, or John Roberts. In November 2012, the millions of Americans who voted in that year's presidential and congressional elections weighed in as well. Had Republican Mitt Romney been elected with a Republican Congress, he planned to move to stop the ACA's implementation. But Obama's victory by about 5 million votes effectively ended the possibility of legislative repeal prior to the implementation of the ACA's main provisions in January 2014.

Nonetheless, the political challenges to the law continued. On October 1, 2013, spurred by Republican senator Ted Cruz, House Republicans induced a shutdown of the federal government in an effort to prevent enactment of the ACA. The move did not accomplish that goal, and it may have even helped the law politically in an unexpected way: the government shutdown helped draw attention away from the disastrous launch of the federal exchange website healthcare.gov. A series of planning and programming failures had produced a website that was almost inoperable at its grand opening.[62]

Late 2013 also saw an uproar over canceled insurance plans. During the debates over the ACA, Obama had repeatedly promised Americans that, "if you like your health care plan, you'll be able to keep your health care plan."[63] But as insurers moved into compliance with the ACA's new standards for insurance plans, they canceled noncompliant plans, leading millions of people to find themselves without insurance just as the ACA was coming into effect. Obama had broken his promise. The Obama administration then backpedaled, allowing the plans to continue through 2014.[64] The website, the shutdown, and the uproar over canceled plans all passed in time. But the ACA was not off to an auspicious start.

Post-Implementation Republican Challenges

Even after the 2014 implementation of the law's main provisions, the ACA faced significant headwinds. In many places, its exchanges created health insurance markets that had high or volatile premiums and narrow plans.[65] But not all the law's wounds were self-inflicted. Republicans and their allies maintained a posture of steadfast opposition to the law and sought to undermine or limit it in a range of venues.[66]

One of those venues was at the state level. By design, the implementation of key aspects of the ACA was dependent on the states, a role that grew larger with the Supreme Court's 2012 decision making the Medicaid expansion optional. Many Republican-controlled states chose not to expand Medicaid.[67] These states also did little to promote the ACA's exchanges as an option for their residents.[68]

Another such venue was Congress, where the ACA's complexity continued to give its opponents opportunities to undermine it. For example, Republican senator Marco Rubio slipped a provision into a 2014 spending bill that limited "risk corridor" payments to insurance companies—which were designed to encourage them to offer policies on the exchanges—in what the *New York Times* deemed "quiet legislative sabotage."[69] (Risk corridor payments were intended to incentivize insurance companies to participate in the exchanges by making payments to insurers who wound up paying too much in claims or earning too little from premiums.) At the same time, the Republican-controlled House of Representatives voted to repeal or undermine the ACA dozens of times in the period between 2011 and 2016, safe in the knowledge that so long as the Democrats had the presidency, such efforts were largely symbolic.[70]

Legal challenges continued too. The *King v. Burwell* case—resolved by the Supreme Court in 2015—was another example of the ACA's unusual legislative birth leading to legal liabilities down the road.[71] *King* was premised on the observation that the ACA's text authorized subsidies on marketplaces "established by the state."[72] The plaintiffs thus held that insurance could only be subsidized on the exchanges that were state-run, and they sought to end subsidies for the majority of states that used federal exchanges.[73] The challengers thus sought to undermine the law by exploiting what seemed to be a drafting error. The Supreme Court would decide against the challengers in this case, but the law's complex structure and reliance on a range of political actors continued to make parts of it highly vulnerable.

Trump-Era Challenges and Changes

Despite these rearguard actions, the most straightforward pathway to ACA repeal remained through winning Congress and the presidency simultaneously. It's Lawmaking 101: if the House and Senate both pass a piece of legislation, it becomes law once it is signed by the president. During the Obama presidency, there was no chance of legislative repeal of the ACA. But Donald Trump's 2016 election made legislative repeal of the ACA through Congress a distinct possibility. Many Republican lawmakers had been elected in the preceding years after campaigning to repeal the law, and after dozens of symbolic votes, GOP lawmakers were finally in a position to make good on those promises.

That said, repealing a law as extensive as the ACA was never going to be easy, and existing Senate rules made it harder still. The original ACA had passed through normal Senate procedures requiring sixty votes to end debate and proceed to vote on a bill. It had done so in 2009–2010, during the only Congress since the 1970s in which either party held at least sixty seats. But the Republicans controlled just fifty-two Senate seats after the 2016 election, and they knew from the outset that they would never win the eight Democratic votes needed to repeal Obama's signature law. They were also committed to maintaining the Senate's existing rules for ending debates, known as "cloture" (with the noteworthy exception of Supreme Court nominations). As a result, the GOP set out to repeal the ACA through Congress's reconciliation process, which is designed to facilitate the passage of budget-related bills by requiring only fifty votes in the Senate. But it also meant that key ACA regulations without direct budgetary implications couldn't be repealed.

We should not let discussions of congressional procedure obscure the GOP's more fundamental problem: the party was divided about just how much of the ACA to repeal. Symbolically, the GOP in the period between 2010 and 2016 had consistently committed to repealing Obamacare, but just how much of it had to go? As we saw earlier, the ACA was an intricate contraption designed to make insurance accessible for people with preexisting conditions through regulations, subsidies, and an expansion of Medicaid. The GOP could not repeal the law without undoing some of its positive features, like the protections for people with preexisting conditions. Republicans couldn't cut the taxes that funded the ACA and still fund or subsidize millions of new health insurance plans, whether through the exchanges or Medicaid.

Some ACA provisions, like those protecting people with preexisting conditions, were known to be quite popular. In fact, key Republican figures had committed to keeping such protections. After comedian Jimmy Kimmel made a televised plea for universal insurance that would cover treatment for conditions like his newborn son's heart condition, Republican senator (and doctor) Bill Cassidy promised that GOP repeal efforts would "pass the Jimmy Kimmel test" of covering those with serious, expensive medical conditions.[74] What's more, by 2017 the list of states that had expanded Medicaid included not just solidly Democratic states but key states represented by Republican senators, such as Nevada, Arizona, Arkansas, Louisiana, Alaska, and Kentucky. To end the Medicaid expansion was to take insurance away from many thousands of people in those states, and also to pull dollars out of those states' health care systems. The Republicans did prioritize ACA repeal when Congress convened in January, but their first offensive was short-lived. On March 24, 2017, House Speaker Paul Ryan pulled his repeal bill from the House floor when it was clear that it did not have the votes; for some Republicans, Ryan's repeal plan didn't go far enough; for others, it went too far. Ryan declared that "Obamacare is the law of the land" and would be "for the foreseeable future."[75]

Just two months into Trump's presidency, many in the Trump administration and the GOP leadership were not ready to throw in the towel. On May 4, 2017, the Republican-controlled House passed a repeal bill known as the American Health Care Act (AHCA), with a 217–213 vote, and sent the legislation to the Senate.[76] The AHCA repealed core elements of the ACA and included tax cuts and large cuts in Medicaid, with funding going to states in the form of block grants. It repealed the mandate that most individuals have health insurance. It also allowed states to get waivers on the ACA's requirements that health history not influence premiums and that insurers cover a basket of essential health benefits.[77] However, it fell short of full-scale ACA repeal.

The passage of the AHCA in the House shifted the focus to the Senate, where Majority Leader Mitch McConnell could lose only two Republican votes and still pass any repeal bill. Senate Republicans then began a period of pitched negotiations about just how much of the ACA to repeal. They faced the same intractable dilemmas that House Republicans had faced, but had less of a margin for error. Defections from any three Republican senators would sink the endeavor.

An adage holds that politicians "campaign in poetry, but govern in prose." That seems an apt description of the GOP's challenge when it came to repealing the ACA. In campaigning to repeal the ACA, the GOP had ignored the trade-offs inherent in health policymaking. And even as repeal was well underway, key Republican figures promised that no significant costs would be incurred in repealing the ACA. In the Rose Garden celebration of the House's passage of the bill repealing the ACA, for example, President Trump said, "Yes, premiums will be coming down; yes, deductibles will be coming down."[78] However, the GOP's primary policy goals—to repeal the ACA, lower taxes, end or scale back the Medicaid expansion, and shutter the exchanges—would result in millions losing health insurance while protections for those with preexisting conditions weakened substantially. It proved easy to unify the GOP around a slogan of repealing the ACA when the details of that repeal were left ambiguous. But it was far harder to commit the party to the particular trade-offs that repeal required. It's no surprise that GOP senators continued to wrangle over the contours of ACA repeal in the late spring and summer of 2017 in what seemed like an endless series of palace intrigues about which senators would support what policies. In late July, Senate Republicans, who had still not coalesced behind a repeal plan, instead opted to punt by proposing a "skinny repeal" that would set up a conference committee with the House.

Even after the dramatic early-morning vote described in this chapter's introduction, when John McCain joined with Susan Collins and Lisa Murkowski to vote against "skinny repeal," Republicans continued to hope that the ACA might still be repealed. In September 2017, with the budget bill that enabled repeal via reconciliation set to expire at the end of the month, GOP senators Lindsey Graham and Bill Cassidy promoted their own variant of ACA repeal. Their plan, dubbed "Graham-Cassidy," would have reduced health care spending and given states more authority in its use.[79] Graham lobbied for the bill, saying it posed a "choice for America: federalism or socialism."[80] But that effort also collapsed under the weight of conflicting policy goals. Graham and Cassidy were never able to win over enough of their Senate colleagues to pass their bill.

After the failure of Graham-Cassidy, legislative repeal efforts largely subsided, with one important exception: in a December 2017 tax bill, Republicans did agree to eliminate the individual mandate as of 2019 by reducing the penalty for not having health insurance to zero dollars. In the 2008 campaign, Barack Obama had opposed a health insurance mandate, only to reverse himself and sign one into law in 2010. In 2012, the individual mandate had been at the center of the Supreme Court case that threatened to end with the ACA being ruled unconstitutional. Five years later, the mandate was eliminated with relatively little fanfare—and with modest impacts on health insurance enrollment.[81] Had experts not convinced Obama that the individual mandate was integral to achieving his policy goals, the history of the ACA might read quite differently.

Executive Actions and Legislation in the Wake of 2017

Despite Paul Ryan's statement that the ACA was the law of the land, even the failure of repeal efforts did not end Republicans' attempts to weaken the ACA. Through actions and inaction, the Trump administration worked to do through the executive branch what it could not do via Congress: weaken the ACA.[82]

For one thing, the Trump administration reduced outreach efforts to promote enrollment via the ACA's exchanges.[83] It also suspended the "cost sharing reduction" payments to insurers that subsidized lower-income enrollees in 2017, forcing insurers to go to court to seek the subsidies.[84] The ACA's payments to insurance companies were clearly seen as a political Achilles' heel—and so a ripe target—by the law's Republican opponents. The Trump administration also approved state Medicaid waivers allowing work requirements in states like Arkansas.[85] The cumulative effect of the Trump administration's policies had raised the fraction of uninsured Americans from a low of 11.4 percent in 2015 to 13.7 percent in 2019.[86]

Upon taking office in 2021, the Biden administration, moving to reverse key Trump-era decisions, suspended the Medicaid waivers allowing states to impose work requirements on Medicaid recipients and bolstered ACA outreach.[87] The American Rescue Plan, passed early in the Biden administration by Democrats in Congress, aimed to further shore up the ACA as part of its Covid relief package: it provided incentives for holdout states to expand their Medicaid programs while increasing the subsidies available to customers purchasing insurance on the exchanges.[88]

The year 2021 also saw what one Supreme Court justice termed "the third installment in our epic Affordable Care Act trilogy"—a 7–2 case in which the Supreme Court dismissed a challenge to the ACA's constitutionality.[89] In the *California v. Texas* challenge, Republican attorneys general and governors built their legal case against the ACA from the Supreme Court's 2012 decision: if the constitutionality of the ACA hinged on the individual mandate being a tax, then the repeal of the individual mandate, they argued, rendered the law unconstitutional. Lower-level federal courts had agreed with the plaintiffs, putting the law's constitutionality in question yet again. But the Supreme Court set aside the challenge and, in referring to *California v. Texas* as the third installment in a trilogy, suggested that it might be the last.

Conclusion

In this chapter, as a first step in understanding how the public thought about the ACA—and the extent to which political elites were able to reshape that thinking—we have sought to understand the ACA as a complex bundle of policies. We have also detailed the political travails of its first decade. If we do not know the saga through which the ACA became a law, or what the ACA actually did, our understanding of public perceptions of the law will necessarily be incomplete. We have seen that the ACA emerged as a large-scale but incremental reform to an already patchwork system of health insurance. The law was highly complex, and it relied heavily on backdoor regulations and private provision to increase the availability of affordable, comprehensive health insurance.[90] Such features could limit its impacts on public opinion, as citizens' experiences with the law are likely to vary markedly. Many of its core provisions operated far from public view.

Still, an in-depth study of public opinion may illuminate at least some of the dramatic twists and paradoxes in the elite-level battles over the ACA. Consider the individual mandate and its prominent supporters and opponents. In 2006, Massachusetts governor Mitt Romney signed a statewide health reform law that was widely seen as a precursor to the ACA, complete with a mandate that residents obtain health insurance. Some advisers thought it would position him well to run for president in 2008.[91] A few years later, when campaigning for president, Barack Obama distinguished himself from his Democratic rival Hillary Clinton by *opposing* such a mandate nationwide.[92] But in 2010 Obama signed a federal health care law that included just such a mandate to purchase health insurance, and the law was so closely associated with him that it became commonly known as "Obamacare." In his 2012 campaign for reelection, Obama found himself defending that law against none other than Mitt Romney, the GOP presidential nominee, who promised to repeal it. On one of the defining issues of the last decade, leaders from both parties had changed their positions markedly. Such shifts give a hint of the intense pressure the issue placed on politicians from both sides of the aisle. But did that pressure arise from public opinion or from other parts of the political system? To answer that question, we turn in the next chapter to the public's reaction to the ACA.

In Shakespeare's *Twelfth Night*, a knight approves of a challenge his friend has written, saying, "If this letter move him not, his legs cannot." Similarly, if any political saga in recent years has been capable of moving American public opinion on a major issue, the ACA would seem to be it. As we have seen here, it was a high-profile story with sabotage, betrayal, and dramatic, late-night turns of events. At different moments, it hung in the balance as a parade of individuals (from Scott Brown and Ben Nelson to John Roberts and Susan Collins) shaped its course. The health insurance of millions of Americans—and the taxes and regulations imposed on millions more—hung in the balance. The drama stood to have profound effects on health insurance options and costs nationwide. How the public responded—and whether it responded at all—is the topic of chapter 3.

CHAPTER 3

The Stability of Public Opinion

THE PREVIOUS CHAPTER narrated the tumult that characterized the ACA's first decade. How did the public respond to the saga's seemingly endless plot twists? As this chapter shows, the public response was something closer to a flatline, especially relative to the elite-level drama. For the most part, the elite machinations left little imprint on public opinion. It was almost as if the audience spent the performance chatting in the lobby and caught only occasional echoes of the yelling onstage. Even the implementation of the ACA's main provisions in 2014 did little to alter the trajectory of ACA attitudes. But one event did lead the public to reevaluate the law: the election of Donald Trump in 2016.

By explaining the ACA's core provisions, the previous chapter provided a benchmark against which to make sense of public (mis)perceptions. After all, we cannot fully understand public opinion toward a policy if we do not first understand that policy in some detail. In particular, chapter 2 underscored the law's complexity, which has critical implications for public opinion formation and mobilization.

To set the stage for the empirical analyses of over-time trends in ACA attitudes, it is valuable to first have some background on how scholars and commentators have commonly conceived of public opinion. Thus, the next section draws hypotheses from prior work on public opinion in general. We then look at over-time evidence from a panel survey and a rolling cross-sectional survey before turning to open-ended questions that allow us to track opinion with greater nuance. Before its conclusion, the chapter also reviews evidence on specific elements of the ACA and details a survey experiment on status quo bias.

Questions about the public's political knowledge—and thus about the public's ability to hold politicians accountable for their actions in office—have recurred across generations of social science scholarship. The portrait of public opinion that emerges in this chapter charts something of a middle course with respect to prior arguments. On the one hand, the evidence presented here clearly dissents from the depictions of public opinion as hollow non-attitudes: public opinion on the ACA proved markedly more stable, coherent, and textured than many recent accounts would suggest. On the other hand, the evidence is also inconsistent with the calculating, utility-maximizing depiction of *homo economicus* that is the starting place for many rational choice models.[1] When explaining their attitudes toward the law, few members of the public highlight its impacts on them personally, and in aggregate the public seems unresponsive to all but the biggest changes in the law. Such a citizenry was not well positioned to adjudicate the more specific disputes that dominated ACA policymaking in the years after its enactment. What's more, the public's limitations are very likely to be exacerbated by today's highly complex, fragmented policymaking landscape.[2]

Coherent Opinions on Complex Policies?

Throughout the twentieth century, prominent voices have argued that American citizens are unable to track political events with anything approaching the understanding needed to reliably hold politicians accountable for their actions.[3] For scholars in this vein, Walter Lippmann is something of a patron saint. In their book's introduction, Christopher Achen and Larry Bartels quote from Lippmann's *Public Opinion*: "The real environment is altogether too big, too complex, and too fleeting for direct acquaintance. We are not equipped to deal with so much subtlety, so much variety, so many permutations and combinations."[4] In this view, social and political reality is at once too distant and too complex for citizens to follow it closely. Achen and Bartels add that "Lippmann remains the deepest and most thoughtful of the modern critics of the psychological foundations of the folk theory of democracy."[5]

But Walter Lippmann published *Public Opinion* in 1922, and it is important to acknowledge just how different the country was a century ago. For
one thing, health care had dramatically less to offer. Penicillin, for example,
had not yet been invented, and as of 1930, life expectancy in the United
States was fifty-eight for men and sixty-two for women.[6] Total federal
spending that year was just 3.5 percent of GDP, with health care accounting
for a tiny sliver of that spending.[7] Lippmann contended that the public was
unprepared to deal with the complexity of political life a century ago. But
today's U.S. government is a vastly larger and more complex enterprise. The
federal government now spends a significantly larger share of GDP on health
care alone—almost 8 percent—than it spent *across all spending areas* in 1930.[8]
And that is not to mention state and local governments, through which
many American public policies are delivered.

The growing complexity of the American government casts concerns like
Lippmann's in a new light. Debates about whether citizens have the political
sophistication necessary to ensure that their policy preferences are enacted
typically focus on one side of the equation—on what citizens know and
whether they draw on that knowledge when participating in politics. Scholars in this tradition ponder why an increasingly educated population seems
unable to meet certain minimum conceptions of engaged citizenship. But
since Lippmann's day, the public policy arena has become vastly more complex, raising the demands made of an informed citizenship even higher.[9]
Whereas Lippmann's critique was akin to a complaint about a third-grader
failing a multiplication test, his modern-day descendants lament a high
school senior's lackluster calculus exam. The task itself has changed.

As the prior chapter made clear, the ACA alone is extraordinarily complicated, to say nothing of the American system of health care more generally. The law relied on a wide range of provisions touching different actors
in the health care system. Some citizens might have been directly affected
by specific provisions, but many others may have been only indirectly
affected (if they were affected at all). If a person experiences a spike in her
premiums or has to trade a limited health insurance plan for a more comprehensive but expensive one, should she attribute those changes to the
ACA? Maybe, but maybe not. To this day, economists and public health
experts debate the causal effects of the ACA in academic journals.[10] And
some of those effects differ from what the ACA's architects initially expected.
For example, despite being a political lightning rod for the law, the individual

mandate was estimated to have done little to increase insurance uptake in its first years in force.[11] If the impacts of the law have become clear to health policy experts only after years of accumulating evidence and careful study, it seems altogether unlikely that citizens would have been in a position to confidently assess the net impacts of a complex bundle of reforms in real time.[12]

Lippmann's Descendants: Inattention and Partisan Rationalization

Lippmann wrote a century ago, but his intellectual descendants make related arguments today. For instance, a powerful vein in contemporary public opinion research argues that citizens have little information about politics, even on issues as salient as the Obama administration's signature policy issue. Writing in 2016, Arthur Lupia noted that, "when it comes to political information, there are two groups of people. One group understands that they are almost completely ignorant of almost every detail of almost every law and policy under which they live. The other group is delusional about how much they know. There is no third group."[13] If voters were largely unaware of the ACA's central provisions, they would not have been able to identify how those provisions were likely to affect them. And they certainly would not have been likely to connect their personal interests with their overall assessments of the ACA, to say nothing of their vote choices in future elections.

This line of thinking was exemplified by a widely viewed 2013 clip in which late-night television host Jimmy Kimmel asked Los Angeles pedestrians whether they preferred Obamacare or the Affordable Care Act.[14] The video seemed to confirm a half-century of research on public opinion: when Americans aren't familiar with a political issue, they often guess at the answer, especially when the question wording prompts them in certain directions.[15] In Kimmel's words, "as you may know, 'Obamacare' is just a nickname for the Affordable Care Act—they're the same thing. But lo and behold, we found people who did not know that, and that didn't stop them from weighing in on it." In the clip, one pedestrian explained the putative difference by saying, "One you—you pay, and then the other one is, Obama pays for you." Another stated that they preferred the ACA "'cause I don't like Obama."[16]

In 2016, in a similar vein, reporter Sarah Kliff found Trump supporters in Kentucky who relied on coverage through the ACA but were convinced

that Trump would not take away their health insurance. "There was a per-
sistent belief," Kliff wrote, "that Trump would fix these problems and make
Obamacare work better."[17] In actuality, Trump encouraged and celebrated
GOP efforts to repeal the law.

Quotations such as these give weight to a related argument: perhaps
public opinion on the ACA is little more than partisan rationalization.[18] Just
as fans of sports teams can develop strongly held beliefs about questions as
arbitrary as weighing a football or banging a trash can, it is plausible that
many citizens use partisan cues to form judgments about the ACA. All that
some need to know is whether the law was backed by Obama or rejected
by Trump. Some researchers have challenged this argument, contending
that such thoughtless partisanship is partly an artifact of surveys or other
low-consequence environments; when people are faced with consequential
decisions, they may not act as reflexive partisans.[19] But in the case of the ACA,
partisanship's influence is sufficiently profound that it shaped even Americans'
decisions about whether to enroll in health insurance.[20] Partisanship, to
repeat the Twitter refrain, seems to be a hell of a drug.

Public inattention and partisan rationalization may also help explain how
and when the public is responsive to messaging from elites. Absent strongly
held prior views, citizens may be more open to elite persuasion or other
avenues of elite influence than those with well-defined attitudes.[21] Yet, as
explanations go, public inattention and partisan rationalization are often
incomplete on their own, because neither explanation is well positioned to
make sense of over-time dynamics. Constants can't explain variables. To
understand their promise and limitations, we now analyze those over-time
dynamics empirically.

Tracking the Same Respondents over Time

As we saw in chapter 2, the elite-level battles over the ACA were volatile and
dramatic; the successive years saw the implementation of some major ACA
provisions, high-stakes court decisions, a botched rollout of the federal website, congressional Republicans' repeal attempts, and so much else.[22] How
did the public respond?

Most surveys, including even high-quality telephone and in-person surveys, rely on different samples of the population at different points in time.
As a result, they may be subject to shifting biases in who responds over time.

Figure 3.1 Support for Repealing the ACA over Time, by 2008 Partisanship, 2012–2020

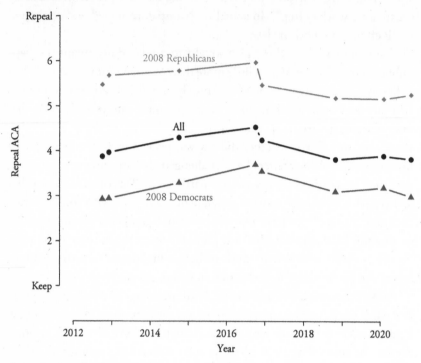

Source: Institute for the Study of Citizens and Politics (ISCAP) panel, 2012–2020 (Hopkins and Mutz 2022).

Such concerns have grown especially acute in the wake of the 2020 election, amid the growing underrepresentation of independent and conservative citizens in polls. It's valuable, then, to start by using a panel that interviews the same respondents over time. Specifically, we draw on the Institute for the Study of Citizens and Politics (ISCAP) panel, a long-running panel survey fielded via a population-based sample. Administered by Knowledge Networks (KN)/GfK/Ipsos, this unique panel tracks a nationally representative, probability-based sample recruited through address-based sampling and random-digit dialing.[23]

In figure 3.1, we illustrate the average response on the seven-point scale for each wave of the panel between 2012 and 2020 for all respondents as well as Democrats and Republicans. Overall, attitudes show stability. Notably, there was not much change—and certainly no pro-ACA change—between 2012 and 2014, when the law's main provisions came into effect.

That said, there were meaningful shifts over time, even at the individual level. Average support for repeal rose from 3.9 in October 2012 to 4.5 in October 2016 ($p < 0.001$), where 4.0 represents someone saying, "Only parts of the 2010 health care reform law should be kept." But support for repeal then dropped sharply, to 4.25, in the November-December 2016 survey, just after Trump's election. A t-test confirms that this drop is highly statistically significant ($p < 0.001$). Support for repeal fell further, to 3.8, by late 2018, and it then stabilized at roughly that level through 2020.

Such evidence is highly instructive. Prior research has illustrated that public opinion often acts like a thermostat, adjusting to present conditions by pushing in the other direction.[24] If a room gets cold, a thermostat will turn on the heat, just as the public reacts to a policy push to the left or right by shifting in the opposite direction. But is this thermostatic response a reaction to actual policy shifts, or can it be induced by the mere threat of such shifts?[25] The evidence here suggests the latter. The election of Trump alone was sufficient to move Americans' views markedly against repeal, even before any concrete repeal plan had taken shape. Simply knowing that Trump and the GOP would be in a position to repeal the law was enough to build support for it. As a thermostat, the public does not need to wait for policy to shift but can adjust its views in anticipation of looming shifts.[26]

Figure 3.1 also allows us to see over-time trends by respondents' 2008 partisan affiliation. (By using 2008 partisan affiliation, we can track the same individuals over time and avoid conflating shifts in partisanship with shifts in attitudes.) It's no surprise that, overall, Republicans were quite favorable toward repealing the ACA, with responses varying from 5.2 to 6.0 over this period.[27] But what is more surprising is that the post-Trump decline in anti-ACA views was most pronounced among Republicans—on average, they dropped by more than 0.4 points in a matter of weeks in late 2016 ($p < 0.001$), more than twice the drop among Democrats ($p = 0.006$). So while both Democrats and Republicans reacted to Trump's election by becoming more pro-ACA, the softening of GOP opposition to the law was especially notable. In other words, in aggregate, the GOP base was becoming less convinced of the need to repeal the ACA at the same time that GOP politicians were finally positioned to follow through on their promises to do just that.

Figure 3.2 Favorable Attitudes toward the ACA over Time, 2010–2020

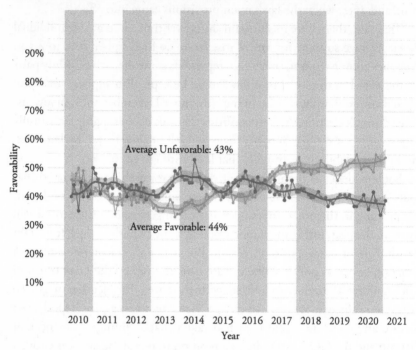

Source: Kaiser Family Foundation (KFF) Health Tracking Poll (Kaiser Family Foundation 2022).
Note: Vertical shading illustrates years. Dots show the fraction of survey respondents reporting favorable or unfavorable views. Smoothing lines and associated 95 percent confidence intervals are also included.

Over-Time Survey Evidence from the Health Tracking Survey

For researchers studying public opinion toward the ACA, the Health Tracking Poll (HTP) is an unparalleled resource. It is a rolling cross-sectional survey administered by the Kaiser Family Foundation (KFF) in most months beginning in 2009; here we focus on the 111 separate polls administered between April 2010 and February 2021. The survey has been primarily administered by phone, and starting in 2021, it was administered online as well. The samples in specific surveys usually number more than 1,000 respondents, and over the full period studied here, the total sample size is more than 130,000. In each of those surveys, the HTP asked Americans their views about the "2010 health reform law."[28] Figure 3.2 illustrates the weighted results by month, depicting both the actual results and smoothing lines (and associated 95 percent confidence intervals).

Figure 3.2 confirms the broad story we saw with the panel data in figure 3.1: there is little evidence of volatility in the public's ACA attitudes. For the most part, those attitudes held stable, with only a few periods when the fundamental trajectory changed.

The ACA's favorability was underwater almost from enactment; negative views basically always outpaced positive views from 2011 to 2016. Attitudes actually became more negative in late 2013 and early 2014, a striking fact given that this was precisely the time when some of the ACA's core benefits became available to millions. The problems with the rollout of the exchanges and the cancellation of noncompliant plans seemed to dwarf any positive impacts of opening the exchanges or implementing the Medicaid expansion in January 2014. Some have suggested that the delayed implementation of the law's core provisions until almost four years after passage left the law politically vulnerable, since many of its key benefits were not available until 2014. But that viewpoint does not fit the data. Far from being a life buoy, the opening of the ACA's exchanges appeared to be more like an added weight dragging down public views of the law. Negativity toward the law did subside slightly by 2015, perhaps as memories of the exchanges' rocky rollout and the cancellation of noncompliant plans receded. But unfavorable attitudes remained more common than favorable attitudes through most of 2016.

Ultimately, it proved to be political rather than policy-related events that led to a durable reassessment of the ACA. An election and its aftermath, not any changes to the policy itself, drove the shift. The inflection point came in late 2016. Almost as soon as Trump won the presidency that year, unfavorable attitudes started to decline and favorable attitudes ticked up. By early 2017, when the Republicans began their repeal attempts in earnest, favorable opinions surpassed unfavorable opinions for the first time since enactment, and the gap in favorability then continued to grow slowly but surely from 2018 to 2020. By the time of the most recent survey included here—one from early 2021—54 percent of respondents were favorable toward the law versus just 39 percent who were unfavorable. (That was just one percentage point lower than the all-time high in favorability of 55 percent recorded in October 2020.) In a conversation with Barack Obama himself, journalist Ezra Klein noted that the ACA "survived the Republican attempts to gut it. It did become popular." And Obama replied, "I thought it was going to happen a little bit quicker, but it didn't."[29] But what explains the law's initial lack of popularity, and how the shift Obama had been counting on belatedly came about?

In Their Own Words: Explaining Support and Opposition

Most survey analyses focus on overall opinions toward policies, typically measured via closed-ended survey questions like those mentioned earlier. These closed-ended questions often lead to reductive conclusions about the public's ideology or lack of political knowledge.[30] By contrast, scholarship that relies on in-depth interviews typically paints public opinion in a more nuanced, reflective light.[31] Here we seek a middle ground by using open-ended survey questions to probe the reasons Americans supported or opposed the ACA. By reporting evidence from such questions, we allow respondents to express their own views of and associations with the law. Respondents can say anything they wish, so finding over-time stability in responses to less structured questions would constitute strong evidence that the American public has coherent, meaningful attitudes toward the ACA.

Specifically, in fifteen surveys conducted between 2009 and 2018 by five firms with different sampling frames, either by telephone or online, respondents were asked why they were favorable or unfavorable toward the ACA.[32] First, respondents were asked a closed-ended question about the "health reform bill signed into law in 2010." Then, based on their answers, they were asked why they held that view: "Could you tell me in your own words what is the main reason you have a favorable/unfavorable opinion of the health reform law?" The answers offer an unparalleled window into the rationales people gave in support of their views. And unlike questions related to overall support or opposition, no single response was the "right" answer from a partisan viewpoint, freeing respondents to express themselves. Analyzing these responses and their shifts over time has the potential to show whether respondents' ACA attitudes were shaped by recent political rhetoric or by their own experiences—or if they held non-attitudes, to use Converse's phrase for non-opinions.

After the surveys were conducted, I worked with undergraduate research assistants to annotate each of the 33,006 responses along multiple dimensions, using the codebook in appendix A. The first survey was a Pew Research survey in the summer of 2009; the final survey was the fall 2018 wave of the

Figure 3.3 The Prevalence of Arguments in Favor of the ACA, 2009–2018

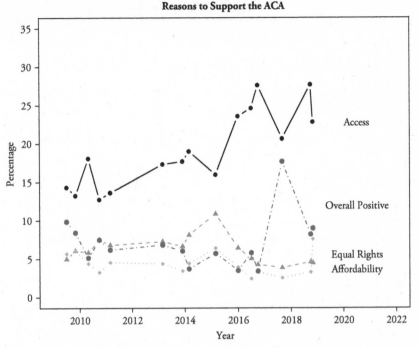

Reasons to Support the ACA

Source: Annotated open-ended arguments from various surveys, 2009–2018.

ISCAP panel, which ended on November 5, 2018. One primary task was to classify the types of arguments given for and against the ACA, as illustrated in figures 3.3 and 3.4. Doing so may provide insights into public opinion that are likely to be invisible to close-ended questioning.

For supporters, the single most common argument in favor of the ACA was its role in increasing access to health care. In this vein, one 2009 respondent said, "There's too many people that don't have health insurance, and they are sitting and dying because they can't afford doctors and medicine." Even before the law was enacted, in the summer of 2009, 14 percent of all respondents who provided a rationale cited increasing access to health care as a reason to support the proposal, a figure that remained above 20 percent in all surveys after 2015. The fact that so many mentioned "access" even before the proposal had been finalized or enacted is instructive, as it speaks to the extent to which the debate fell into the grooves of preexisting rhetorical

Figure 3.4 The Prevalence of Arguments against the ACA, 2009–2018

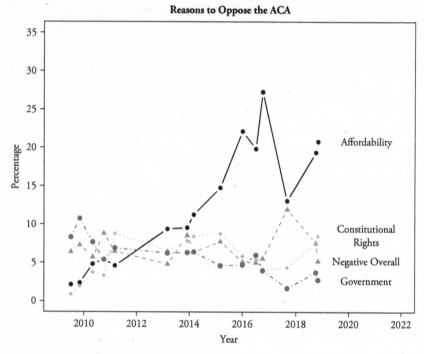

Reasons to Oppose the ACA

Source: Annotated open-ended arguments from various national surveys, 2009–2018.

frames or narratives. Americans did not think of the ACA as some entirely novel policy; instead, they saw it as part of an ongoing debate about the American health care system, and they drew on those narratives to explain their views toward the law.[33] To some degree, these responses may even echo rhetoric from prior health care debates.

The second most common supportive category was that of generically positive responses. Such answers averaged 7 percent of responses over the decade, with no evidence that they tailed off over time as Americans became more familiar with the law. In fact, generic positive responses spiked in 2017, perhaps in response to GOP repeal efforts that year.

No other arguments in support of the law are as prominent. Despite the word "affordable" in the law's name, only 4 percent of respondents on average mentioned affordability in a positive light. One example came from a respondent to an online SSI poll, who said in 2017, "It saved my life, without it I would not have been able to afford medications that I will need every day for the rest of my life."

Former Iowa Democratic senator Tom Harkin famously termed the ACA a "starter home" because it could serve as a starting point for broader reforms.[34] A January 2016 ISCAP panel respondent gave voice to this view, stating: "It's a start to something better than we have had. Needs work, but it's a start." But on average just 4 percent of respondents mentioned backing the ACA because it was a step in the right direction, though this fraction did seem to have increased in 2017, when the law was threatened with repeal. Similarly, only 2 percent of respondents on average argued for the law because of its benefits for specific social or economic groups, like women, senior citizens, or low-income households. These replies included comments like, "it helps the middle class," as one March 2015 KFF respondent put it.

Just 0.2 percent of respondents cited Obama or another politician in their explanation for why they liked the law, in what we term "pro-ACA opinion leadership." One 2009 Pew respondent made this argument, replying simply, "I trust Obama." Such evidence provides one hint of the limits of elite influence. Other potential influences also seem to have little impact. For example, just 0.2 percent on average pointed to economic benefits (such as increased labor mobility) or issues related to abortion in explaining their support.

What about reasons for opposing the ACA? Here we see some consistency over time but also some evolution. As figure 3.4 illustrates, a lack of affordability was not originally a major source of opposition to the ACA. But it then came to be the single most common reason given for opposing the law, with a marked uptick in 2015 and 2016. Overall, 12 percent of all responses cited affordability-related concerns, with more than 25 percent of respondents saying so in late 2016. One respondent in 2016 explained that "the law has caused the cost of insurance premiums to skyrocket, the deductible to balloon beyond reason, and a significant decline in medical services." This trend probably reflects reactions to the law's implementation, at least in part, and the shift toward practical concerns that comes with implementation. Generic rationales for holding unfavorable attitudes were common as well, with 7 percent of all respondents falling into this category by offering responses such as, "That's just how I'm feeling about it." Conservative arguments against government overreach also loomed large throughout this period, with an average of 6 percent of all respondents arguing that the ACA was unconstitutional or violated constitutional rights and another 6 percent of respondents seeing the government as overstepping its role. To some extent, these two expressions of opposition are substitutes for each other, as the more generic claim that the ACA was government overreach was supplanted by the more specific claim that it was unconstitutional. It is noteworthy that the Supreme Court's June 2012 *National Federation of Independent Business v. Sebelius* decision finding the law's key elements constitutional did not do much to blunt that concern.

One respondent said, "Anything that makes us more reliant on the government is scary," while a second said, "It was done illegally and is unconstitutional." A third respondent was more colorful, noting, "The government has no business requiring its citizens and noncitizens to buy or use any product. What's next? Maybe a mandatory purchase of a gallon of milk per week? This president is out of control." A fourth person made a related point, saying, "[I] don't want the government telling me what doctor I can and cannot use." The consistent concerns about government overreach are also noteworthy in light of the widespread resistance, beginning in 2020, to mask mandates and other policies put in place to reduce the spread of Covid-19.[35] Others have argued that the well of American resistance to perceived government intrusion is deep, and such results are consistent with that conclusion.[36] In a related vein, 12 percent of respondents opposed a would-be health reform law based on concerns about rising taxes, a concern that declined as the proposal developed. (In point of fact, the ACA did entail substantial new taxes, but they fell chiefly on a small fraction of high-income taxpayers.)[37]

Other concerns were raised less frequently. On average, about 3 percent of all respondents cited access issues as a reason to oppose the ACA, while another 3 percent mentioned fairness concerns. On fairness, one 2015 respondent explained, "I don't think it's fair for me to have to pay for other people who want to [sit] on their butt and not work."

Two percent shared the sentiment about government ineffectiveness of one 2011 respondent who said, "If the government can't run a post office, then how are they going to run a health reform law?" Another 2 percent complained about the process through which the bill passed, although such concerns waned over time.

Smaller fractions cited a range of other reasons for opposing the ACA, including the concerns of some respondents about coverage for unauthorized immigrants or for abortions and the preference of others for a single-payer system. Given that one of the final hang-ups before the House of Representatives passed the ACA was related to members' concerns about abortion—and given the general power of anti-abortion politics—it's noteworthy that this so rarely emerges as a reason for opposition. In fact, opposition to abortion is mentioned by just 0.3 percent of all respondents. This, too, is evidence of the disconnect between the issues that animate elite divisions and those emphasized by the public. Overall, across various categories, we see evidence of significant stability, not only in Americans' overall assessments of the ACA but also in their underlying reasoning for those assessments.[38]

The Salience of Personal Experiences and Social Groups

As this book unfolds, it will interrogate a variety of explanations of public opinion, including those focusing on personal experiences with the ACA (chapters 4 and 5) and the role of salient social groups (see especially chapter 6). In figure 3.5, we briefly set the stage for those inquiries by examining two facets of the open-ended data: the extent to which respondents mentioned their own personal experiences, and their references to salient social groups.

As the left panel of figure 3.5 illustrates, on average, 11 percent of all responses made reference to individuals' personal experiences with the law. The absence of a clear trend over time is highly instructive. Though the law's main provisions came into effect in January 2014, roughly as many people cited personal experiences in 2011 as in 2016. The health care system is extraordinarily complex, so one explanation for these patterns is that those with positive or negative opinions of the ACA are likely to be able to construe personal experiences to justify their attitudes.[39]

Salient social groups were mentioned in about 10 percent of all responses, with seniors (19 percent), the poor (17 percent), and the uninsured (9 percent) most commonly mentioned in that subset. It's noteworthy that overall 2.3 percent of responses across surveys mentioned assisting social groups in a positive light—that is, they were given as a reason to support the law. On the flip side, 2.0 percent of responses mentioned social groups explicitly as a reason to oppose the law.

Immigrants came up in 5 percent of responses citing specific groups, while African Americans came up in 0.1 percent. It's hard to discern a clear

Figure 3.5 The Prevalence of Mentions of Personal Experience and References to Salient Social Groups in Public Opinion about the ACA, 2009–2018

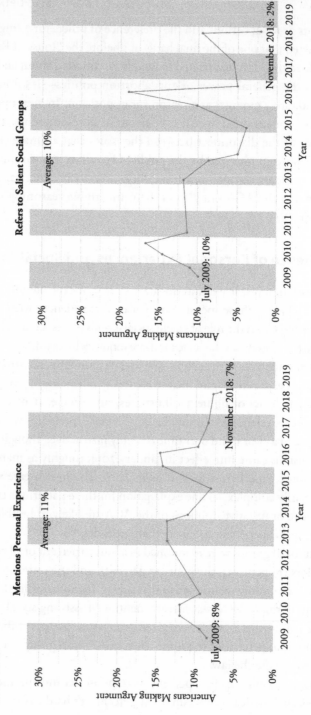

Source: Annotated open-ended arguments from various national surveys, 2009–2018.

pattern over time, although, with the exception of one survey of activists in mid-2016, specific groups appear to have been invoked less often in the later parts of the decade. Given these results, it is plausible that group-based thinking is one of several stabilizing elements of public opinion. We will explore that question in more depth in chapter 6.

The Whole Is Not Equal to the Sum of the Parts

We are now well positioned to understand another key aspect of Americans' attitudes toward the ACA: the surprising disconnect between their evaluations of the law's key parts and their views of the law as a whole.[40] In January 2010, even before the law's enactment in March of that year, the KFF surveyed Americans about different elements of the law.[41] Overall, the public was equally divided on the law, with 42 percent supporting it and 41 percent opposed. With that said, 31 percent of respondents strongly opposed the law, a figure that dwarfed the 19 percent who strongly supported it. Intensity was on the side of the opponents.

But there was a catch. The same survey also found that many of the law's core elements were actually quite popular. Sixty-three percent of respondents said that the law's prohibition against insurance companies denying coverage or raising premiums for people with preexisting conditions made them more likely to support the law. Fifty-seven percent said that the law's provision of subsidies for those whose incomes were below 400 percent of the federal poverty line made them more likely to support it, and 67 percent said the same about the creation of health insurance exchanges. Likewise, 62 percent reported that the law's expansion of Medicaid would increase their support. Even the provision to raise income taxes won 59 percent support. There was good reason to think that if the ACA did pass, awareness of key provisions would increase and support might grow. This is probably what Nancy Pelosi meant when she said in a March 2010 speech, "We have to pass the bill so you can find out what's in it, away from the fog of controversy."[42]

Still, despite a set of popular provisions, the KFF poll also showed that the law had an obvious Achilles' heel. Just 22 percent of respondents said that a provision requiring "nearly all Americans to have a minimum level of health insurance or else pay a fine" made them more likely to support the law; 62 percent said that it made them less likely to support it. To the extent that the public focused on the individual mandate—the part of the law people liked least—support for the law would remain tepid. And the ACA's complexity seems key: it enabled citizens to see in the law whatever their partisan and ideological predispositions foregrounded. Some saw the law's strengths, and others focused on its liabilities. For millions, the law's complexity allowed it to become synonymous with whatever they found to be its least popular provision.

Status Quo Bias: From Bane to Boon?

It's widely agreed that in politics and policymaking the burden is on would-be reformers—it's vastly easier to defend existing policies than to introduce new ones. But this systemic bias toward the status quo could have multiple sources. It could emerge from institutional forces: the proliferation of veto points (especially in American government) certainly advantages those defending existing laws and systems.[43] The political tendency to preserve current arrangements might also be grounded to some extent in voters' psychology. Indeed, one possible explanation for the public's pro-ACA shift after Trump's election is the public's bias toward the status quo.[44]

Status quo bias—a preference for the current state of affairs—is a general aspect of psychology in which loss-averse people (read: people) prefer to avoid change.[45] Strongly rooted at the individual level, this sort of bias is likely to operate within groups of people as well. Although some of the initial tests were conducted in the realm of consumer finance, status quo bias also appears to operate in politics: in initiatives and referendums put before voters, they frequently default to preserving the status quo.[46] In the period between the ACA's 2010 enactment and the GOP's 2017 repeal efforts, the ACA shifted from a disruptive reform to part of the established health care system. It is possible that the GOP's 2017 repeal efforts made that transition concrete in many citizens' minds, thus reinforcing support for the ACA. In 2010 the Republicans were the defenders of the status quo; in 2017 they undertook the harder task of overturning it.

Chapters 4 and 5 consider at length one mechanism that may underpin this shift: after its enactment, citizens came to benefit from the law in tangible ways. Nevertheless, here we consider whether psychological biases toward the status quo might help explain the pro-ACA shift in attitudes we observed. I administered a survey experiment via Survey Sampling

International (SSI) between September 26 and September 28, 2017, just as Senate Republicans' final serious repeal attempt in that year, the Graham-Cassidy proposal, was drawing headlines. (It was also days before the start of the new fiscal year would set GOP repeal efforts back considerably by requiring GOP legislators to start the legislative process from scratch.) Eight hundred forty-two randomly selected respondents saw text describing efforts to repeal the ACA as "returning the health care system closer to where it was in 2010," making the baseline the pre-ACA status quo. In that framing, status quo bias should work *in favor* of repealing the ACA. But another 789 randomly selected respondents instead read that the Republican plans sought to make "significant changes to the health care system." This second condition instead makes the ACA the status quo and so should harness status quo bias in its favor.

As figure 3.6 illustrates, status quo bias did seem to be at work to some extent. Those who heard repeal efforts described as returning to the pre-ACA status quo averaged 2.37 in their favorability toward repealing the ACA, where a score of 1 indicates very unfavorable views and a score of 4 indicates very favorable views. But when the ACA was itself the status quo, repeal's favorability dropped to 2.26, a significant difference ($p = 0.03$, two-sided test). That difference, 0.11, is 10 percent of the dependent variable's standard deviation, making the effect meaningful but not overwhelmingly large. (By way of benchmarking, the average difference between Republicans and Democrats is 1.25.) Still, whether the public thinks of a policy as the status quo can clearly affect its assessment of that policy. Having passed and enacted the ACA, the Democrats finally found themselves swimming downstream as the Republicans tried to repeal it.

Conclusion

Chapter 2's narrative about the ACA's elite-level politics and policymaking can be summarized in one phrase: years of sparring over a complicated law. This chapter's account of aggregate public opinion, however, can be summarized even more succinctly with a single word: stability. In that respect, this chapter joins a long tradition of research showing that aggregate public opinion is often stable and responsive primarily to shifts in the direction of government policy.[47] That political opinions are often characterized as less stable than behaviors like voting or vote choice makes the stability and

Figure 3.6 Favorability toward ACA Repeal When the Program Is Presented as the Status Quo and When It Is Not, September 2017

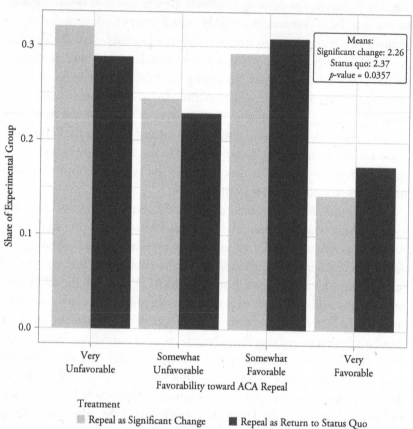

Source: Author's survey via Survey Sampling International (SSI), September 26–28, 2017.

predictability detailed here even more noteworthy. Although research focusing on individual citizens commonly concludes that Americans' attitudes on specific policies do not reflect consistent ideological thinking and can be incoherent, research focusing on the public as a whole tends to reinforce characterizations of public opinion as stable.

Together, these two dueling characterizations underscore the disconnect between elite-level actions and public opinion on the ACA. After all, very few elite-level actions concerning the ACA—the adoption of new arguments, the implementation of the law's key provisions, even Supreme Court decisions—left any imprint on public opinion whatsoever. In that respect, the elite-level actors were playing to an empty house. With that said, the election of Donald Trump and the possibility of the ACA's repeal prompted the public to shift quickly in ways that thermostatic accounts would expect.[48] This account of public opinion is consistent with a public that pays little attention to the specifics of policymaking but is nonetheless responsive to possible policy changes at the broadest level.

In another respect, the law's complexity and the stability of public opinion may actually reflect two sides of the same coin. The complexity of the law enabled citizens to focus on very different elements when they evaluated it. To the law's opponents, the law was commensurate with the individual mandate and constituted an unnecessary government intrusion into private enterprise. To its supporters, on the other hand, the ACA was a set of concrete benefits: the Medicaid expansion, the exchanges, and protections for people with preexisting conditions. In short, the ACA's complexity allowed different citizens to fixate on very different aspects of the law.

From its 2010 enactment until the end of 2013, the public experienced the ACA largely as an abstraction. But with many states expanding Medicaid in January 2014, and with the opening of the exchanges and the imposition of the individual mandate, it was possible that public opinion could have shifted at this point, at least among the small group of Americans most directly affected. Whether and to what extent it did is the topic of the next two chapters.

CHAPTER 4

Public Opinion and the Medicaid Expansion

JOHN JACOBS IS a veteran of the second Iraq War who credited the ACA with keeping him out of prison. The son of a police officer, Jacobs was imprisoned after pawning stolen electronics to feed his drug addiction. But because he was released in 2014 in West Virginia—months after the state expanded Medicaid—Jacobs was able to participate in a drug treatment program. As he explained, "I was fortunate to get Medicaid because I was getting [treatment] for free for three months through the [Veterans Administration] and then I got to pay for the rest of it."[1] This chapter focuses on citizens' political responses to the Medicaid expansion that Jacobs found so vital.

In chapter 2, we saw that one of the ACA's central pillars was the expansion of Medicaid, a means-tested program that provides health insurance to qualifying low-income individuals. In participating states, the expansion raised the income ceiling for Medicaid eligibility while also extending coverage to adults without children. For those who receive it, Medicaid provides substantial economic support: an average of $5,736 was spent per enrollee in 2014.[2] That is an extraordinarily large benefit for most Americans, and especially for those with incomes low enough to qualify. Medicaid improves lives: those eligible for it utilize more health care, have better mental health, and accumulate less medical debt.[3] Receiving Medicaid is also associated with a decreased risk of low-birthweight children and infant mortality, as well as improved educational outcomes for children.[4] While vice president, Joe Biden famously referred to the ACA as a "big f——ing deal," and for Americans who were newly eligible for Medicaid, it's easy to see why.

Despite eliciting a hot-mic moment from the vice president, the implementation of the ACA's main provisions did not induce a corresponding shift in public opinion overall, as we saw in chapter 3. In February 2013, roughly a year before the implementation of the Medicaid expansion and other key provisions, 42 percent of Americans had unfavorable views of the ACA. In June 2016, more than two years after implementation, the figure was almost unchanged, at 44 percent.[5] For the vast majority of Americans, however, the ACA did not affect the source of their health insurance. So beneath that aggregate stability in public opinion, it's possible that attitudes *did* shift among the fraction of Americans like John Jacobs who benefited substantially and straightforwardly from it.

Among the ACA's various elements, the Medicaid expansion is what political scientists term a "most-likely case" for a policy feedback on public opinion—if policy feedbacks operate anywhere, they should operate in this example. Mass-level policy feedbacks refer to political processes in which personal experiences with a policy shape subsequent political attitudes and behaviors, and so are closely related to self-interest.[6] Not only were the benefits for new Medicaid recipients large, but there were millions of new beneficiaries. Between late 2013 and 2020, the number of Americans insured by Medicaid increased by 14 million, a number that understates the total number of people who relied on Medicaid for a spell of time during that period.[7] Medicaid rolls grew further during the Covid-19 pandemic with the suspension of rules on removing people who became ineligible.[8] To date, the Medicaid expansion has done more than any other element of the ACA to increase insurance coverage for Americans.[9] Unlike the ACA's exchanges (the topic of chapter 5), the Medicaid expansion also involved the direct provision of health insurance by the state, providing increased clarity to beneficiaries that the insurance was in fact provided by the government.[10] Prior studies indicate that although self-interest is rarely a central driver of political attitudes, it is most likely to matter in cases where the stakes are high and interests are clearly defined.[11] If any part of the ACA could reshape public opinion by playing to its beneficiaries' self-interest, the Medicaid expansion seems like a promising candidate.[12] This chapter thus examines the interplay of public opinion and the Medicaid expansion while also addressing more general questions. For one, at a time of pronounced political polarization and nationalization, can political elites use social policy to durably shift public opinion?[13] With some policymakers discussing further extensions of government-provided health insurance—such as single-payer health care like "Medicare for All"—these analyses can also provide insights into how the members of the public who would benefit most directly might respond.

By design and definition, studies of policy feedbacks on citizens examine the impacts of a policy *after* it has been implemented, meaning that policy feedbacks do not reflect the total political impact of passing a policy.[14] More narrowly, policy feedbacks reflect the effects of direct experience with the policy.[15] But the ACA was signed into law in 2010, and years passed before the Medicaid expansion or other key provisions were actually implemented. There was ample time for citizens to learn about the law and its potential impacts and for the parties to message aggressively on that very topic (see chapter 7). Given that delay and those debates, it is worth considering a second possibility: perhaps those most likely to benefit became more positive toward the ACA even before Medicaid was expanded in their state. If so, such anticipatory effects might mask any policy feedbacks, although they nonetheless suggest a clear pathway through which political elites can build support for their policies and perhaps their parties. To provide a comprehensive account of the political impacts of enacting a policy, then, we need to consider the effects of the law both before and after its implementation.

To do so, this chapter exploits cross-state variation in whether, when, and how the Medicaid expansion was implemented. The 2012 Supreme Court ruling in *National Federation of Independent Business v. Sebelius* allowed states to opt out of the expansion. That decision significantly limited the law's impacts by leaving a coverage gap in many states for people whose incomes were too low to qualify for subsidies via the exchanges (see chapter 2).[16]

Seven states whose governors and legislatures initially declined to expand Medicaid put the question to their voters via ballot measures. Despite being mostly Republican-leaning states, including Utah, Idaho, and Missouri, voters in six of these states opted to expand Medicaid. Through in-depth analyses of the votes in Maine and Oklahoma, this chapter initially studies whether communities with larger fractions of residents who would benefit from the Medicaid expansion had higher levels of support for it. In short, is there aggregate-level evidence that self-interest might have been at work even prior to the Medicaid expansion's implementation?

In a book that leans heavily on survey data, these analyses of election results also provide a critical counterweight. Although survey data allow researchers to know who within a population holds particular views, it is critical to also examine how Americans behave when they can act on their ACA views directly. Surveys are sometimes misleading about the overall levels of support for a policy in the electorate, and attitudes toward a policy may sour in the wake of sustained attacks during a political campaign.[17] To our knowledge, researchers have not previously studied any of these initiatives.

This chapter's second section considers the impact of the Medicaid expansion on people's assessment of the law by comparing survey respondents living in expansion states with similar respondents living elsewhere. Americans in states that expanded Medicaid subsequently became more favorable toward the ACA, an effect concentrated among the lower-income Americans more likely to be eligible for the Medicaid expansion. Substantively, the effect is equivalent to moving about 3 percent of the distance from being "very unfavorable" (1) to being "very favorable" (4), or about 0.1 on a 1–4 scale. Such effects are surely meaningful, but not large enough to reshape the electoral landscape.

The chapter's third section considers a most-likely case for policy feedbacks: when a valued policy is threatened by repeal. Loss aversion and the endowment effect are well-documented psychological tendencies that lead people to react especially negatively to losing things they already have.[18] Given these facets of human psychology, a highly visible repeal effort is a most-likely case in which a policy's beneficiaries might come to recognize the policy's effect on their lives and become more supportive of it. To test this hypothesis, we analyze the pro-ACA shift in attitudes after Trump's 2016 election, paying special attention to respondents on Medicaid as well as those reliant on the exchanges.

In concluding, we underscore three other factors that limit policy feedbacks from the Medicaid expansion. First, as of 2019, the total fraction of the U.S. population insured through either Medicaid or CHIP was 21 percent.[19] On the one hand, that is a larger number of people than the entire population of the United Kingdom. Even at 21 percent, however, Medicaid recipients are still a minority of the American population, meaning that such personal experiences are limited to a small subset of the electorate. The second factor is the long-observed reality that voter turnout levels are low among those on Medicaid relative to other demographic groups.[20] This further dampens the political impacts of the policy feedback effects uncovered in this chapter, since these attitudinal shifts are occurring among less consistent voters and so are less likely to be influential at the ballot box—or in the minds of elected officials.

The third limitation also pertains not to policy feedbacks but to their broader political import. This chapter focuses on attitudes toward the ACA and votes in favor of or against expanding Medicaid. Those who stand to benefit personally from the ACA are more likely to shift their views on the law itself than to change other, more remote attitudes or predispositions.[21] So even if the Medicaid expansion helped build support for the ACA, it does not follow that Democrats would necessarily be rewarded in subsequent elections, which may well have been fought over different issues. It is a long way from influencing someone's attitudes on a specific issue to influencing their vote choice at the next election.

In the wake of Donald Trump's unexpected 2016 victory, and then again after his narrow loss in 2020, some commentators faulted the Democratic Party for not prioritizing the lower-income Americans who had been central to their victories in earlier years.[22] In the words of the Democratic strategist David Shor, "College educated people have taken over the branding and issue prioritization of the Democratic Party, at the expense of working class white people who were in the party and working class non-white people who are in the party, and that's driving people away."[23] But the ACA was a top Democratic priority, and it was a large-scale policy that provided sizable economic benefits and security to many of those same lower-income citizens. So the question is not so much about why the Democrats did not target this group, but about why the ACA did not do more to win over those voters.

Maine's 2017 Medicaid Expansion Initiative

Even before the Medicaid expansion's implementation, is there evidence that the people and communities most likely to benefit concretely from it were especially supportive of it? To address that question we first analyze town-level election results from a 2017 initiative on Medicaid expansion in Maine known as Proposition 2. Maine is a valuable state in which to study the interplay of self-interest and support for the Medicaid expansion. Demographically, Maine swung toward the Republicans in 2016, with Donald Trump losing the state by a surprisingly close margin of under three percentage points. Maine is home to a sizable number of the white, non-college-educated voters thought to find Trump's identity-infused appeals compelling.[24] However, these same voters are the ones most likely to benefit from redistributive policies such as the ACA.[25]

Proposition 2 went to voters in November 2017, just months after the failure of Senate Republicans' efforts to repeal the ACA through the Graham-Cassidy bill. Some eighty thousand Mainers were thought to be eligible for expanded Medicaid, and the federal government was committed to footing at least 90 percent of the bill.[26] Supporters argued that expanding Medicaid "would help financially fragile rural hospitals, create jobs and provide care for vulnerable people who have long gone without it."[27]

Maine's governor at the time was Paul LePage, a Republican and Trump ally whose brash, combative approach to politics was sometimes seen as a precursor to President Trump's. On five occasions prior to the 2017 vote, the Maine legislature had passed legislation to expand Medicaid only to see LePage veto the expansion.[28] The governor justified his opposition in language that connected Medicaid with welfare, noting that "it's free health care paid for by the taxpayers, and it's got to be said that way. It's pure welfare. If you don't want to call it welfare, call it an entitlement."[29]

But not all voters saw the expansion the same way LePage did. In chapter 3, we saw that voters' views on the ACA depend in part on the specific element of the ACA under discussion. The individual mandate, for example, was consistently unpopular before its effective repeal in late 2017. By contrast, the ACA's Medicaid expansion proved unexpectedly popular, even in many states that chose not to adopt it. Illustrating this, in a 2017 KFF survey 84 percent of respondents said that it was somewhat or very important that "a replacement plan makes sure states that received federal funds to expand Medicaid continue to receive those funds."[30] In light of such surveys, we might expect the Medicaid expansion to pass.

And it did. On election night in November 2017, Proposition 2 won almost 59 percent of the vote.[31] But beyond the overall outcome, it is critical to know which cities and towns were more or less supportive of expanding

Medicaid. Were they the towns with higher shares of poor residents who were likely to see more concrete benefits, or did support come from more affluent or highly educated towns that had been trending Democratic? These are ecological inferences about collections of people, and as such require caution.[32] To say that a town with a higher poverty rate backs the Medicaid expansion does not imply that poor voters drove the shift. Still, these aggregate results represent one piece of evidence in the broader puzzle and are especially useful as a counterweight to individual-level survey data.

Empirically, our goal is to identify the types of towns that were more or less likely to back Proposition 2 and to isolate trends above and beyond political partisanship. (Towns are the smallest geographic unit for which the necessary data are available.) To do so, we merge municipality-level election returns from the 2017 initiative and prior elections with demographic and employment data from the American Community Survey.[33] The total number of cities and towns in our analysis is 485. We then estimate linear models in which we regress the share of total votes cast that backed the Medicaid expansion as a function of political and demographic measures.[34]

The key independent variable of interest is the fraction of each town or city likely to benefit directly from expanding Medicaid. We measure this in multiple ways. The primary measure is the share of the population with public assistance income from means-tested programs like Temporary Assistance for Needy Families (TANF, sometimes referred to as "welfare") and the Supplemental Nutrition Assistance Program (SNAP, known colloquially as "food stamps"). Given that Medicaid is a means-tested program, the share of a community with public assistance income from other means-tested programs is a strong proxy for communities with more prospective beneficiaries from Medicaid expansion.[35]

Table B.1 displays the results. The two measures of prior Republican voting—the percentage backing LePage in 2014 and Trump in 2016—are both strongly negatively associated with support for Proposition 2. But once we condition on those measures, Maine cities and towns with larger shares of people reporting public assistance income were only somewhat more likely to back Proposition 2. The coefficient is 0.255 with a standard error of 0.108. Substantively, this relationship between economic need and support for Proposition 2 is not large, as figure 4.1 illustrates: holding other variables constant, a shift of two standard deviations (0.068) is associated with a

Figure 4.1 Support for Medicaid Expansion in Maine as a Function of Share of Town with Public Assistance Income, 2017

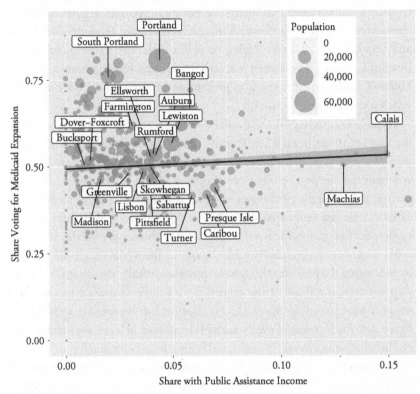

Source: American Community Survey (ACS), Maine Secretary of State (U.S. Census Bureau 2020).

1.7-percentage-point increase in support for the expansion. From this test, self-interest does not seem to be a primary driver of Proposition 2's electoral success.[36] There is also no evidence that communities with rural hospitals were more supportive.[37] In short, measures of economic need and deprivation are associated with support for Proposition 2 in the expected ways, but the associations are substantively modest.

Oklahoma's 2020 Initiative

The results of voting in any one state could be driven by idiosyncratic factors of time or place. So after Oklahoma voters narrowly backed the Medicaid expansion through their own initiative on June 30, 2020, we ran parallel county-level analyses on those results. As in Maine, supporters of the Medicaid expansion pointed to the struggles of rural hospitals. One reporter summarized the campaign by noting supporters' arguments about "how Medicaid expansion would increase health care access in Oklahoma and help save the state's struggling rural hospitals after a run of closures."[38] But unlike Maine, Oklahoma is a very Republican-leaning state—in 2016, Hillary Clinton failed to crack 30 percent support or win a single one of the state's seventy-seven counties.

In table B.2, we report the results of linear regression models predicting the share of voters in each Oklahoma county backing the Medicaid expansion. We use counties for a straightforward reason, as counties are the unit at which the election results were readily available. It is unsurprising that partisanship is highly predictive: counties with higher levels of 2016 Trump support were less supportive of the Medicaid expansion. Still, there is some suggestion that economic need is associated with support for the Medicaid expansion. For comparability with the results from Maine, model 1 begins by presenting the positive (though not quite statistically significant) relationship between the share of the county with public assistance income and support for expanding Medicaid—a relationship depicted graphically in figure 4.2. An increase of two standard deviations in a county's share with public assistance income is associated with a four-percentage-point uptick in the share backing the Medicaid expansion on average. This meaningful but moderately sized relationship is bolstered by models 2 and 3, which illustrate that counties with lower median incomes (model 2) or higher fractions of residents below the poverty line (model 3) were also more supportive of expanding Medicaid. In Oklahoma as in Maine, there is evidence that places that stood to benefit concretely from the Medicaid expansion were somewhat more supportive of it. But such effects were substantively small, and not the main story behind the initiative's passage.

When voters in Maine and Oklahoma were asked to weigh in on the Medicaid expansion, they were favorable. But these analyses do not show much evidence that the Medicaid expansion could prospectively reconfigure political support in either state. The votes largely appear to have followed expected partisan divides, albeit with a relatively uniform pro-expansion shift. Keep in mind that these initiatives allowed voters to weigh in directly on Medicaid, making them a most likely case for economic self-interest to operate above and beyond existing political divides. As we saw in the states'

Figure 4.2 Support for Medicaid Expansion in Oklahoma as a Function of Share of County with Public Assistance Income, 2020

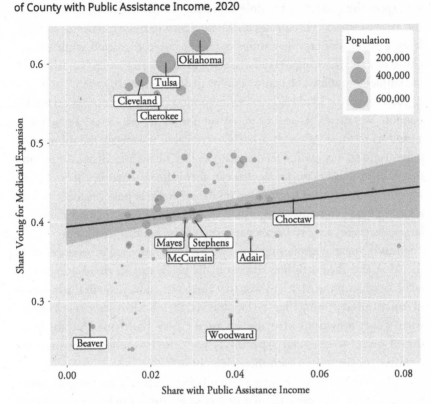

Source: ACS, Oklahoma State Election Board (U.S. Census Bureau 2020).

2016 presidential elections, when Maine and Oklahoma voters had to assess not just the ACA but a broad range of policies and personalities all at once, the outcomes were substantially less favorable to the Democrats. At least prospectively, before these states had expanded Medicaid, it does not appear that the possibility of Medicaid expansion produced dramatic shifts in the communities that tended to support it.

Policy Feedbacks from the Medicaid Expansion

If the prospect of the Medicaid expansion was not sufficient to meaningfully disrupt the existing geography of political loyalties and win any significant amount of additional support in poorer communities in Maine or Oklahoma, what about the actual implementation of the Medicaid expansion? Shouldn't we expect the impact of tangible experiences with insurance to outweigh the mere prospect of obtaining it? We now turn to those questions, gaining leverage from the fact that some states expanded Medicaid while others chose not to. The long delay between the ACA's enactment in 2010 and the implementation of its core benefits makes it especially useful to investigate whether the Medicaid expansion produced policy feedbacks on public opinion. Was the ACA's anemic public support in the years after its enactment a product of those delays? It is likewise critical to investigate the substantive magnitude of any policy feedbacks: the fact of such feedbacks does not necessarily put them on a scale that can alter existing dynamics of two-party support. Prior research has focused on the existence of policy feedbacks, but assessing their substantive magnitude is crucial as well, as only substantively large effects are likely to help a party expand its political coalition.

Already, there is scholarship linking Americans' personal experiences with the ACA and their attitudes toward it. By using a panel survey, Lawrence Jacobs and Suzanne Mettler show that there was an increase in the number of Americans reporting that the law affected their health care access in 2014, when its key provisions were implemented.[39] Also, Katherine McCabe finds that Americans' personal experiences with the law, whether positive or negative, are associated with their views of it.[40]

Still, prior research also suggests that policy feedbacks are far from automatic. Instead, they depend on a variety of factors, from how the policy is designed and implemented to questions of public perception and stigma.[41] Programs such as cash assistance have design features that can be disempowering, partly because recipients can be subject to the whims of street-level bureaucrats.[42] Medicaid is a complex, means-tested program that requires recipients to periodically verify their income, so it too may have disempowering effects.[43] Also, Medicaid is often provided through nongovernmental actors under different names; in southeastern Pennsylvania, for example, Keystone First is a Medicaid-managed care plan run by Blue Cross/Blue Shield. Indirect provision may dampen its visibility as a government program.[44] That being said, customer satisfaction with Medicaid is relatively high, with 75 percent of those on Medicaid reporting satisfaction with how the health system is working.[45]

What's more, the archetypal examples of policy feedbacks, whether the GI Bill or Social Security, come mostly from policies enacted in earlier eras, at a time when partisanship was less of an anchor on public attitudes.[46] The ACA in particular has been highly salient and divisive from its inception, so it is something of a lightning rod for polarization during an already polarized time.[47] If citizens already have well-formed views of the ACA that are shaped by their partisanship, they may disregard information or experiences that undercut those views.[48] Also, policy feedbacks research finds more consistent impacts on political participation than on public opinion, both generally and for the Medicaid expansion specifically.[49] Given the competing predictions about the impact of the Medicaid expansion, it provides a critical test case for the impact of policy feedbacks on public opinion—and for the possibility that contemporary political elites can expand their political coalitions through public policy.

The evidence presented earlier in this chapter makes it clear that the support for the Medicaid expansion was not driven primarily by places that might benefit disproportionately from it—or by anticipatory shifts in support prior to the expansion's implementation. So we turn now to estimating the effects of the expansion once implemented. Note that our research design isolates effects only on the fraction of Medicaid beneficiaries whom the ACA had made newly eligible. To do so, we present and extend evidence detailed at more length in an earlier work.[50] Specifically, we turn to the KFF's rolling, cross-sectional telephone surveys between January 2010—when the KFF first asked about favorability toward the ACA—and October 2018. The data set includes 124,164 respondents interviewed in ninety-five separate surveys.[51] We focus on 90,473 respondents who were under sixty-five, since older respondents typically had Medicare coverage and were less likely to be affected by the Medicaid expansion.[52] We separate respondents living in one of the thirty-one expansion states plus the District of Columbia from those in the nineteen non-expansion states (as of our study's 2018 endpoint).[53] When a state expanded Medicaid after the bulk of states had done so on January 1, 2014, we code that state as having expanded only for surveys after its state-specific expansion date.

Figure 4.3 (left panel) illustrates that the Medicaid expansion had a sizable impact on Medicaid receipt in the expansion states: the share of respondents receiving Medicaid increased by 4.9 percentage points. However, only 8.9 percent of survey respondents under sixty-five in an expansion state reported receiving Medicaid even after the expansion took place.[54] That means that only a small fraction of the respondents were likely to have had recent

Figure 4.3 Proportion of Medicaid Recipients and Favorability toward the ACA before and after Expansion

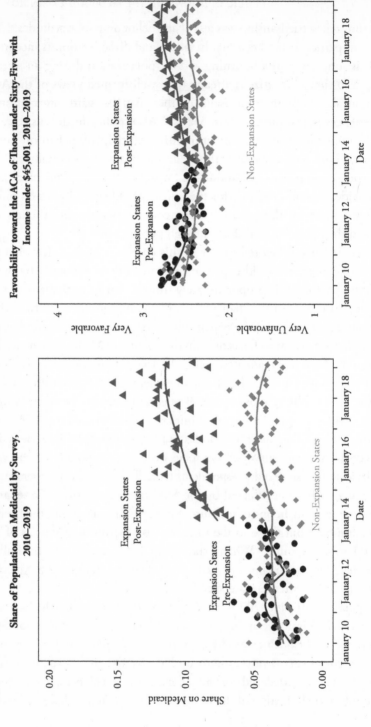

Source: KFF Health Tracking Poll (Kaiser Family Foundation 2022). Figure reprinted with permission from Hopkins and Parish 2019.

personal experiences with Medicaid. The median respondent on Medicaid reported an income of less than $20,000, although some recipients may have had higher incomes, especially those with larger families.[55]

If the expansion shaped attitudes through recipients' self-interest, we would expect its effects to be strongest among low-income survey respondents who were likely to be eligible for Medicaid. For that reason, we focus on non-elderly survey respondents making less than $45,001 annually.[56]

States that accepted the Medicaid expansion may have differed in various ways even before its implementation. To provide an initial assessment while addressing that concern, figure 4.3's right panel presents a dichotomized measure of ACA favorability among respondents making less than $45,001 for three groups of states. The first group comprises states that expanded Medicaid after each survey was conducted, while those that expanded Medicaid before each survey make up the second group. The third group includes states that did not expand Medicaid at any point in this time period.[57] The figure uses smoothing lines to highlight trends.

Respondents' attitudes in the two groups of states trend in the same direction before the expansion, suggesting that the dynamics are roughly similar and that analyses comparing them are appropriate. Certainly, respondents in states that participated in the Medicaid expansion were slightly more favorable toward the ACA even prior to expansion. Those differences grew after January 2014, however, as the residents of expansion states began to experience the benefits of Medicaid directly. Specifically, before the ACA's January 2014 implementation, the difference between states that would and would not later expand is 7.5 percentage points. After January 2014, it grew to 9.7 percentage points. It is also noteworthy that after January 2014, even attitudes in the non-expansion states grew very slightly more favorable (by 0.1 percentage points).[58]

To formally estimate the effect of the Medicaid expansion we employ "difference-in-differences" estimation, a statistical approach that compares the differences across two groups, one of which experienced a treatment at a certain point in time.[59] This method adjusts for time trends evident in the control group—and so requires the assumption that absent the treatment, the treatment group's trajectory would have followed the control group's. This estimation strategy accounts for any fixed differences in ACA favorability between states that expanded Medicaid and those that did not, as well as any over-time shifts in attitudes that are common across states. Practically, we specify linear regression models that isolate the differential change in ACA attitudes among respondents in some states (those states that expanded their Medicaid program) in a specific time period (after the expansion took place).

To estimate the effect of a state's Medicaid expansion on ACA favorability while accounting for individual-level differences we employ a variety of covariates. Our models include measures of respondents' education, income, gender, age, race, Hispanic ethnicity, and political identification as Republicans or independents.[60] To help rule out the possibility that the differences we observe are actually a product of differences across states or time periods we also include fixed effects for each survey as well as the respondents' states.[61]

Table B.3 reports the fitted ordinary least squares (OLS) models of the four-category favorability measure for three groups: all respondents, low-income respondents, and high-income respondents. In each case, the key estimate is the interaction between living in an expansion state and being in the post-expansion period. To benchmark effect sizes, note that the dependent variable in these analyses has a range of 3 and a standard deviation of 1.19. The estimated effects are substantively small and indistinguishable from zero for high-income respondents, indicating no discernible effect of the expansion. For low-income respondents, however, the effect is 0.101 (SE = 0.024, $p < 0.001$), meaning that those in expansion states averaged 0.101 higher on the 1–4 favorability scale after the expansion took place. The effect for low-income respondents is meaningful but not large; it is equivalent to moving 3 percent of the distance from "very unfavorable" (1) to "very favorable" (4). These results prove quite robust, as we discuss in more detail elsewhere.[62] They are also pronounced among Democrats and independents but not strong among Republicans. These results are thus consistent with an influence of self-interest filtered through the prism of partisanship and related group attachments.[63]

In recent decades, those who identify as Republicans or Democrats have been increasingly likely to adopt political attitudes consistent with their party's elites.[64] Such sorting has the potential to disrupt the channels through which policies influence public opinion. Here, however, we have shown that the Medicaid expansion had discernible effects on public opinion in the states that undertook it. It induced moderate positive effects on ACA favorability among low-income Americans. Put differently, the Medicaid expansion induced larger effects among the fraction of Americans who were more likely to be Medicaid-eligible. The impacts of the Medicaid expansion are also more apparent among nonwhite and Democratic respondents than in other groups.

Here we have employed a research design that allows us to differentiate the effects of the Medicaid expansion from self-selection into Medicaid. And we have found effects that are meaningful, but not politically transformative.

How Did Trump's Election Shift Attitudes?

As we saw in chapter 3, the election and inauguration of Donald Trump corresponded with a sizable pro-ACA shift in Americans' attitudes. But was the attitude shift an immediate response to Trump's election or a reaction to Republicans' concrete attempts to repeal the ACA in 2017? To assess to what extent policy feedbacks were at work, it is vital to investigate whether the post-Trump shift was driven by large shifts among those most likely to be affected personally or by smaller shifts in a broader swath of the population. If Trump's election made citizens more aware of the extent to which they personally benefited from the ACA, we might expect the increase in support to be concentrated in the groups that unambiguously benefited from the ACA, including those on Medicaid and those purchasing insurance through the exchanges.[65] It is also possible that Trump further polarized attitudes toward the ACA, meaning that increases in support may have been concentrated among Democrats.

We start by examining those on Medicaid and the question of whether Medicaid respondents were especially likely to become more supportive of the ACA after Trump's election. To do so we turn back to the HTP, the rolling cross-sectional phone survey of different American adults, and fit linear regression models of ACA favorability separately for each available month from early 2010 to late 2018. In all, 88,240 respondents are analyzed here. The factors we account for in these models include various basic demographics, such as identifying as Asian American, black, Hispanic, or male. They also include three functions of age and indicators for different levels of education, income, and political partisanship. The key covariates of interest, however, are those for respondents' type of health insurance coverage. Although we include indicator variables for coverage through Medicare, employer-provided insurance, and having insurance, we are principally interested in respondents who were insured by Medicaid—after all, this group had an especially clear, unambiguous interest in the ACA's survival. Note that we do not condition on respondents' state, both because our estimates within many surveys would be imprecise for most states and because we are interested in the association between Medicaid receipt overall and ACA favorability.

As a reminder, coefficients tell us the average change in the outcome given a one-unit change in the independent variable. In figure 4.4, we plot the coefficients for being insured through Medicaid for groups of three consecutive surveys from the ACA's passage in 2010 through late 2018. The coefficients are generally positive throughout this decade, indicating that, on average, those who received Medicaid were more supportive of the ACA than demographically similar Americans who did not. And these coefficients are on average somewhat larger in the period after Trump's inauguration (mean = 0.14) than in the period between 2014 and 2016 (mean = 0.08). Yet, the overall shift in ACA favorability in that period was a sizable 0.18. With just 7 percent of our post-implementation respondents reporting being on Medicaid, these estimates jointly imply that less than 1 percent of the overall shift in ACA attitudes post-Trump can be accounted for by changes among those receiving Medicaid.

If we restrict our analyses to the post-implementation period, we can also evaluate the effect of enrolling via the exchanges. Accordingly, in table B.4, we approach this estimation another way: we use multilevel models with the same covariates as well as an indicator for using the exchanges to predict four-category ACA favorability. We fit separate models for respondents during the 2014–2016 period and then for respondents during the 2017–2019 period. In the earlier period, the ACA had been implemented, but Obama was president and able to veto measures seeking to repeal it. In the later period, Trump, then president, pursued plans to repeal and replace the law.

If the threat to the ACA had a greater impact on those on Medicaid or those using the exchanges, we should expect the corresponding coefficient to grow in the second period. And it does—but only from 0.162 (SE = 0.030) to 0.168 (SE = 0.030), a difference that is not statistically significant (p-value = 0.45, one-sided). What's more, the coefficient for those insured through the exchanges actually decreases, from 0.421 (SE = 0.041) to 0.293 (SE = 0.044). The bulk of the movement in favorability after Trump's inauguration cannot be explained by those on Medicaid or those

Figure 4.4 Relationship between Medicaid Receipt and ACA Favorability over Time

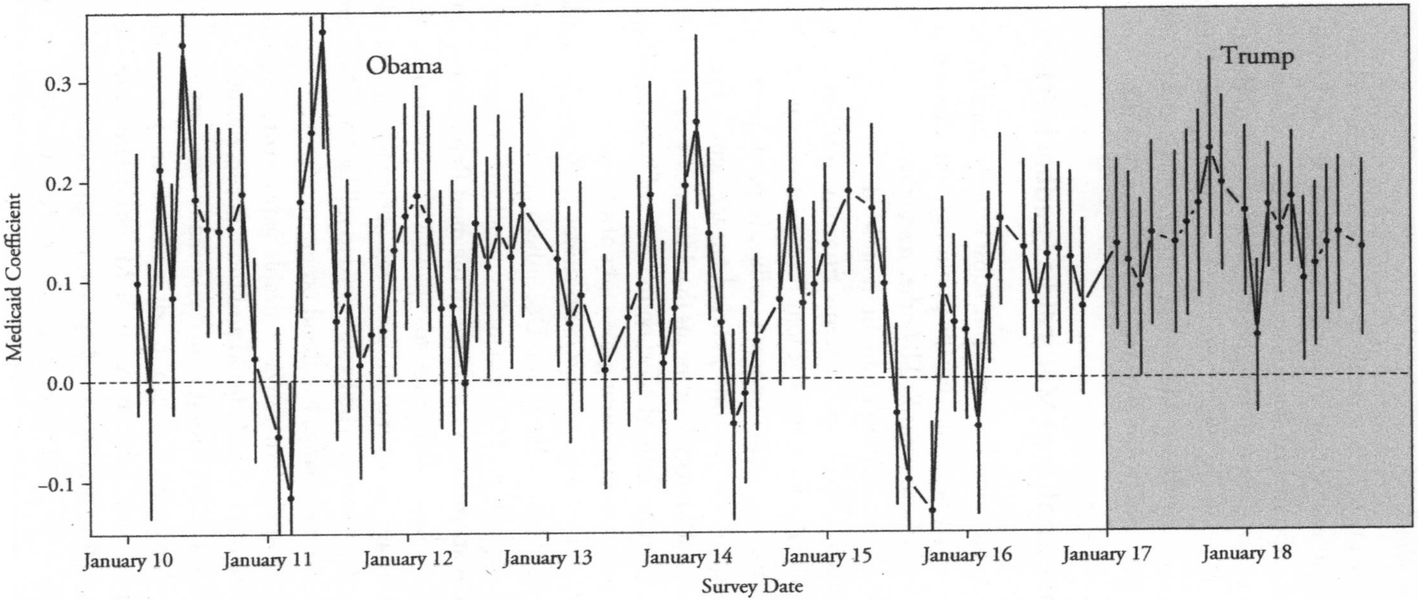

Source: KFF Health Tracking Poll (Kaiser Family Foundation 2022).

using the exchanges. (These results remain similar when including state fixed effects, suggesting that they are not driven by associations between Medicaid receipt and respondents' state of residence, either.) The pro-ACA shift in opinion does not appear to have been driven by some of the constituencies most dependent on the law.[66] Instead, it was a more general political shift, one driven more by the significant majority of Americans who *did not* come to rely on Medicaid or the exchanges after the expansion.

Secondary Limits on Medicaid's Feedback Effects

This chapter has identified real but substantively small policy feedback effects of the Medicaid expansion on public opinion, effects that are broadly consistent with those identified by other researchers.[67]

Still, there is another important limit on Medicaid's capacity to generate policy feedback effects, and it stems from unequal voter participation. Americans with low incomes have long been shown to vote at lower rates[68]— and while Medicaid enrollment can influence participation, it often does so in contexts of low baseline political engagement.[69] From the vantage point of electoral strategy, that means that influencing the views of Medicaid recipients has a more limited effect on the views of voters, as many Medicaid recipients are not always among the ranks of voters.

Consider, for example, a 2015 KFF survey of Kentucky residents conducted between November 18 and December 1 of that year, just after voters had elected Republican Matt Bevin.[70] Kentucky is a critical state in which to study ACA attitudes, as it was one of the most Republican-leaning states to establish its own exchange and to expand Medicaid. In backing Bevin by a nine-percentage-point margin over Democrat Jack Conway, Kentucky voters elected a governor who had pledged to roll back the ACA and shutter the state's Kynect exchange Medicaid program.

In the KFF survey, there was a sizable gap in voter registration rates between those receiving Medicaid and those not receiving it: 83 percent of respondents not on Medicaid were registered to vote versus just 61 percent of those on Medicaid. The gap in self-reported turnout in 2015 was even starker: 47 percent of those not receiving Medicaid voted, but just 19 percent of those receiving Medicaid did so. Although those on Medicaid were markedly more favorable toward the ACA, they were also decidedly less likely to have voted.[71] The overall political effects of the Medicaid expansion were thus further dampened.

Conclusion

As the ACA evolved in the decade after enactment, the Medicaid expansion came to be its central pillar, insuring significantly more people than the exchanges. The Medicaid expansion also directly provides a major benefit—health insurance—to low-income Americans. If there was any element of the ACA that was likely to help build public support for the law, the Medicaid expansion was it.

This chapter has considered three related questions about personal experiences and attitudes toward the Medicaid expansion. The first relates to support for the Medicaid expansion before its implementation: Did the people and places who stood to benefit directly support Medicaid expansion at disproportionate levels when they were able to vote on it? The short answer is yes, but only somewhat. By analyzing initiatives on expanding Medicaid in Maine and Oklahoma, we have seen that community-level partisan loyalties were strongly correlated with support for expanding Medicaid. The Maine and Oklahoma communities that were more supportive of expanding Medicaid were principally those that were more supportive of electing Democrats. Yes, low-income communities were somewhat more favorable toward the Medicaid expansion than you might expect based on partisanship alone, but partisanship seems to be the main driver. So there is not much evidence that self-interest was a primary engine behind support for the Medicaid expansion.

That said, our evidence indicates that once the Medicaid expansion came to a state, its low-income residents did grow demonstrably more supportive of the ACA. There was a clear policy feedback at work. Its political impact was muted, however, both by the fact that many states opted not to expand Medicaid and by relatively low levels of voter registration and turnout among Medicaid recipients. And shifting ACA attitudes do not necessarily mean shifting vote choices.[72]

Chapter 3 made clear that while the American public's attitudes toward the ACA were quite stable, the election of Donald Trump in November 2016 and the subsequent push to repeal the ACA by the Republican Congress did produce a rapid and marked uptick in support for the law. It is possible that those who had come to depend on the ACA were especially threatened by its repeal. But in this chapter's penultimate section, we saw that those on Medicaid were not behind the pro-ACA shift. So even though Medicaid recipients in general are quite pro-ACA, and the expansion made low-income Americans a bit more pro-ACA, the most pronounced system-level attitude change came from the broader population.

Of course, the Medicaid expansion was just one element of the ACA. In the next chapter, we consider the exchanges and associated policies like the individual mandate. Does the mode through which the government backstops individuals' health insurance make a difference in its political impacts?

CHAPTER 5

The Offsetting Effects of the Exchanges

With William R. Hobbs

IF THE ACA could win the loyalties of anyone, it was likely to be couples like the Recchis. Interviewed in Steven Brill's *America's Bitter Pill*, Ohio residents Sean and Stephanie Recchi were Republicans, sure, but Sean had been diagnosed with cancer in 2012, and he knew firsthand the costs of going without comprehensive health insurance. When Sean sought cancer treatment in Houston, he had to first wait for his $83,900 check to clear.[1]

Even so, when the ACA exchanges opened in the fall of 2013, the Recchis were not initially interested. Stephanie explained that "I hear a lot of bad things," referencing "television ads and some politicians talking on the news." At Brill's urging, Stephanie did check out the options on Ohio's health insurance exchange, the statewide marketplace established by the ACA and run by the federal government. But like many Americans, Stephanie was stymied by the website's interminably long delays. The Recchis subsequently enlisted an insurance broker to help them navigate the complexities of the post-ACA health care landscape, though they told the broker point-blank that they "don't want any part of Obamacare." The broker's reply: they could see what was available on the "Ohio exchange."[2]

Stephanie and Sean's story provides insights into the rollout and politics of the ACA exchanges. For families like theirs, the exchanges offered the promise of comprehensive health insurance that could serve as a critical financial backstop in the case of a major illness or accident. The value of the

ACA's insurance subsidies alone could reach thousands of dollars a year per policy. But in their early years, the exchanges operated in a highly polarized and nationalized political environment that heightened Republicans' suspicions of the program.[3]

On the other hand, the ACA's array of complex backdoor policy levers obscured the government's role in facilitating the health insurance options available on the exchanges. As with many market-based policies in recent decades, this indirect provision was born of policymakers' dueling aims to expand social protection without (appearing to) expand the government—and without disrupting private insurance markets.[4] The ACA's indirect mode of provision gave the Recchis' broker an opening to peruse their health insurance options without calling attention to the exchanges' connection to Obama. Yet by clouding any sense of linkage between those options and the ACA, the law's complex design also dampened the political implications of any positive experiences with the exchanges. Such is the irony of indirect provision: the same policy design that cloaked the role of government and so helped the ACA win support in the Senate may have undercut its ability to generate political support among citizens.

As chapter 2 detailed, the ACA was meant as a patch for a fragmented system, with the limited goal of providing insurance to groups not well served by the preexisting, employer-based system. Still, when the ACA was drafted in 2009 and 2010, the law's architects assumed that the launch of health care exchanges—not the expansion of Medicaid—would be the law's central vehicle for increasing insurance coverage. In fact, they expected that roughly 75 percent of all the gains in health insurance enrollment would come from the exchanges.[5] That same assumption pervaded the 2012 Supreme Court decision in *National Federation of Independent Business v. Sebelius*, the judicial compromise in which the individual mandate to obtain health insurance was preserved while the Medicaid expansion was ruled optional.[6] Yet, as of 2020, the Medicaid expansion accounted for 60 percent of that year's ACA enrollments, even without being implemented in more than a dozen states.[7]

Why the exchanges failed to insure as many people as planned is a critical policy question, but not the focus here.[8] Instead, this chapter probes the political impacts of the exchanges and associated market-based policies, such as the individual mandate, on would-be customers. The exchanges were potentially pivotal in political as well as policy terms since they were designed to serve a predominantly middle-class constituency and so could have fostered a cross-class coalition backing the ACA in combination with the Medicaid expansion.[9]

As we have seen in prior chapters, political scientists have long studied the ways in which public policies might reconfigure the political landscape at the elite and mass levels through feedback effects.[10] Policies that are delivered directly by governments commonly generate feedback effects on public opinion.[11] For example, chapter 4 provided evidence that the Medicaid expansion improved ACA favorability among low-income Americans in expansion states. This finding demonstrates that direct government provision of a major benefit can change attitudes. However, policies like the exchanges that rely on indirect mechanisms—such as private markets, regulations, or the tax code—often do not generate feedback effects, in part because policies provided indirectly are often less publicly visible and less easily politicized.[12] Even their beneficiaries may not link their personal experiences back to government action.

The ACA is similar to other indirect policies in that it relies heavily on incremental and individually low-salience measures.[13] As chapter 2 explained, the law is highly complex, as it includes a wide array of regulations and subsidies targeting insurers, employers, and consumers. The public was unlikely to be aware of most of those provisions, and that is why the Recchis needed a broker to help them navigate the post-ACA landscape. One straightforward expectation, then, is that the exchanges and associated policies will fail to produce policy feedbacks.

Yet there are also reasons to think that complex policies will produce complex feedback patterns that require us to study various provisions separately. Having been extensively covered by news media, the ACA's exchanges and other provisions may have been more visible to citizens than most policies that are provided indirectly, a topic we take up in chapter 7.[14] Indeed, the exchanges and associated policies may have produced different effects on different groups of people, a heterogeneity that may be masked by solely considering these policies' impacts on the population overall. For many, the ACA had substantial downsides extending well beyond the notorious website malfunctions in 2013: the law also led directly to the cancellation of approximately 2.6 million health insurance plans in 2013.[15] What's more, during its first five years, the law imposed fines on those who did not purchase health insurance.[16] Even those who received subsidies to purchase health insurance faced stiff tax penalties if their incomes rose, leading the Recchis' broker to suggest to some families that they reduce their overtime or take a month off at the end of the year: "If not, they could get hammered with huge tax bills that they never expected."[17] The ACA also relied on state-level exchanges, which varied markedly in pricing and the menu of options available.[18] And of course, since people differ dramatically in their health care needs and consumption, they differ in the extent to which they benefit from being insured. The ACA produced clear losers alongside winners. Thus, for the fraction of Americans who were directly affected, the package of policies supporting the exchanges and individual markets—including the mandate and subsidies—may well have produced offsetting feedback effects better characterized by heterogeneity than invisibility.

Prior research on the ACA's political impacts has focused primarily on its Medicaid expansion or on its overall effects.[19] To date, research examining the impacts of the exchanges or associated policies has been more limited.[20] Still, studying the exchanges and associated regulations may shed light on critical theoretical questions: Can a salient but complex policy relying heavily on indirect provision generate policy feedbacks on public opinion? If so, do such effects depend on citizens' personal situations?

The more general question underpinning this book is the extent to which political elites can exert influence on public opinion via policymaking. Given how heavily contemporary American public policy relies on complex public-private arrangements in a range of policy areas, the political impacts of the exchanges are likely to be instructive about elites' capacity to build support via policy feedback effects well beyond health care.[21] Chapter 4 may have tempted advocates of single-payer health care to conclude that direct government provision is a tried-and-true path to political support. Readers coming to any such conclusion will find this chapter less sanguine, as it provides major warnings about the political palatability of disrupting existing health insurance markets.

Chapter Roadmap

This chapter inherits the complexity of its subject. Drawing on and extending my article with William R. Hobbs, it first sketches how the exchanges operate and then uses prior research to develop theoretical expectations.[22]

The subsequent empirical section opens with descriptive analyses using the KFF's rolling cross-sectional survey. These analyses aim to provide a big-picture assessment of the correlations between personal experiences and ACA attitudes. Those who purchased their own insurance became more favorable toward the ACA at precisely the moment when the exchanges opened. At approximately the same time, those without insurance became less favorable toward the ACA. There is suggestive evidence, then, that at least some of the citizens with a direct stake noticed and reacted to the opening of the exchanges. Given that the ACA's implementation varied substantially from state to state, we also investigate these relationships in the bellwether state of Kentucky. Kentucky is a Republican-leaning state that was quick to open its own ACA exchange, so we report similar patterns in a survey of that state's residents.[23] Together these descriptive results hint at policy feedbacks from the exchanges and mandate—and so at the potential for elite influence through policy. But that influence can be negative as well as positive.

Nonetheless, those patterns could well be the product of selection bias. Like the Recchi family, political views might have influenced who sought out insurance under the ACA rather than the reverse.[24] Accordingly, this chapter next presents results from a population-based panel survey that reinforce the prospect of a causal relationship by showing that those who lost insurance between 2016 and 2018 became more negative toward the ACA. These findings are consistent with prior research by Jacobs and Mettler, and they reinforce the evidence of negative policy feedbacks, at least for those who became uninsured after the ACA's implementation.[25]

Government policies provided indirectly have the potential to generate offsetting patterns of policy feedback. It is critical, then, to test specific ACA provisions alongside more overarching estimates of citizens' reactions. Given that, we focus on three specific elements of the ACA that are especially informative. In the first, we link administrative data on exchange pricing to geo-coded survey respondents to show that respondents who used the exchanges and whose local exchanges experienced price shocks became more anti-ACA as a consequence. The ability of these consumers to politicize their experiences constitutes additional evidence of negative policy feedbacks.

The second test focuses on a group especially likely to benefit from the ACA's individual markets: those just below age sixty-five, like Sean Recchi.

People in this group face higher average health care costs than younger cohorts but do not yet enjoy Medicare's coverage and protections (for which they will be eligible starting at sixty-five). Moreover, among its other regulations, the ACA limited the premiums that insurers could charge older customers relative to younger customers and banned discrimination based on preexisting conditions.[26] These factors together make those in their early sixties a likely case for positive feedback effects. In keeping with this expectation, our analysis demonstrates positive attitude changes among those in their early sixties after the newly capped premiums.

In these two cases, the ACA's indirect policies do produce feedback effects, albeit in opposite directions. However, a third case—people in their twenties who lose eligibility for coverage through their parents' insurance—reveals no significant change in attitudes.[27] Such null effects are more typical of prior studies of indirect or market-based policies.[28] Even within the ACA, different provisions produce quite different effects.[29]

Overall, these results suggest that some Americans sometimes shifted their attitudes in response to the ACA's perceived benefits and costs. That implies that, at least at times, they did attribute certain personal and local experiences with health insurance to the ACA. The feedback effects, however, canceled each other out in aggregate, owing to concentrated perceived costs and backlash among those likely to be uninsured. In other words, the ACA's complexity did not preclude policy feedback effects. Effects were instead complex themselves, varying across places, people, and specific policy levers. Backlash was real and meaningful.[30] Elite policymaking can move subsequent public opinion, but when the policy is targeted and complex, its impacts on mass opinion are likely to be offsetting and substantively small overall.

Indirect Policies and Policy Feedbacks

Rather than provide health insurance directly, as Medicare does, the ACA's exchanges and associated policies sought to use indirect levers to increase the public's uptake of health insurance through private markets. Prior research indicates that such indirect policies do not generally produce policy feedback effects on public opinion.[31] This section briefly recaps basic information about the exchanges' design. It then develops the hypothesis that if indirect and complex policies are sufficiently salient, they may still be able to shape public opinion, albeit in cross-cutting and circumscribed ways.

The Exchanges

As we saw in chapter 2, one of the ACA's core elements was the creation of exchanges on which individuals could purchase private health insurance. The law aimed to keep insurance prices down by fostering competition and subsidizing the insurance of lower-income Americans whose incomes left them ineligible for expanded Medicaid. In 2016, 6.1 million American households received this credit, with a mean subsidy of approximately $4,000.[32] Households with incomes up to 400 percent of the federal poverty line qualified for the subsidy, but those whose incomes rose past this threshold had to repay the government. The exchanges are simply a market-place: once customers are enrolled, their primary interactions are not with government but with a private insurer. After the exchanges' opening year, customers could automatically re-enroll, meaning that for many, the government's role in facilitating the exchanges might have become an increasingly distant memory.[33]

Well-functioning markets require many buyers and many sellers—that's Economics 101. And insurance markets risk what economists call "adverse selection": if those who are more likely to need insurance are more likely to acquire it, prices can soar. For example, if only people who anticipate high health care costs buy insurance, premiums will need to be very high to keep insurance companies from going out of business. To limit prices, the ACA used sticks as well as carrots—that is, the law compelled as well as enticed. Specifically, as enacted in 2010, the ACA included an individual mandate that required most Americans to have insurance or else pay a fine. In 2016, 5 million tax returns included such payments, with a mean payment of $727.[34] The individual mandate was subsequently repealed by Republicans in 2017. But even while the individual mandate was in force, the exchanges in many states fell short of the standards of well-functioning markets.[35] In late 2013, the federal website serving thirty-six states launched to weeks of delays.[36] And as we discuss later, many exchanges saw rapidly rising prices, few affordable choices, and/or plans with narrow networks in the years following their establishment.[37]

One study that considers whether indirect policy levers can produce feedback effects on public opinion is Kimberly Morgan and Andrea Campbell's analysis of the 2003 Medicare Modernization Act (MMA).[38]

The MMA was a prescription drug benefit enacted by congressional Republicans and signed into law by President George W. Bush a year before he stood for reelection in 2004. Like the ACA, the MMA was a health policy reform that relied on indirect mechanisms—in this case to reduce prescription drug costs. Known as Medicare Part D, the prescription drug benefit is provided through private companies, with both the federal government and citizens assuming some of the costs. Republican strategists argued that the law was essential to shore up political support for Bush among seniors. However, the MMA's impacts on public opinion turned out to be limited: the policy's implementation did not lead beneficiaries to support more market-based policies generally, nor did it improve perceptions of Republicans' handling of health policy.[39] Research on other indirect government policies—such as those provided via tax deductions—reinforces the claim that they are unlikely to have sizable feedback effects on public opinion, as such policies are difficult to trace back to government actions.[40]

There is good reason to think that the ACA's exchanges might follow this same pattern. The government's role in facilitating the provision of insurance is not a salient feature of the exchanges' design, which may reduce citizens' capacity to trace elements of their insurance back to government action or to link the exchanges' various benefits (and costs) to the same underlying policy.[41] Citizens may not be aware of the links between different elements of the ACA, such as the way the individual mandate was intended to limit adverse selection and keep premiums down.[42] Prior research also concludes that feedback effects are more readily detected on political participation than public opinion.[43] Such findings further dampen any expectation that the exchanges had feedback effects on ACA attitudes.

The ACA's Salience and Complexity

The ACA differs from other indirect policies in key respects. The visibility of the law was heightened by the sustained, salient political battles over it that lasted for years after implementation.[44] This high level of media coverage may have helped overcome the barriers that often prevent citizens from connecting their experiences to their evaluations of indirect government policies. The law's salience might also help explain why exchange usage was unusually politicized relative to most other policies.[45] Republicans proved less likely to enroll through the exchanges than Democrats or independents.

Indirect policies are typically less visible to citizens, but that was not true of the ACA.

The exchanges and associated policies also stand out for the extent to which they were likely to generate heterogeneous responses. Receiving health insurance can have sizable impacts on people's lives; it can increase health care access, reduce debt, and even improve mental health.[46] For those receiving tax credits like the Advance Premium Tax Credit in particular, the financial subsidies for purchasing insurance can be large—and generous benefits are one likely source of policy feedbacks.[47]

The experiences of those who used or were otherwise affected by the exchanges are likely to differ dramatically depending on their health care utilization, their eligibility for subsidies, the quality of their state's exchange, and the options available in their market (including whether their previous plan remained available).[48] Having the same insurance does not mean having the same health care needs or experiences. A person who is forced to buy comprehensive coverage she does not need or, conversely, to pay a lot for insurance that still leaves her exposed to significant costs may well sour on the ACA. But someone with a serious preexisting condition who can get heavily subsidized insurance is likely to be much more positive. As discussed later, prices on the exchanges vary dramatically across the country: similar people can pay very different premiums depending on where they live. Plans also differ in the breadth of their networks, meaning the number of local providers they cover. For example, in 2014 an Indiana resident had to spend five months looking for a primary care doctor who would take the silver-level insurance she purchased on the exchanges.[49]

Such heterogeneous impacts may well have been exacerbated by the ACA's complexity. Campbell notes that policy feedbacks are more likely when the policy's beneficiaries are concentrated in ways that encourage them to identify as a coherent group and act on their shared interests.[50] The archetypal example is Social Security, with its payments to seniors who amassed credits through their work history.[51] But because of the ACA's complex, multifaceted design, key beneficiaries have a stake only in specific, often disparate provisions. This complexity may keep the beneficiary population fragmented and reduce the law's capacity to generate a cohesive identity.[52] Issues of timing may also dampen the ability of beneficiaries to act collectively in support of the policy. People often do not know how their health needs are going to change down the road, and so they cannot anticipate when, or even if, specific ACA provisions will matter to them.

The ACA's design might also have inadvertently heightened the salience and traceability of one of the law's least popular elements: the individual mandate.[53] In general, people are prone to negativity biases—that is, they are disproportionately influenced by negative information and events.[54] The tangible and immediate negative costs associated with the individual mandate might well have outweighed any inchoate sense that the exchanges' other features produced benefits.

These points jointly suggest that experiences with and responses to the ACA are likely to be individualized and variable. Only small subpopulations of Americans were unambiguously affected by the exchanges and associated policies in this period, whether for good or ill. As a consequence, it would be surprising if the ACA's exchanges had consistently large, positive feedback effects. But for the most affected subpopulations, the salience of the ACA's exchanges may enable them to trace their experiences back to the law. Even an indirectly provided public good may generate policy feedback effects under certain conditions—just not the consistently positive policy feedbacks that the ACA's architects had hoped for.

Evaluating Policy Feedbacks: Research Design and Data Sets

To evaluate the prospect that the ACA exchanges generated different political responses from different groups, it is critical that we consider the full package of policies designed to make the exchanges functional. This package includes not only the exchanges but the individual mandate and other associated regulations, as well as the various subsidies to help customers pay for insurance. We begin with descriptive analyses. Certainly, we must be mindful of the very likely prospect of selection bias; people do opt into or out of being insured for reasons related to their political views. Correlation does not always equal causation. However, substantively meaningful causal effects often generate correlations in observational data. Moreover, when political elites assess the political impacts of a policy, they rely heavily on such correlations, which are often the only evidence available to them. These initial analyses also help identify subpopulations that were especially

Figure 5.1 Distribution of HTP Respondents by Health Insurance Source before and after the ACA's January 2014 Implementation

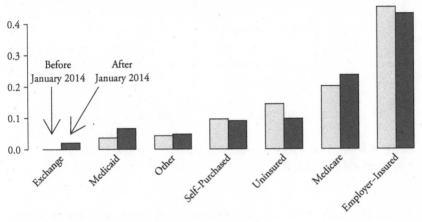

Source: KFF Health Tracking Poll (Kaiser Family Foundation 2022).

affected by the exchanges and the mandate, pointing to subsequent causal analyses that target specific ACA provisions.

A Primer on ACA Exchange Users and Their Attitudes

The primary data source for our descriptive analyses is the Health Tracking Poll, the rolling cross-sectional telephone survey by the Kaiser Family Foundation of adults' health policy attitudes that has anchored analyses in prior chapters.[55] As in chapters 3 and 4, this survey's extraordinary sample size provides a unique opportunity to observe the evolution of Americans' ACA attitudes as well as the trajectories of ACA attitudes among key subgroups.

To understand the exchanges' impacts on public opinion, it is helpful to first identify who actually used them. Figure 5.1 illustrates the distribution of types of health insurance before and after the ACA's primary provisions came into effect. For example, it shows the decline in the uninsured rate from 14.4 percent before January 2014 to 9.7 percent afterwards.[56]

Overall, however, the changes in the distribution of insurance were marginal. At the population level, the basic contours of health care provision in the United States remained much as they were before the ACA.

Figure 5.2 ACA Favorability by Health Insurance Status and Source, 2010–2018

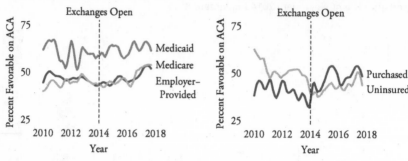

Source: KFF Health Tracking Poll (Kaiser Family Foundation 2022). Figure reprinted with permission from Hobbs and Hopkins 2021.

What's more, the share of U.S. adults who reported using the exchanges averaged only 2 percent of the surveyed population. Categories of insurance that were less overtly affected by the ACA—employer-provided insurance and Medicare—remained far and away the largest sources of insurance. These patterns place important limits on the ACA's direct policy feedback effects: people in the parts of the insurance market most influenced by the ACA represent a small minority of citizens.[57]

The ACA was rightly touted as a once-in-a-generation health policy reform—which says as much about the limits of large reforms as it is does about the breadth of the transformations wrought by the ACA.

Figure 5.2 presents the trends in a binary measure of ACA favorability by insurance type. As the left side shows, respondents insured through Medicaid are always more favorable toward the ACA than those insured through Medicare or employers: 61 percent of Medicaid recipients report favorable attitudes versus 47 percent of those with employer-provided insurance and 45 percent of those on Medicare. The over-time patterns for these groups are roughly similar, with growing favorability between 2016 and 2018 in the face of GOP repeal efforts, although the smallest group (Medicaid recipients) is understandably more variable.

In the right-hand panel of figure 5.2, we see the trends for the respondents in insurance categories for whom the ACA's exchanges and mandate are especially impactful: those who lack insurance, those who buy insurance themselves, and those who buy insurance via the exchanges. Here the over-time dynamics differ, quite possibly owing to selection bias. Before the ACA's 2014 implementation, those without insurance were consistently more favorable toward the ACA than those purchasing insurance on the individual market. In the pre-implementation period, the average ACA favorability for those without insurance was 52 percent, compared to 41 percent among the self-insured. But these groups switched places almost immediately after implementation. Favorability among the uninsured dropped sharply in the run-up to implementation and averaged just 42 percent in post-implementation surveys. By contrast, favorability among those on the individual market rose, averaging 47 percent after implementation.[58]

Such changes are likely to reflect selection processes as the composition of who is insured or uninsured changed. The ACA's core elements shifted the composition of groups such as the insured in critical ways. The law enabled many with preexisting conditions to purchase insurance, and at the same time it raised costs for some who did not anticipate needing comprehensive insurance, especially if they were ineligible for subsidies. In anticipation of the ACA's new requirements, insurance companies ended noncompliant plans, sending millions of cancellation notices in late 2013. Still, it is possible that such changes reflect people's experiences too, as those without insurance faced a new tax penalty and those needing to self-insure enjoyed a range of new options and protections, alongside subsidies in some cases.

The HTP also gives us a direct measure of Americans' perceptions of the ACA's impacts. Several surveys between 2010 and 2014 included a separate question about whether the respondent and her family had benefited from or been harmed by the law. As figure C.1 shows, both responses increased notably in 2014, a finding consistent with the prospect that citizens recognized the changes and responded in heterogeneous ways. (It is also noteworthy that more than 40 percent of survey respondents reported harm or benefit, a fraction that is significantly larger than the share directly affected by the exchanges, insurance cancellations, and Medicaid expansion.) Elsewhere we reported that separate KFF surveys of those without group-based insurance uncover generally similar relationships.[59] Those who bought insurance on the exchanges—and especially those who received a subsidy—were more positive toward the ACA than similar citizens who did not.

Attitudes in Kentucky, 2015

Residents of specific states with unique post-ACA trajectories are an especially instructive group. Kentucky was one of the few Republican-leaning states to create its own health insurance exchange, known as Kynect, as well as expand its Medicaid program. Post-ACA, Kentucky saw one of the largest increases of any state in the percentage of insured residents—but in late 2015 its voters elected Republican Matt Bevin as governor after he had promised to shut down Kynect.

At the time of Bevin's election, the KFF conducted a poll of Kentucky residents and asked various questions about respondents' attitudes toward the ACA and health insurance.[60] Even in Kentucky, a state that opened its own exchange without difficulty, the survey data indicate that only 10 percent of adults under sixty-five had insurance they purchased themselves, and just 21 percent of those respondents reported having obtained their insurance through Kynect.[61] What's more, only 13 percent of adults who purchased their own insurance—and just 2 percent of adults under sixty-five overall—reported receiving a subsidy to help with their insurance premiums.[62] Some of the groups of clear-cut ACA beneficiaries are not large in number.

Table C.4 reports linear regression models in which we analyze ACA favorability (measured on a 1–4 scale) as a function of a variety of standard demographic measures as well as respondents' sources of insurance.[63] In some models, we include a measure for whether the respondent used Kynect while in the others we do not. People who purchase their own insurance are not noticeably different from other Kentucky respondents, as the regression coefficients are substantively small and inconsistent in their signs. Nor is there evidence that people who used the Kynect exchange were more favorable—there the coefficients are −0.20 (SE = 0.15) or −0.24 (SE = 0.15).[64] Regression coefficients report the expected change in the outcome for a one-unit change in a given independent variable. Substantively, these results mean that those who purchased insurance via Kynect had levels of favorability that were on average 0.24 lower on the 1–4 favorability scale than other respondents, but they are not statistically significant.

We observe too few people receiving subsidies to estimate their correlation with ACA attitudes precisely, but it is noteworthy that the coefficient in the regression is substantively very large, at 0.32 to 0.46.[65] As best as we can tell, receiving a subsidy is associated with a substantial boost in ACA favorability, even conditional on income, education, and indicators for respondents' racial and ethnic backgrounds. So while there is little evidence that exchange users were more positive toward the ACA, those receiving subsidies might have been.

Panel-Based Estimates of Trends in ACA Attitudes by Insurance

We now return to the population overall. As we saw in figure 5.2, around the time of the ACA's implementation, the relationship between people's insurance status and their ACA attitudes shifted: people who purchased their own insurance became more favorable toward the ACA, and the uninsured became less so. But such relationships at least partly reflect selection bias, as individuals who already felt favorably or unfavorably toward the ACA may have shifted their insurance status accordingly.

Panel data provide one way to address this challenge. With their repeated observations of the same individuals, panels enable us to hold all of respondents' fixed characteristics constant, and so to isolate the effect of changes in insurance status on changes in attitudes.[66] Here we draw on the 2012–2018 waves of the ISCAP panel (introduced in chapter 3) to evaluate Americans' attitudes toward the ACA over time.

Becoming uninsured is not randomly assigned, so even in these analyses nonrandom selection remains a concern. In a given period of time, however, some number of people will lose their insurance unexpectedly, possibly because they or their family members lost jobs. This research design analyzes whether their ACA attitudes change in those circumstances, and it holds respondents' fixed characteristics constant (like their political ideologies or general health). For that reason, panel analyses offer one piece of the broader puzzle.

Few respondents fell into the self-purchased or uninsured categories. Of the 639 panelists who completed both the October 2016 and October 2018 waves, only 44 (7 percent) reported in January 2016 that they purchased their insurance themselves and did not use the exchanges. Another 36 panelists (6 percent) reported being uninsured at that time, an estimate lower than the 2016 national benchmark of 11 percent.[67] On their own, these numbers are yet another reminder that the populations most directly

Figure 5.3 ACA Attitudes among Respondents to the 2012–2018 ISCAP Panel Who Completed the November–December 2016 and October 2018 Waves

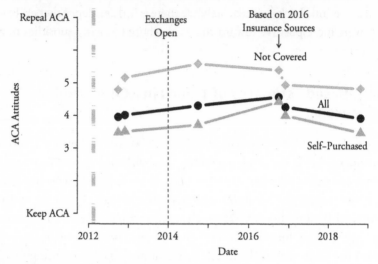

Source: Hobbs and Hopkins 2021. Reprinted with permission.

Note: N = 589. Insurance status is as of January 2016, the first wave in which it was measured. The gray horizontal lines on the left report the distribution of the outcome variable for the October 2012 survey. The November–December 2016 and October 2018 waves were conducted through GfK's Knowledge Panel.

affected by the ACA were small relative to the total population of American adults. Selection bias may also still be at work if it unfolds dynamically—for example, if those whose ACA attitudes improve then subsequently purchase insurance.

Even with these small, selected samples, however, the panel allows us to observe how these respondents' attitudes shifted relative to the population overall, partly because panel analyses can isolate changes within individuals, thus offering far more statistical precision than analyses across different individuals. In these analyses, our outcome measure comes from the following panel prompt: "Some people think the health care reform law should be kept as it is. Others want to repeal the entire health care law. Still others are somewhere in between." Respondents could reply on a 1–7 scale, with 1 indicating the "health care reform law should be kept as it is" and 7 indicating that "the entire health care law should be repealed."

As figure 5.3 illustrates, the groups defined by insurance status in 2016 differed at the baseline but moved roughly in parallel. There is no evidence that those who purchased insurance themselves differed markedly in the trajectory of their ACA attitudes compared to other insured groups. Overall, there is little evidence that respondents who purchased their own insurance in 2016 evince distinctive over-time patterns, as we might expect had there been a sizable policy feedback effect for that group. However, support for ACA repeal declined less among those without insurance between 2016 and 2018 relative to people in other groups.[68]

We next analyze the relationship between shifts in insurance status and changes in ACA attitudes statistically. Certainly, those who became uninsured between 2016 and 2018 were likely to be quite different from those who were uninsured before the ACA's implementation. Those who were choosing to become uninsured in the years after 2014 were less likely to qualify for subsidies or to have preexisting conditions or other reasons to anticipate major health care needs. In short, they were a population for whom the ACA was not as good a deal. So by examining changes in insurance status between 2016 and 2018, this approach may offer a conservative test of the effects of such changes on ACA attitudes—that is, a test that understates the full effect.

More formally, we use an estimation strategy, sometimes called difference-in-differences, in which we regress the change in respondents' support for repealing the ACA between the fall of 2016 and the fall of 2018 on various measures, including changes in three types of insurance status that are closely connected to the ACA (lacking insurance, purchasing one's own insurance, and being on Medicaid).[69] As table C.6's first model illustrates, someone who loses insurance is on average 0.64 points (SE = 0.36, p = 0.07, two-sided) more supportive of repealing the ACA, a very sizable effect even on a 1–7 outcome scale. By contrast, while the coefficients for a change in being self-insured or on Medicaid are positive, they are substantively small and quite uncertain.[70] For evidence of the robustness of these results, see the additional analyses presented in figure C.2 and table C.7.

Given that losses and gains are asymmetric—an asymmetry known to exist with health care attitudes—it is also valuable to differentiate those who gained insurance from those who lost it.[71] We see the expected asymmetry in table C.6's right column: while those who gained insurance became very slightly more favorable toward the ACA (0.16 points lower on the repeal scale), that result is far from statistically significant (SE = 0.62, p = 0.80). By contrast, losing insurance is associated with a marked 0.94-point increase

(SE = 0.45, p = 0.04) in support for repealing the ACA. These estimates imply that it would take more than five newly insured people to outweigh the negative effect of one person who lost insurance. The evidence that the ACA had negative effects on at least some Americans is certainly reinforced by such over-time changes.[72] The fraction of Americans who became uninsured well after the ACA's implementation was small. But as a consequence, those people became demonstrably more negative toward the ACA, and more supportive of repealing it.

Testing Specific ACA Features

Price Spikes on the Exchanges

Prior research on indirect policies suggests that they are unlikely to shape attitudes, as citizens do not commonly attribute personal experiences to them. The correlations detailed here, however, suggest that the exchanges and associated policies may have been an exception—they may have had different effects on attitudes depending on the personal circumstances of those seeking insurance. In particular, negative experiences with the exchanges and the mandate may have durably shaped attitudes. Consider the case of Loralea Grey, an Oregon resident whose family had a limited "catastrophic" plan before the ACA but then faced a premium increase of nearly 40 percent for 2017 alone. "How is this possible or allowable?" Grey wondered. "When I contacted the Oregon insurance commissioner, I received a response back telling me I should feel free to shop around; as if I wasn't smart enough to have already done that?"[73]

Given experiences like Loralea's, it is valuable to consider a most-likely case for negative policy feedbacks: price shocks on the exchanges. Specifically, in light of negativity biases and the sizable price increases on some exchanges, we examine whether people who purchase insurance on the exchanges became more negative toward the ACA if local prices spiked. During the period in question between 2014 and 2017, the average benchmark premium rose by 32 percent.[74] But with extensive subsidies, customers may have been insulated from those price spikes—or they may not have linked them back to the ACA. To test those possibilities, we combine a geo-coded version of the HTP with administrative data on exchange pricing to estimate the effects of local price changes on ACA favorability.[75] We then estimate the attitudinal effects of price changes on local markets.[76]

Table 5.1 Multilevel Models Fit to KFF Respondents from 2015, 2016, and 2017, with Insurance Market Conditions (and Other Independent Variables) Predicting ACA Favorability, Measured on a 1–4 Scale

	Dependent Variable			
	ACA Favorability			
	Nonmarket	Market	Uninsured	Market
	(1)	(2)	(3)	(4)
Number of plans (logged, in standard deviations)	0.001	0.07	0.004	0.08
	(0.01)	(0.06)	(0.03)	(0.07)
Mean premium (in standard deviations)	0.004	0.04	0.05	0.04
	(0.01)	(0.07)	(0.03)	(0.07)
Mean change in premium (in standard deviations)	0.001	0.19	0.02	0.17
	(0.01)	(0.07)	(0.04)	(0.08)
Mean change in benchmark premium				0.0003
(in standard deviations)				(0.002)
Observations	15,987	442	1,772	438
Month fixed effects	Y	Y	Y	Y
County-level demographics	Y	Y	Y	Y

Source: KFF Health Tracking Poll (Kaiser Family Foundation 2022).

Relatively few respondents used the exchanges—the annual sample sizes for exchange users are 157, 134, and 151. So we fit a multilevel model to borrow strength across the three years and estimate the effects of price shocks jointly. In other words, we feed data for all three years into a single model, affording us more observations and more statistical power. This model accounts for the total number of plans available on each market as well as the mean premium for that year and the mean change in premiums from the prior year.[77] The model also includes random effects for each of the three years as well as individual- and county-level covariates. (In multilevel or hierarchical models, "random effects" are additional group-level parameters; in this case, they are constrained to follow a normal distribution. They capture the possibly differing effects across years.)

Shown in table 5.1 (and in full in table C.8 and the supplemental information for Hobbs and Hopkins 2021), the model suggests that rising average premiums on the ACA exchanges are associated with sizable declines in ACA favorability among respondents who actually used the exchanges.[78] The estimated coefficient is 0.19 (SE = 0.07), meaning that an increase of one standard deviation in the mean monthly premium change ($33) is associated with a 0.19-point drop on the 1–4 ACA favorability scale. This shift is substantively quite meaningful. Importantly, this relationship does not hold for other respondents or for the uninsured, as the additional columns on the left side of table 5.1 demonstrate. These findings indicate that we are detecting the effects of experience with the markets and not simply spurious county-level associations.[79]

The finding of a price effect is especially noteworthy given that most consumers on the marketplaces have government subsidies—and the APTC's design should shield subsidized customers from price spikes to a significant degree. As of 2017, 84 percent of the 12.2 million exchange enrollees nationwide received the APTC to help cover the cost of their premiums.[80] Undeniably, some people experienced sharp jumps in prices. But since others were insulated by the subsidies, these effects could reflect perceived prices or result not only from actual price spikes but also from associated changes in health plans.[81]

For instance, rising premiums may force customers to switch plans or choose a less preferred plan. The size of the subsidies are tied to the second-cheapest silver plan, but which plan that is may change from year to year. Future expectations may also influence customers' attitudinal feedbacks. Since the APTC is tied to income, those with unexpected positive income shocks may have to repay a portion of the subsidy. In 2016, 5 million people had to make such payments, with a mean payment of around $700.[82] Uncertainty about possible future subsidies may induce price sensitivity too. Whatever the mechanism, in the case of the exchanges, indirect policies can generate negative attitudinal feedbacks.

The Discontinuity at Age Sixty-Five

The ACA used various policy levers to bolster the exchanges and increase the availability of health insurance, so we now examine another most-likely case: the law's overall impact on Americans in their early sixties. This group has higher health costs than younger groups, and yet people this age are not old enough to participate in Medicare; its members were especially vulnerable pre-ACA. But the ACA provided valuable new opportunities and protections for those in their early sixties. It created exchanges on which non-elderly adults could purchase insurance—sometimes with subsidies—while also mandating that insurers not discriminate on the basis of preexisting conditions. The ACA also limited premiums for older customers to no more than three times the premiums of younger customers, creating an effective subsidy if health care costs for older customers exceeded that ratio.

We need a separate group of people who can serve as a baseline against which to compare those in their early sixties. Here we focus primarily on those just above sixty-five, in part following prior research.[83] The most common source of health insurance for Americans age sixty-five and older is Medicare; 68 percent of HTP respondents in that age bracket reported that their health insurance came through Medicare. These respondents were potentially affected by messaging on the ACA, but their Medicare eligibility made them less likely to be personally affected by the exchanges, individual mandate, or cancellation of noncompliant plans. To the extent that the ACA's 2014 implementation affected Americans directly, it was substantially more likely to affect those just under sixty-five.[84]

Figure 5.4 shows average ACA favorability separately for sixty-four- and sixty-five-year-olds before and after the 2014 implementation. Favorability is noticeably lower among the sixty-four-year-olds prior to January 2014, but slightly higher afterwards—mean favorability among sixty-four-year-olds jumps from 2.16 to 2.40, while among sixty-five-year-olds it hardly moves (2.33 to 2.35). These trends are consistent with the claim that changes in attitudes are driven more by shifts among those just under sixty-five. From the trend lines, we see that the effect emerged only months after the January 2014 implementation, suggesting that some combination of the exchanges' rocky rollout, an open-enrollment period spanning several months, delays in the actual use of health insurance, and other factors may explain the timing of the shift. Still, the figure also clarifies that by late 2014, ACA favorability among sixty-four-year-olds was often higher than it was among sixty-five-year-olds, a pattern rarely observed just before the ACA's implementation.[85]

We next estimate the ACA's impacts on those just under sixty-five (just below the threshold for Medicare) as compared to those just above it.[86] There is a precedent for this research design. Studying the period before the ACA's full implementation, Amy Lerman and Katherine McCabe sought to understand whether Americans' experiences with publicly provided insurance through Medicare changed their health policy attitudes.[87] But whereas that study examined the effects of becoming Medicare-eligible at

Figure 5.4 Smoothed Favorability Ratings for Sixty-Four-Year-Olds and Sixty-Five-Year-Olds, 2010–2018

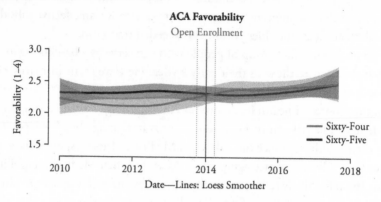

ACA Favorability

Date—Lines: Loess Smoother

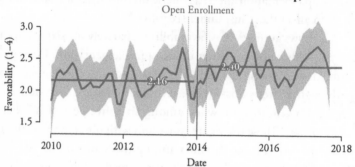

ACA Favorability: Sixty-Four (Treatment Group)

Lines: Loess Smoother Approximating Quarterly Moving Average

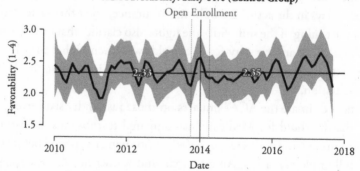

ACA Favorability: Sixty-Five (Control Group)

Lines: Loess Smoother Approximating Quarterly Moving Average

Source: KFF Health Tracking Poll (Kaiser Family Foundation 2022). Figure reprinted with permission from Hobbs and Hopkins 2021.

Note: The top panel displays a loess smoother (default span = 0.75), while the bottom two panels display loess smoothing using roughly quarterly spans. The horizontal lines in the bottom panels indicate pre- and post-2014 means. Shading indicates 95 percent confidence intervals.

one point in time, we use those who are sixty-five or older as a benchmark to understand the changing attitudes of those in their early sixties in response to the ACA.[88]

Our goal is to estimate the difference in ACA attitudes associated with Medicare eligibility before and after the ACA's full implementation and then to compare the estimates. To do so we return to the HTP. We first calculate the optimal bandwidth, so our initial analyses include respondents ages sixty-two to sixty-eight, enabling us to isolate the shift in attitudes between sixty-four- and sixty-five-year-olds with more precision.[89] We begin by confirming that key variables do not differ across the discontinuity (see table C.9). We then regress the four-category measure of ACA favorability on several variables, including measures for time trends; respondents' age in years; Medicare eligibility via age; levels of education; self-identification as male, black, Hispanic, or Asian American; income; and a five-category measure of partisan identification.

In the pre-implementation surveys, we find that being under sixty-five and not yet eligible for Medicare produces a coefficient of −0.12 (SE = 0.06) (see table C.10 for the full fitted model). Substantively, this result means that someone who is not quite Medicare-eligible rates the ACA −0.12 lower on average, which amounts to 10 percent of that variable's standard deviation. Lerman and McCabe attribute this difference to positive experiences with Medicare, since a majority of Americans shift their insurance status at sixty-five, when they become eligible for Medicare.[90] However, our key estimate is not simply the change in ACA attitudes at sixty-five, but the extent to which the ACA's implementation reduced any differences in attitudes at age sixty-five. Did the pro-ACA attitudinal bump at age sixty-five persist, or did the ACA's implementation improve experiences for those in their early sixties and so close the gap? We thus estimate a parallel OLS model for respondents after the ACA's January 1, 2014, implementation, shown in figure 5.5. The impact of being under sixty-five shrank to just 0.01 (SE = 0.06). Post-implementation, those who were under sixty-five and therefore more directly affected by the ACA were essentially no less supportive than people just slightly older.

For our purposes, the key question is the extent to which the effect declined after the ACA was implemented, and figure 5.5 presents that estimated difference using dots. Similarly, using triangles, figure 5.5 shows the comparable estimates via an estimator that does not condition on

Figure 5.5 Change in HTP Respondents' ACA Attitudes Associated with Turning Sixty-Five Pre- and Post-ACA Implementation

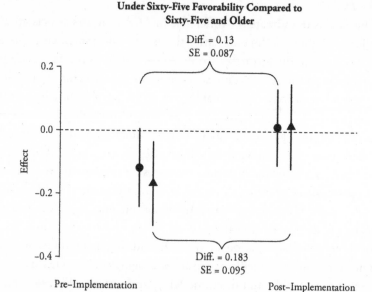

Source: Hobbs and Hopkins 2021. Reprinted with permission.

Note: Those just under sixty-five were especially likely to benefit from the exchanges' price caps after their 2014 implementation. Dots indicate estimates from models conditioning on various potential confounders; triangles indicate estimates from models without such controls.

any variables beyond age. In both cases, the estimated difference is positive, varying from 0.13 (SE = 0.087) with controls to 0.183 (SE = 0.095) without controls. In short, ACA implementation had a detectable but small overall impact, closing the gap between those who were and were not Medicare-eligible. This result is compatible with the hypothesis that the ACA would have a larger effect on the small groups most affected by the law. Given various ACA policies and their age and guaranteed issue regulations, this group was likely to have been more positively affected than others.[91] Indirect policies typically do not produce policy feedback effects on public opinion, but in some specific cases, such effects are possible. (Whether such effects will persist in the years to come, when those in their sixties no longer have experienced the pre-ACA health insurance markets, is an open question.)

Remaining on Parents' Insurance until Age Twenty-Six

Under some conditions, indirectly provided policies can shape attitudes, although not always in ways the policies' architects would have wanted. Still, the ACA was highly complex, and the examples studied here were chosen precisely because they were unusual cases in which policy feedbacks were especially likely. In this section, we consider another age-based ACA regulation: the 2011 requirement that private insurance plans cover dependents until they turn twenty-six.[92]

The ACA took a piecemeal approach to increasing health insurance access by targeting provisions to specific demographic groups. The requirement that private insurers cover dependent children until age twenty-six was one such provision, and it had a clear impact on insurance rates. In the HTP, after the ACA's implementation, 83 percent of twenty-five-year-olds reported having health insurance, a figure that dropped to 76 percent for twenty-six-year-olds. But it is a regulation that simply increases the availability of private insurance, and it may not be visible to the young adults who are its principal beneficiaries.

Indeed, this particular regulation is more representative of backdoor policies than the subsidies and price caps for those in their early sixties. Those in their twenties tend not to use much health care (with the important exceptions of pregnancy and childbirth), and they are not in the habit of discussing health policy with their parents either.[93] For a policy feedback to operate, people in their early twenties would need to have positive experiences with health insurance and to attribute those experiences to a regulation that is low-salience (even if the overall law is not). That's a tall order.

Insurance rates prove markedly higher among twenty-five-year-olds than among twenty-six-year-olds, probably as a consequence of the ACA provision mandating coverage up until twenty-six. But that was a lone provision that received comparatively little attention, and it operates indirectly through regulations on insurance companies (as well as through the beneficiaries' parents, making it still more obscure). So did this ACA provision shift young adults' attitudes toward the ACA? Figure 5.6 provides initial evidence by presenting average levels of ACA favorability by age for young adults. There is little that distinguishes the attitudes of twenty-five-year-olds from those of twenty-six-year-olds. At first glance, the policy was effective in insuring young adults, but not in changing their views.

Figure 5.6 Average ACA Favorability among HTP Respondents by Age, 2011–2019

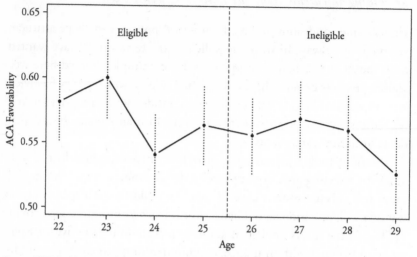

Source: KFF Health Tracking Poll (Kaiser Family Foundation 2022).
Note: The vertical lines are bootstrapped 95 percent confidence intervals.

To estimate the effects more formally, we again use the sharp age cutoff to get empirical leverage by comparing HTP respondents who are just under twenty-six with those just over. Specifically, we focus on 6,431 respondents between twenty-two and twenty-nine.[94] We then estimate the discontinuous effect at age twenty-six on ACA favorability. We find no strong effect: those older than twenty-five (and thus ineligible to stay on their parents' insurance) are just 0.9 (SE = 2.7) percentage points less likely to favor the ACA than those just below that cutoff, a small and insignificant effect that could easily be explained by chance alone. We have now seen indirect elements of the ACA that provoked a backlash, indirect elements of the ACA that did the opposite, and indirect elements that seem to have followed the usual pattern by not shifting attitudes one way or the other.

Conclusion

One theme of this chapter has been heterogeneous experiences. Some people had very positive experiences with the ACA while others had extremely negative ones. In fact, some people could lay claim to both experiences.

Consider Arizona's Natalie McCasling, who was among the citizens most likely to benefit from the opening of the ACA's exchanges. The mother of an autistic daughter, McCasling and her family relied on the exchanges for insurance that provided $50,000 in care and therapy. But in 2016, when Aetna said that it would exit the marketplace, McCasling and her fellow Pinal County residents were left with no options on their exchange. As she explained it, the ACA's initial implementation was "one of the best days of my life, and when we found out [in June] we couldn't, it was one of the most devastating."[95]

This chapter has demonstrated that Natalie McCasling's experiences with the exchanges, combining good and bad, could stand in for those of many Americans. At the time of its enactment, the ACA was expected to increase health insurance enrollment principally through its new exchanges. In fact, the exchanges and the associated individual mandate were sufficiently central to the ACA that Barack Obama had dropped his earlier opposition to health insurance mandates.

The exchanges and the individual mandate embodied an indirect approach to public benefit provision, one that had the potential to leave a faint imprint on public opinion. Yet the ACA was highly salient and contentious, so much so that citizens' partisanship shaped their willingness to enroll via the exchanges. We also saw in chapter 4 that while the Medicaid expansion bolstered pro-ACA opinions, this effect's political impact was dampened by the relatively small proportion of Americans affected and their relative political disengagement. Here in chapter 5 we have employed a range of data sets and analyses to test the exchanges' competing influences on public opinion toward the ACA.

Overall, we find that while the net effect of the ACA's core, indirect features was muted, the exchanges and individual mandate did appear to influence the opinions of those most likely to be affected. In one most-likely case for negative policy feedbacks, we found that local price spikes on the exchanges reduced support for the ACA. In another most-likely case, we investigated the discontinuity at age sixty-five—the eligibility threshold for Medicare—and showed that the ACA's implementation reduced the gap in ACA favorability between sixty-four- and sixty-five-year-olds. Those in their early sixties were among those most likely to benefit from the ACA's exchanges, price caps, and other policies, and the ACA's implementation had a positive effect on their ACA attitudes when compared to their pre-implementation attitudes. In a similar vein, the study's panel data demonstrate that those who became uninsured between 2016 and 2018 also became substantially less favorable toward the ACA.[96]

But showing that the ACA had discernible impacts among highly affected populations still leaves open questions about its capacity to generate policy feedback effects in general. In yet another example—one more typical of many indirectly provided policies—we saw that the policy enabling adult children to stay on their parents' private insurance until age twenty-six increased insurance rates but not ACA favorability. Despite concerns about detecting feedback effects with an indirect and complex policy, we find that a key factor limiting the ACA's mass-level policy feedbacks was the heterogeneity of its effects. That said, there were plenty of ACA provisions (like dependent coverage until age twenty-six) that were invisible. Given the variety of results presented in this chapter, we can be confident that these conclusions are not dependent on any one data set or research design.

Various factors shaped how the ACA was designed, implemented, and challenged, and public opinion was only one of them.[97] Still, by showing that indirect policies can produce complex and self-canceling feedback effects, this chapter's findings help explain why the ACA's exchanges and its mandate were politically vulnerable for years after the law was enacted and implemented. These findings also illustrate the significant limitations facing politicians who wish to build support through public policy: even spending billions of dollars establishing insurance exchanges and subsidizing insurance policies is no guarantee of robust, one-directional feedback effects. What's more, given America's electoral geography, only a small fraction of national programs are likely to land in the most heavily contested jurisdictions.[98]

In 2021, the sometimes-troubled exchanges got a shot in the arm via an infusion of increased federal spending. That March, President Joe Biden signed the American Rescue Plan, a sweeping Covid relief bill that sought to increase uptake of exchange plans by both increasing subsidies for those already eligible and increasing the eligibility threshold for 2021 and 2022.[99] The 2022 Inflation Reduction Act extended those subsidies for three additional years.[100] Although those increased subsidies merit study, the results here suggest that they were not likely to induce any broad changes in public opinion.

These results are relevant even beyond health policy. Relative to other industrialized democracies, the United States relies on indirect policy mechanisms to pursue its social and economic policy goals to an unusual extent, from child care to housing.[101] Key proposals to address climate change have relied on a complex mixture of direct and indirect government provision that resembles the ACA.[102] Here we have shown that indirect policies can be visible to citizens if they are the subjects of extensive political debate—and if they produce tangible effects on people's personal lives. At the same time, indirect policies can generate patterns of feedback across individuals that can be offsetting, in part because negative experiences can powerfully influence attitudes. Put simply, complex, indirect policies can produce feedback effects that are themselves complex.

This book began with a quotation from Bill Kristol about the possibility that the Democrats might reshape public opinion by passing Bill and Hillary Clinton's regulation-first 1993 health care plan. That plan failed, and in the subsequent congressional election of 1994, the Democrats lost control of the House of Representatives for the first time since the 1950s. But the combined results of the past two chapters suggest how unlikely it was that passing health care reform—especially reform that was a complex bundle of regulatory policies—would have fundamentally changed the Democrats' political position.

If policymaking is not a powerful tool of elite influence, is rhetoric? It is to that question that we turn in the coming chapters.

CHAPTER 6

The Indirect Role of White Americans' Racial Attitudes

JONATHAN METZL'S 2019 book, provocatively titled *Dying of Whiteness*, opens with a striking story connecting ACA attitudes to one white American's racial views. A Tennessee man dying with an inflamed liver says, "Ain't no way I would ever support Obamacare or sign up for it. . . . I would rather die. . . . We don't need any more government in our lives. And in any case, no way I want my tax dollars paying for Mexicans or welfare queens." In Metzl's words, that man "voiced a literal willingness to die for his place in this hierarchy, rather than participate in a system that might put him on the same plane as immigrants or racial minorities."[1]

This chapter will show that man to be an outlier in the close connection he made between the ACA and his racial prejudices. But it investigates the question he raises in vivid terms: How do whites' racial attitudes color their views of the ACA? Given that racial cues operate differently for white Americans and for Americans from other ethnic-racial backgrounds, this chapter's focus is primarily on white Americans' views rather than on those of the broader population.[2] Certainly, in an increasingly racially diverse nation, a comprehensive picture of ACA attitudes must include nonwhite groups.[3] The aim of this chapter, however, is to isolate the role of racial attitudes for a group that makes up a sizable majority of the U.S. population and electorate. Of the racial-ethnic groups in America's system of racial stratification, it is white Americans who have historically shown high levels of opposition to policies that disproportionately benefit black Americans.[4]

The chapter's core argument is that whether we term white Americans' ACA attitudes "racialized" hinges on how we define "racialization" and the time frame on which it acts.[5] (By "racialization," we mean the process through which racial attitudes become integrated with attitudes toward other political objects.) If we follow much of the recent research on public opinion by defining racialization narrowly—and so focus on white Americans' reactions immediately after encountering racial cues—ACA attitudes do *not* appear highly racialized. Across seven experiments conducted with a range of samples in varied settings, attitudes prove highly stable; momentary racial primes do little to shift whites' views of the ACA expressed immediately after.

On the other hand, if we understand racialization as a long-term process that shapes policy narratives and integrates partisanship with policy views, evidence of its impact is stronger (albeit more circumstantial). Under the first, contemporaneous conception of racialization, it can explain sudden shifts. Under the second, long-term conception, however, it is a mechanism of over-time stability. In other words, the first conception implies that racialization may be a mechanism of elite influence because elite rhetoric has the potential to prime racial attitudes. By contrast, under the second conception, racialization is more likely to serve to stabilize public opinion—and so to act as a brake on elite influence.

Distinguishing between different conceptions of racialization based on their time frames also helps explain a central mystery of ACA attitudes: How did the Medicaid expansion manage to remain popular and avoid the fate of prior racialized policies, such as welfare in the 1980s and 1990s? As we will see, far from being an anchor dragging the ACA down, the Medicaid expansion proved something closer to a life buoy for the law. And that popularity hints that the role of racial attitudes in shaping whites' views of social policy may be changing too.

These results are also noteworthy in what they mean for the methods that researchers use to study racial attitudes. In recent decades, survey experiments have become the dominant method for such research.[6] But survey experiments overwhelmingly test short-term effects and so are ill suited to illuminate processes that unfold over longer periods of time.[7] In short, the over-time mechanisms through which racial attitudes operate in the case of the ACA are especially difficult for social scientists to detect using today's primary methods. An exclusive reliance on survey experiments may understate the role of racial attitudes in shaping white Americans' views of the ACA. Here we supplement survey experiments with evidence from long-running, population-based panels.

Since its inception, American policymaking has been deeply entangled in racial divisions and the reproduction of racial stratification.[8] In fact, the historical interpenetration between racial divisions and policymaking can make it challenging to know where to start. We thus open this chapter by discussing an ACA element that is prone to racialization: the expansion of Medicaid, a means-tested program. Doing so enables us to study racial divisions and ACA attitudes while also previewing this chapter's core argument about their complex, possibly unexpected relationship. Drawing on research about this relationship in prior decades, the chapter then conceptualizes the varied ways in which a policy might be racialized. It subsequently turns to a range of empirical evidence, including observations from the ISCAP panel as well as seven novel survey experiments conducted via different modes and samples. When analyzed over broad swaths of time, ACA attitudes show clear signs of racialization. But when looking at responses to more momentary primes—of the kind political elites might employ—they do not.

The Medicaid Mystery

As we saw in chapters 2 and 4, the Supreme Court's 2012 *National Federation of Independent Business v. Sebelius* ruling allowed states to decide whether to accept the ACA's Medicaid expansion, producing a landscape in which, by 2021, only twelve states had not expanded Medicaid. Those states were disproportionately those with large black populations and Republican political leadership, among them Texas, Florida, North Carolina, Georgia, Alabama, and Mississippi.[9] In fact, eight of the twelve states that had not adopted the Medicaid expansion had been part of the former Confederacy.

Beyond the opening quotation from Metzl's book, there is good reason to suspect that whites' racial attitudes and their views of the ACA may be integrated.[10] The ACA was the signature domestic policy achievement of the nation's first African American president, even taking on his name through the moniker "Obamacare."[11] In West Philadelphia at least, a version of Obama's 2008 campaign logo could be seen in pharmacy windows advertising

ACA enrollment years after the law's enactment. As Jamila Michener points out, the law itself was explicitly designed to reduce health inequalities based on race and ethnicity and made extensive reference to "disparities," "discrimination," "racial/race," and "ethnicity/ethnic."[12] The ACA ultimately helped reduce racial gaps in health insurance coverage and health care access, especially in its early years.[13]

The extent to which racial attitudes shaped white Americans' *perceptions* of the ACA is a related but separate question. Prior research shows that Americans' views on redistributive policies generally are shaped by their racial attitudes.[14] In an analysis of public opinion on government spending from 1992 to 2000, Paul Goren finds that there are two clusters of attitudes: views on welfare and food stamps (which are associated with racial stereotypes) and views on other social programs (which are not).[15] As we saw in chapter 2, the ACA was certainly redistributive, as it used taxes on high-income Americans to expand insurance access principally for Americans with low incomes. One of the ACA's key elements was the Medicaid expansion, itself a redistributive, means-tested program that many white Americans viewed through a racialized lens even prior to the ACA's enactment.[16] What's more, the decade following the ACA's 2010 enactment was defined by other racially inflected issues, including immigration, policing, and criminal justice.[17]

In the 1970s, 1980s, and early 1990s, Republicans used the issue of welfare to reinforce their winning political coalitions, attacking government handouts with racialized rhetoric, including Ronald Reagan's salvo against a "welfare queen."[18] This strategy was part of a broader effort to harness racial prejudice to the GOP's electoral advantage.[19] In a 1981 interview, the Republican strategist Lee Atwater explained the strategy in explicitly and unapologetically racist terms. "By 1968," Atwater said, candidates could not just use the worst of racial epithets in political campaigns: "That hurts you, backfires. So you say stuff like, uh, forced busing, states' rights, and all that stuff, and you're getting so abstract. Now, you're talking about cutting taxes, and all these things you're talking about are totally economic things and a byproduct of them is, blacks get hurt worse than whites."[20]

With Democrats convinced that such attacks hurt them electorally, their 1992 presidential candidate, Bill Clinton, promised to "end welfare as we know it." Clinton made good on that promise in 1996 by signing a sweeping welfare reform bill.[21] The experience of welfare seemingly lent force to the adage that "a policy for the poor is a poor policy," as means-tested programs were thought to be incapable of generating the broad political support necessary to become uncontroversial.[22] Like welfare, Medicaid is a means-tested program, and as chapter 4 detailed, it arguably became the centerpiece of the ACA.[23] Given that, we might well have expected that the ACA would be doomed by the same racially charged political dynamics that led to welfare reform in 1996.

But that is not what happened. Instead, the Medicaid expansion's popularity helped *bolster* support for the ACA when its fate hung in the balance in 2017.[24] In that year, 84 percent of Americans told the KFF that it was important that any GOP plan to replace the ACA ensured that "states that received federal funds to expand Medicaid continue to receive those funds."[25] It is no accident that one of the final attempts by Senate Republicans to repeal the ACA—the "skinny repeal" in late July 2017—omitted the Medicaid expansion entirely. That November, Maine voters backed the Medicaid expansion with nearly 59 percent support—a year after having backed Democrat Hillary Clinton with just 48 percent of the vote. In the years that followed, voters in Republican-leaning states, including Idaho and Oklahoma, would also support the Medicaid expansion, a story we recounted in chapter 4. These observations raise a question: What accounts for the unexpected popularity of the Medicaid expansion?

The Multiple Meanings of Racialization

As we investigate the influence of racial cues and attitudes on whites' ACA views and attempt to make sense of the shift from the 1990s to the 2010s, there is critical historical context to bear in mind. In the United States, activists within the two major political parties came to take different positions on civil rights and other race-related issues as early as the New Deal in the 1930s.[26] By the civil rights era, such differences were entrenched. The 1964 Democratic presidential candidate had signed the Civil Rights Act while his Republican opponent had voted against it.

With the parties taking increasingly clear and divergent stances on race-related issues such as civil rights and busing, the public followed suit, such that citizens who identify as Republicans today have quite different views about the role of the federal government in reducing racial inequality than do Democrats.[27] Evidence suggests that the connection between white

Americans' racial attitudes and political partisanship has grown tighter still since 2008 in the wake of the Obama and Trump presidencies.[28] It is no overstatement to say that differences on race-related questions are among the central dividing lines between Democrats and Republicans today.[29] And through partisanship, racial attitudes can come to be associated with a wide range of attitudes on even ostensibly race-neutral issues.[30]

The tightening relationship between racial attitudes and partisanship also changes the political calculus of explicit racial rhetoric—for both political parties.[31] In the 1980s and 1990s, the sizable number of citizens with liberal attitudes on government spending but more conservative attitudes on race-related issues created clear electoral incentives for Republican politicians to use racialized appeals.[32] However, in the era after 2008 (when Obama was elected), and especially after 2016 (when Trump was elected), the increasingly close connection may have eroded the number of cross-pressured citizens in the electorate who could be won or lost through racial appeals.[33]

Such a history makes it critical to consider the various mechanisms through which racial divisions could influence ACA attitudes, including those that are not direct or that do not act at a single moment in time.[34] Consider an example: In a criminal trial, a defendant might be found innocent for a wide range of causes. Some of them—say, a juror persuades other jurors, or a final witness is compelling—come into play just before the outcome in question. We might term such causes "proximate." But other causes— including the facts of the crime, the way the facts are presented, and even the procedures by which the court operates—can have a causal effect even though their influence comes much earlier in the causal chain.[35] In fact, some influential criminal procedures may be older than anyone in the courtroom.

It is usually easier for an outside observer to identify a causal agent if it acts in close temporal proximity to the outcome. But if we seek to assess the mechanisms that connect racial attitudes with ACA attitudes com- prehensively, we have to consider multiple pathways—including those, like partisanship, that act through backdoor channels or over longer periods of time. Whites' racial attitudes may shape their views of the ACA directly and immediately, as seems to have been the case for the Tennessee man quoted at the outset of the chapter. However, they may also operate through indirect channels by shaping who identifies as a Democrat or Republican, or by shaping the kinds of narratives through which people make sense of politics.[36] To say that a policy is "racialized" can thus have multiple meanings, as racial attitudes and undertones can operate at various points on a causal chain.

For example, when a 2015 HTP respondent said, "I think some of these lazy people should get off their butts and go to work so they can purchase health insurance," they made no explicit mention of race.[37] Yet given the tenacity of negative stereotypes about black Americans' reliance on welfare, it is very plausible that the narrative about people living off the government has persisted partly from its historical connection to race.[38] In this account, race is not to be found at the scene of the crime, but the legacy of racism in the United States is likely to have played a role nonetheless.

As this chapter shows, whether we characterize the ACA as "racialized" hinges on precisely how we define the term.[39] Although whites' racial attitudes are clearly related to their views of the ACA, that relationship is very stable; it does not vary with political events or even experimental primes that heighten the salience of the ACA's black and Hispanic beneficiaries. Racial attitudes can explain some of the broad patterns we observe, even though they cannot explain momentary reactions or over-time shifts.

This model of racialization is of stable, enduring associations—and in this account, racialized issues may be especially stable. The idea is that because race and related attitudes are chronically accessible in many white Americans' minds, they are already so tightly integrated with political attitudes that further increasing their salience will do little to shift political attitudes. In a deluge of racially charged events and rhetoric, why should a single experimental manipulation or a racially inflected TV advertisement change minds? That is especially true if white Americans' beliefs about the role of government and their views about racial and ethnic minorities are already intertwined.[40] Here racial attitudes may operate years or even decades before a particular policy proposal by shaping whites' partisanship and reinforcing narratives about deservingness.[41] In this case, we might expect strong static correlations between white Americans' racial views, their views on the ACA, and their partisanship.[42] And we might also expect that momentary racial cues will not further shift white Americans' ACA attitudes, since those attitudes are already stably integrated. For Edward Carmines and James Stimson, the 1972 election provided evidence of the impact of racial attitudes precisely because those attitudes were associated with vote choice even though the campaign *did not* foreground related issues.[43]

But a policy might also merit the term "racialized" if views on that policy *change* in response to a shift in information that makes the racial element of a policy more salient. In recent decades, there have been extensive investigations into this second, more proximate notion of racialization, in part because it lends itself well to testing through survey experiments.[44]

Because white Americans are so frequently exposed to political rhetoric on race-related issues, the cognitive connections between these issues may be well established, and so racial cues may easily activate cognitive schema or familiar emotions and thus influence attitudes.[45] In this vein, Antoine Banks reports that feelings of anger can activate white Americans' racial attitudes and result in shifts in their views on health care.[46] Anger, in short, can racialize opinion. Similarly, threats to white Americans' status and political power can reduce their support for welfare.[47] Like an overplayed song, racial cues may trigger familiar mental scripts, which in this case means familiar stereotypes about social policies. In this conception, white Americans' racial attitudes will again be strongly associated with their partisanship and their views about the ACA at baseline. But this view also expects racial cues to reinforce such connections immediately after exposure. From this perspective, racial attitudes are a proximate cause of policy attitudes.

Testing Different Conceptions of Racialization

The distinction between the various notions of racialization has critical implications for researchers and those who would like to understand the ongoing role of white Americans' racial attitudes in shaping American politics. Here we empirically test these possibilities using a variety of research methods, some observational and others experimental.

Our first set of tests uncover meaningful evidence of racialization by the static, correlational definition. Specifically, these tests examine perceptions of who benefits from the ACA. White Americans who see the ACA as disproportionately benefiting black people, Latinos, or unauthorized immigrants have more negative views of the law. The second set of tests reinforce this view. Using a unique panel that tracks the same white Americans from 2012 to 2020, we find that racial prejudice is strongly and stably associated with their views on the ACA. That holds true even accounting for political partisanship.

That said, other evidence shows some of the limits of the racialization of ACA attitudes. For one thing, ACA attitudes prove to be more highly correlated with programs like student loans than with more overtly racialized policies like food stamps. Evidence of racialization using the second, change-oriented definition is more limited still. The stability of the associations we detect in the panel suggests that changes in information streams are not serving to racialize or deracialize ACA attitudes at specific moments in time. In short, there is not much observational evidence of racial priming.

What about experimental evidence? To date, and to our knowledge, there have not been studies that test the prospect that varying the perceived beneficiaries of the ACA influences ACA attitudes. We seek to fill this gap by conducting seven survey experiments using different survey modes in different places at different times. The experimental evidence bolsters the claim that the connection between racial attitudes and ACA attitudes is stable and not subject to priming. Across the survey experiments, we find little consistent evidence that making the ACA's black and Latino beneficiaries more salient to respondents shapes their ACA attitudes. Given this evidence, racial attitudes appear to be an upstream influence, one that affects actors' setting and vocabulary more than their momentary decisions onstage. ACA attitudes are racialized because white Americans' public policy views generally are closely connected to their racial attitudes. But ACA attitudes do not evince the particular patterns of the prototypically racialized policies such as food stamps or welfare.

Perceptions of Who Benefits from the ACA

For decades, researchers have reported links between Americans' attitudes toward social policies and their perceptions of who those programs' chief beneficiaries are.[48] Programs such as those known colloquially as "food stamps" or "welfare" are seen as benefiting black Americans disproportionately; as a result, they commonly receive less support from white Americans. What about the ACA? Which groups were perceived as the primary beneficiaries of the ACA?

The ISCAP panel's 2016 post-election wave included a battery of questions about precisely that. Those questions asked whether different groups of people were perceived to have been made better off or worse off by the ACA. The groups in question included blacks, Hispanics/Latinos, and women, as well as "undocumented/illegal immigrants," partisan groups, senior citizens, and the respondent and their family. Between 353 and 356 white

Figure 6.1 White Americans' Perceptions of the ACA's Beneficiaries, 2016

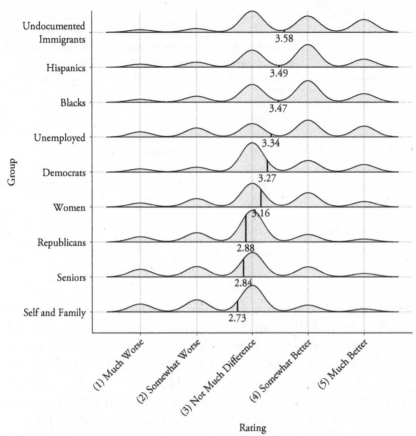

Source: ISCAP panel, 2016 (Hopkins and Mutz 2022).

respondents answered each item. We code the items as ranging from 1 to 5, with 1 indicating that the group was made much worse off by the ACA and 5 indicating that it was made much better off. The scale's midpoint, 3, indicates that the ACA "hasn't made much difference" for that group.

As figure 6.1 illustrates, the group perceived by white Americans as having benefited the most on average was undocumented immigrants (3.58 on average). As a factual matter, such perceptions are false: unauthorized immigrants are not eligible for Medicaid or Medicare, and they are unable to buy insurance through the exchanges. So the number of respondents willing to say that unauthorized immigrants benefited from the ACA should

Table 6.1 Relationships between Group Benefits and ACA Support or ACA Repeal, 2016

Group	Average Perception of Group's Benefit from the ACA	Correlation between Benefit Perception and Support for ACA Repeal	Correlation between Benefit Perception and Favorability toward the ACA
Self and family	2.73	−0.57	0.61
Seniors	2.84	−0.55	0.57
Women	3.16	−0.51	0.51
Republicans	2.88	−0.40	0.46
Unemployed	3.34	−0.33	0.31
Blacks	3.47	−0.26	0.22
Democrats	3.27	−0.19	0.20
Hispanics	3.49	−0.18	0.21
Undocumented immigrants	3.58	0.10	−0.13

Source: ISCAP panel, 2016 (Hopkins and Mutz 2022).

be treated as purely expressive of their views about unauthorized immigrants as well as the ACA. In a similar vein, Hispanics (with a mean of 3.49) and blacks (3.47) were seen as benefiting on balance from the law. That perception of net benefit is true to a lesser extent for the unemployed (3.34), Democrats (3.27), and women (3.16). That women should be perceived to have benefited makes some sense, as the law ended premium discrimination by sex. In sum, groups defined by race or ethnicity are among those that stand out as perceived beneficiaries in the eyes of many white Americans.

Whatever its impact in helping pass the ACA through Congress, the ACA's provision to increase prescription drug coverage does not seem to have led white Americans to perceive the law as benefiting seniors on average; the 1–5 rating for seniors is 2.84, which falls on the "harm" side of the midpoint. Republicans (2.88) and respondents and their families (2.73) were also seen as being harmed on balance. That last finding is especially instructive, as results like that may have fueled Republican politicians' sense that ACA repeal would prove popular.

But if we turn to table 6.1's middle and right columns, we see a somewhat different story. Those columns measure the relationship between each group's perceived benefit and respondents' ACA attitudes via two questions. The middle column presents the Pearson's correlations for support for ACA repeal.[49] These correlations are mostly negative—if a respondent thought that groups benefited from the ACA on average, she was less likely to back repealing the law. The right column presents the (mostly positive) correlations between perceptions of group benefit and ACA favorability.

The group whose perceived benefit is most closely integrated with overall ACA attitudes is respondents and their families: that item has a Pearson's correlation with support for repeal of –0.57 and ACA favorability of 0.61. In fact, it is noteworthy that ACA assessments are much more strongly associated with groups like seniors, women, and Republicans than by groups defined in terms of race or ethnicity. By this metric, the ACA appears less racialized, as ACA attitudes are primarily integrated with white respondents' views of its impact on themselves—and on groups that Republicans tend to see positively, including seniors, women, and Republicans.[50]

Evidence from a Population-Based Panel

What is the relationship between white Americans' racial attitudes and their feelings toward the ACA, and how, if at all, did it change between 2012 and 2020? Charting any over-time shifts in this relationship is key, as doing so may help identify the extent to which political rhetoric or events can temporarily racialize an issue like the ACA. For example, did the end of Obama's presidency reduce the association between racial attitudes and ACA views?[51] Such priming effects have been a major focus of political science research for at least two decades.[52] But while priming effects have been the subject of extensive study via survey experiments, it remains unclear whether they produce meaningful effects in contemporary American political debates.

Given the deep historical connections between partisanship and racial attitudes, it is critical to consider the interplay of partisanship and prejudice as well. Much of the relationship between racial attitudes and opinions on the ACA may flow through the former's connection with political partisanship. Thus, finding that white Americans' prejudices aren't directly associated with ACA attitudes does not necessarily mean that they play no role in the causal chain. Similarly, just because someone was not at the scene of a crime does not absolve them of involvement.

The ISCAP panel is uniquely suited to address these questions, as it is a population-based panel that repeatedly asked the same individuals the same question about their views of the law between 2012 and 2020. This enables us to chart the evolution of their views in reaction to changing events. The question reads, "Some people think the health care reform law should be kept as it is. Others want to repeal the entire health care law. Still others are somewhere in between. Where would you place yourself on this scale, or haven't you thought much about this?" The response options run from 1 ("The health care reform law should be kept as it is") through 7 ("The entire health care law should be repealed"). Note that this item does not include a response option for expanding the ACA; instead, it tracks the broad contours of the political debate between 2010 and 2020, which pitted those who wished to preserve the ACA against those who sought to repeal it or scale it back. Note, too, that using this panel's measure, we are only able to track these relationships beginning in 2012, after the 2010 enactment of the ACA.

Here we focus on 670 respondents who identified as white in 2012 and participated in the November 2012 to January 2013 and October 2020 waves. In any such analyses, the choice of the measure of racial attitudes can be crucial. Our analyses employ measures of anti-black prejudice that have been widely used and validated.[53] Specifically, we first ask respondents to assess white and black Americans with respect to two stereotypes: work ethic and trustworthiness. We then generate a composite measure of prejudice by subtracting stereotypes of black Americans from stereotypes of white Americans. In theory, the resulting scale varies from −1 to 1, with a 1 representing an extremely positive assessment of white people and an extremely negative assessment of black people and a −1 representing the reverse. In our sample, the mean score is 0.07, indicating that the average respondent was notably more willing to apply negative stereotypes (or not apply positive stereotypes) to black Americans than to whites. Overall, 27 percent of respondents scored below 0 (meaning that they rated black people more positively on average) while 60 percent scored above 0 and showed anti-black prejudice. This finding in itself is noteworthy. Even given strong norms against expressing prejudice or racism, a majority of these white panelists scored on the prejudiced side of the scale.[54]

By using a fixed measure of prejudice from 2012 to 2013, we can analyze its (possibly changing) relationship with ACA attitudes measured at various points in time.[55] We can thus assess whether anti-black prejudice was more tightly integrated with views on the ACA when Obama was president as well as whether Trump's 2016 campaign served to racialize attitudes about

Figure 6.2 Regression Coefficients and Confidence Intervals for White Respondents' 2012–2013 Anti-Black Prejudice (–1 to 1) When Predicting Support for Repealing the ACA over Time (1 to 7)

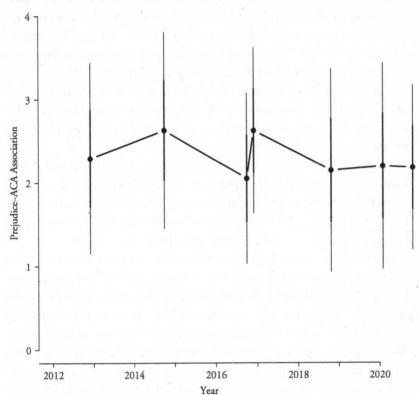

Source: ISCAP panel, 2012–2020 (Hopkins and Mutz 2022).

the law.[56] Accordingly, we fit regression models in which the key independent variable is an anti-black prejudice measure generated by averaging across the October 2012 and November 2012 to January 2013 waves.

Figure 6.2 presents the coefficient for 2012 to 2013 prejudice when predicting support for repealing the ACA while conditioning on a basic set of demographics (including gender, union status, income, education, age, and identification as Catholic or Protestant). The median coefficient is 2.20, meaning that a one-standard-deviation increase in prejudice (0.16) is associated with a 0.35 increase in pro-repeal attitudes. (To benchmark this against other differences, the difference between black and white respondents in late 2012 was 2.01 points, while between Democrats and Republicans it was 2.85. So this shift is 17 percent of the black-white difference and 12 percent of the Republican-Democrat difference.) As the figure makes clear, however, there is little evidence of priming at specific points in time. The coefficients are very stable between 2012 and 2020, suggesting that the relationship between prejudice and ACA views is not bolstered or dampened by specific political events or rhetoric. At least as of 2012, there is no evidence that specific politicians shifted the role of whites' racial attitudes in their ACA evaluations. Quite consistently, white Americans who scored higher on the prejudice score from 2012 to 2013 were more supportive of repealing the ACA.

Certainly, there is a well-documented, long-standing association between racial attitudes and political partisanship among whites, with white Republicans holding more prejudiced or racially conservative attitudes than white Democrats on average.[57] Given that, neither the magnitude nor the consistency of the association here is necessarily surprising.

In table D.1, we thus present coefficients from similar models that also add indicator variables for respondents' October 2012 political partisanship. Doing so sheds no light on the causal relationship between partisanship and prejudice.[58] But it does help us understand how much of the relationship between prejudice and ACA attitudes could be explained by partisanship. And the answer is a lot: controlling for partisanship cuts the median coefficient by more than half, to 1.03. In these models, a one-standard-deviation increase in anti-black prejudice is associated with a 0.16 increase in pro-repeal sentiment.

In sum, accounting for political partisanship reduces the relationship between anti-black prejudice and ACA attitudes markedly, but it does not eliminate the relationship. What's more, this relationship, which is weaker but detectable, is again reasonably stable, with an upward tick in the post-2016 election wave that may or may not be statistical noise. These patterns are consistent with the claim that more highly prejudiced white Americans are more likely to want to repeal the ACA because they are more likely to be Republicans. At the same time, these patterns suggest that the integration of prejudice and ACA attitudes is generally stable and not very responsive to political rhetoric or events. In other words, the racialization of ACA attitudes is not a time-varying relationship—and thus does not appear to be subject to politicians' rhetoric or even major political events.

In recent decades, the relationship between racial attitudes and political views has been a central preoccupation of political science. Political scientists often employ the concept of priming to explain how political events and rhetoric can tighten or relax the ways in which white Americans' racial attitudes are integrated into their views on policies and politicians.[59] This research tests the hypothesis that events and the information streams they produce can influence the cognitive accessibility of racial attitudes and so become more or less influential in subsequent policy evaluations. Certainly, priming research fits well with the discipline's emphasis on experimental testing. But the observational evidence here indicates that in the case of the ACA there is little evidence of racial priming: white respondents' racial prejudice was consistently associated with their ACA views. In other words, one of political science's principal tools for understanding racial attitudes does not do much to explain the stable relationship between racial prejudice and views of the ACA. Such patterns are instead consistent with the prospect that racial attitudes are chronically accessible and therefore stably integrated with political beliefs.[60]

To an important extent, the prejudice-opinion relationship emerges from the structure of American political divisions, in which race-related issues are among the enduring dividing lines between Democrats and Republicans.[61] From the evidence here and elsewhere, racial prejudice seems to imbue the language of deservingness with an exclusive, punitive edge, and it sets the stage for bitter divides over the ACA through its influence on partisanship.[62]

The ACA and Other Issues

Gwen Hurd, a New Hampshire resident who purchased insurance through the exchanges, saw the ACA as fundamentally unfair. "It seems to me that people who earn nothing and contribute nothing get everything for free," she told the *New York Times*. "And that the people who work hard and struggle for every penny barely end up surviving."[63]

Ms. Hurd was certainly not the only person to think about the ACA as a program that gave some people benefits they had not earned. Similar ideas come up in Theda Skocpol and Vanessa Williamson's 2016 book, in which they note: "Health care reform was portrayed by GOP leaders as a threat to Medicare and an expensive new entitlement that would force hardworking and hard-pressed citizens and businesses to pay higher taxes to provide health insurance to younger, less well-to-do, and often 'undeserving' people—including illegal immigrants, it was claimed."[64] Journalist Darlena Cunha's conversation with a Florida resident about health care policy mirrors this sentiment. As she tells it, "The conversation took an unexpected turn when he went on to rail against universal health care. He didn't want to pay for other people to get help. He didn't have health insurance and told me he once duct-taped a cut on his arm because he couldn't afford stitches." In the man's own words, "I'd rather take care of my own self with tape than be stuck in a system where I pay for everyone else."[65]

When Americans think about a complex policy like the ACA, there are a great many frames that they can invoke. The notion of hardworking people paying for undeserving free riders is a prominent one, and it has been used in a variety of social policies for decades.[66] It is also a narrative that gains strength and emotional force from racial stereotypes, although as the case of Gwen Hurd in New Hampshire reminds us, this narrative can surely be active in heavily white communities as well.[67] And the ACA did have a redistributive element, as it imposed new taxes on high earners to fund a major expansion of Medicaid, a means-tested program. But those were hardly the only features of the law, and that was far from the only frame that Americans could use when making sense of it. Other elements of the ACA were regulatory in nature, including the creation and oversight of the exchanges and the mandate that all Americans obtain insurance. Indeed, the ACA's complexity makes it important to ask a straightforward question: What are some other policies that divide the public in ways similar to the divisiveness of the ACA? Are ACA attitudes more highly correlated with attitudes toward redistributive programs, social insurance, market subsidies, or regulatory policies? Since policies vary in the extent to which they are racialized, answering that question gives us leverage to understand racial attitudes and the ACA.

Accordingly, we included a battery of survey questions designed to tap respondents' attitudes toward different types of policies on a fall 2018 survey conducted through SSI/Research Now. The sample includes 1,945 total respondents, 1,366 of whom were white. Specifically, randomly chosen subsets of respondents to both surveys were asked about their views on a number of different policies that were chosen for being analogous to different aspects of the ACA. For instance, some respondents were asked whether they supported increased or decreased spending on food stamps, an item designed to tap their views on another redistributive policy targeting low-income Americans.

To get more texture to respondents' thoughts about each program, we also asked an open-ended question and present replies to it via word clouds in figure D.1. If many Americans think about the ACA in the same way that Gwen Hurd did, we might well expect their attitudes toward the law to be strongly related to their views on food stamps, a well-known redistributive policy that respondents discussed using words like "needs," "hungry," and "work."

Some respondents were asked about their support for spending on disability insurance, a policy that mirrors those elements of the ACA that provide social insurance for health-related issues. Here keywords included "need," "help," "people," and "work," reinforcing the role of work in shaping perceptions of deservingness for assistance. The survey also included a question about respondents' views on unemployment insurance spending, which should tap views on social insurance outside the health-related arena. Commonly used words here were "need," "job," "money," and "work." Respondents were sometimes asked about their support for increased regulation of the student loan industry, a policy with consumer protection elements that parallel aspects of the ACA. Keywords on this issue included "advantage," "loan," "people," and "debt." It is noteworthy that questions about beneficiaries' ability to work, so prominent for other attitudes, are not at play with respect to student loans.

Which of these attitudes were most closely associated with our survey respondents' views on the ACA? To gauge that, we estimated Pearson's correlations between white respondents' views in each policy area and their favorability toward the ACA. We report the results graphically in figure 6.3 (for white respondents) and figure 6.4 (for all respondents). In both years, respondents' favorability toward the ACA was positively associated with more liberal positions in almost all cases, as we would expect. Still, the substantive magnitude of the correlations is not especially strong, ranging from −0.01 to 0.36. In spite of the litany of quotations, like those here, from Americans describing the ACA in redistributive terms, the correlation between views on food stamp spending and the ACA is only 0.13 (for white respondents) or 0.12 (for all respondents). In other words, the positive association between ACA favorability and food stamp spending is relatively modest: knowing someone's views on food stamp spending is mildly

Figure 6.3 Variable Correlations for White Respondents, 2018

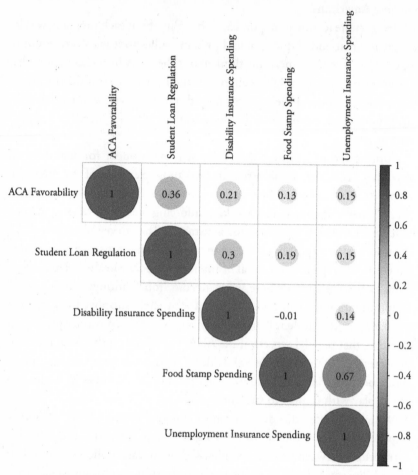

predictive of their views on the ACA, but the two attitudes are far from coterminous.[68]

In a similar vein, it is noteworthy that ACA support is also not very highly correlated with support for unemployment insurance spending, a social insurance policy with a redistributive element. For white respondents, the correlation is 0.15, while for all respondents it's 0.10. The correlation between ACA attitudes and disability insurance is just a touch higher, at 0.21 for white respondents and 0.18 overall. Respondents' support for

Figure 6.4 Variable Correlations for All Respondents, 2018

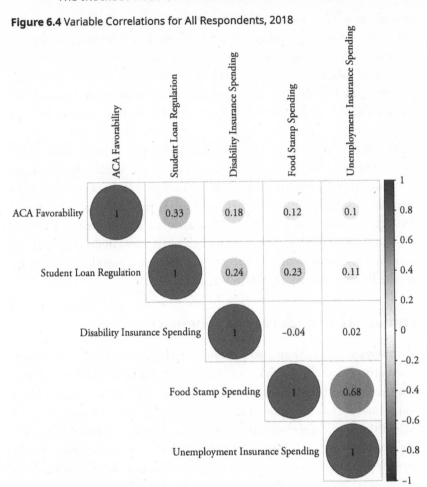

Source: SSI Survey, 2018.

spending on different types of social insurance is only tangentially connected to their ACA attitudes.

Instead, the attitudes most highly correlated with ACA attitudes are those about regulating the student loan industry. In that case, the correlations rise to 0.36 (white respondents) and 0.33 (all respondents). For these respondents at least, the ACA is perceived in ways that are most similar to student loan regulations. Correlations between 0.33 and 0.36 are not enormous—ACA attitudes do not track attitudes on any of these issues closely. But of these issues, ACA attitudes appear most closely connected to questions about how involved the government should be in regulating the economy.[69] While student loans have become a higher-profile issue in recent years, their salience has not approached that of the ACA. This correlation is likely to be a product of the underlying similarity between student loans and the ACA: both foreground the question of government intervention in the economy.

The ACA is highly complex; some of its pieces run parallel to auto insurance regulation, tax policy, or consumer protection, while other elements are more explicitly redistributive. This evidence makes clear that while ACA attitudes are integrated with racial attitudes, the ACA was not viewed through the same lens as programs that are closely associated with people of color, such as food stamps. The public's assessments of different policies are grounded partly in the specifics of that policy area, limiting the capacity of elite rhetoric to reshape public attitudes.

Priming Race via Survey Experiments

The analyses here paint a mixed portrait of the influence of white Americans' racial attitudes. ACA attitudes are durably related to which social groups are perceived to benefit from the law, as well as to prejudices against black Americans. But at the same time, the relationship between prejudice and ACA attitudes did not change between 2012 and 2020, suggesting that priming was not a key mover of attitudes during that period, despite racially explicit and implicit appeals from elites like Trump. What's more, ACA attitudes are not closely correlated with views on spending on food stamps or unemployment. In fact, ACA attitudes are more closely related to respondents' views on student loan spending, a spending area that is not as explicitly connected to black Americans. That evidence weighs strongly against the possibility that our panel analyses miss racialization because it took place before 2012.

Here we test the second definition of racialization—the impact of heightened salience just prior to rendering an evaluation. Specifically, we detail the results of seven separate survey experiments designed to probe whether white Americans view the ACA differently when they have just been reminded of the law's black and Latino beneficiaries. Because any one survey experiment might raise concerns about generalizability, our goal is to avoid generalizing conclusions from a single experiment by deploying survey experiments with varied samples conducted using multiple modes at different points in time.[70]

Experiments Embedded in Exit Polls

Survey experiments are commonly conducted with opt-in samples so they may not generalize to real-world samples if most voters are less attentive to or knowledgeable about politics.[71] Accordingly, we conducted two experiments embedded in exit polls, which allow us to test for racialization in real-world populations of voters. Despite the theoretical prominence of claims about the impact of perceiving a program's beneficiaries as being disproportionately black Americans or other ethnic-racial minorities, there are surprisingly few experiments that test this causal link[72]—and none that we are aware of on ACA attitudes. Here we present the results of seven separate experiments designed to probe the link between perceptions of who benefits from the ACA and overall assessments of the law.[73]

Alabama is one of the GOP-dominated states that had not expanded its Medicaid program as of 2022 and where a sizable fraction of those who stand to benefit from it are black. It is thus a likely case for identifying a relationship between whites' perceptions of ACA beneficiaries and attitudes toward the law. In December 2017, we had a unique opportunity to conduct just such a test.

In that month, Alabama voters went to the polls in a special election that would transform federal politics: the solidly Republican state sent a Democrat, Doug Jones, to the Senate over GOP nominee Roy Moore. In that election, Michele Margolis and I distributed exit polls to 234 white voters at two polling sites in Calhoun County in the eastern part of the state. We randomly distributed two versions of the surveys. In one, respondents first answered a standard question, "A health reform bill was signed into law in 2010. Given what you know about the health reform law, do you have a generally favorable or generally unfavorable opinion of it?" There were four response categories, from "very favorable" to "very unfavorable." In the second version, respondents were first asked whether the 2010 health reform law had made different groups better or worse off, and they were asked to assess five groups: themselves and their families, their communities, whites, blacks, and Hispanics. The items asking about "Whites," "Blacks," and

Figure 6.5 ACA Favorability among White Voters in Calhoun County, Alabama, by Experimental Racial Prime and Presidential Preference, 2017

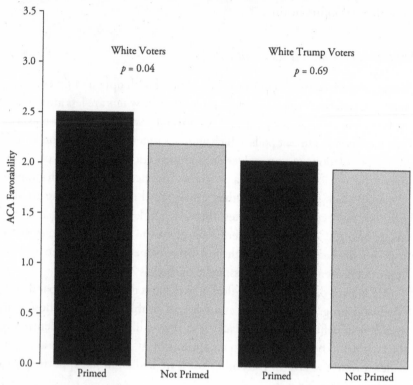

Source: Alabama 2017 exit poll.

"Hispanics" appeared immediately before the question about the respondent's favorability toward the ACA. This version of the survey questions may have primed views of the ACA's personal impact, but it should also have primed views of its racial impacts. Did encouraging people to think about the ACA's impacts on different racial and ethnic groups change their favorability toward the ACA?

In Alabama, the answer appeared to be yes, but not in the expected direction. As figure 6.5 illustrates, the average score for favorability toward the reform was 2.50 for the 122 voters who first assessed the ACA's impacts on different racial-ethnic groups, while for the 112 who did not it was *lower*, at 2.19 ($p = 0.04$). So that certainly is not evidence of that form of racialization. It is possible, for example, that this version's priming of people to think about how their families or communities benefited outweighed the racial prime. It is also possible that racial attitudes are stably integrated with these respondents' views of the ACA and not subject to influence from subtle primes. But to be sure, it was one survey experiment conducted in one Alabama county, and so it bears replicating.

In 2019, Alabama and West Virginia were both among the states with the ten highest poverty rates. Unlike Alabama, West Virginia is both a heavily white state and one that expanded its Medicaid program. For those reasons, we chose it for a follow-up experiment.

In May 2018, West Virginia held primaries, including in the race for a U.S. Senate seat held by Democrat Joe Manchin. I joined three other researchers—Brielle Harbin, Michele Margolis, and Kalind Parish—in West Virginia to conduct the same exit poll experiment among white voters that Margolis and I conducted in Alabama, with respondents either assessing the ACA first or doing so after assessing its impacts on the five social groups. This time, however, there was no overall effect: favorability was 2.48 among the 107 respondents in the control group and slightly lower, at 2.37, for those in the treated group ($p = 0.45$). Among voters in the Republican primary, the 1.80 favorability among treated voters was similarly indistinguishable from the 1.72 average favorability in the control group. From the exit polls alone, the results are inconclusive, but they certainly do not suggest that calling attention to the law's black and Hispanic beneficiaries dampened support among white voters.

Experiments with Online Samples

Experiments embedded in exit polls have key advantages, one of which is that they enable researchers to reach a broader population that includes more low-engagement citizens than experiments with online, opt-in samples.[74] There are many Americans who will take an exit poll but would never sign up for an online survey panel.[75] Still, the exit polls' sample sizes are limited, and the results may be shaped by the particularities of the places or people we interviewed. Given that, we now turn to similar experiments conducted with online samples.

In the fall of 2018, we ran one such experiment that utilized an SSI sample, which had been recruited for a separate survey by physician Emily Gregory and was principally on issues related to patients' health and health care

Figure 6.6 ACA Favorability among White Voters in Online Patient Survey by Experimental Racial Prime, 2018

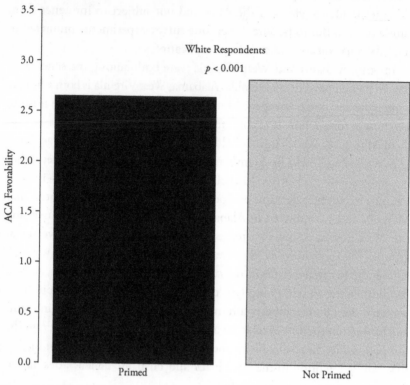

Source: 2018 Health Utilization Survey.

utilization. At the end of the survey, respondents were randomly assigned to answer two groups of questions. Some respondents first reported their favorability toward the ACA, the survey's first question about politics. As in the exit polls, they then answered five questions about people who may have been made better or worse off by the ACA, with "Whites," "Blacks," and "Hispanics" listed alongside "you and your family" and "the community where you live." The treated group, by contrast, answered the questions about who benefited first.

We restrict the sample to the 1,350 respondents who reported "White" as among their racial identities. For this group, priming ACA beneficiaries clearly had a downward impact on their views of the ACA (see figure 6.6). In the control group, ACA favorability was 2.83 on a 1–4 scale, bringing it closer to "somewhat favorable" than to "somewhat unfavorable." Among those who first assessed groups benefiting from the law, however, ACA favorability fell to 2.65. The associated p-value for a two-sided t-test is less than 0.001. One downside to this treatment is that it is a composite treatment, meaning that we cannot know which of the group assessments was especially influential. But one upside is that respondents had been answering questions unrelated to politics so they may not have been thinking in partisan terms when these questions came along. Put differently, this experiment's evidence is consistent with the prospect that priming may be more impactful when people are not already thinking about politics.

We also replicated the experiment in a separate fall 2018 SSI survey, although in that survey we expanded the primed racial categories by increasing the number of groups we asked respondents to assess to twelve, with the final four being "Hispanics/Latinos," "Undocumented immigrants," "Blacks," and "Whites."[76] Of the 1,366 white respondents, 696 first answered the questions about groups while the remaining 670 first reported their favorability toward the ACA.

As figure 6.7 illustrates, the white respondents overall land almost exactly in the middle of the scale, whether they were primed (2.50) or not (2.49), and the difference is statistically indistinguishable ($p = 0.87$). The 659 Republican identifiers, on average, were much less favorable toward the ACA, with 2.11 average favorability (just above "somewhat unfavorable") among the treated and 2.05 among the control group. Again, the difference is not statistically significant ($p = 0.46$). So far, our experimental evidence on racialized attitudes points in contradictory directions.

The Impact of Priming Black and Hispanic Beneficiaries

In a separate set of experiments, we used an experimental design with a treatment designed to remedy some of the limitations of the treatments in the experiments already described. We asked all respondents about their views of "the 2010 health reform law" on a scale from "The 2010 health reform law should be repealed and not replaced" (1) to "The 2010 health reform law should be expanded" (4). But in the preface to the question, we told a randomly assigned control group, "Experts recently estimated that the 2010 health reform law has allowed approximately 18 million non-elderly adults to get health insurance." For the treatment group, we added that

Figure 6.7 ACA Favorability among White Voters in SSI Survey by Experimental Racial Prime and Political Party Identification, 2018

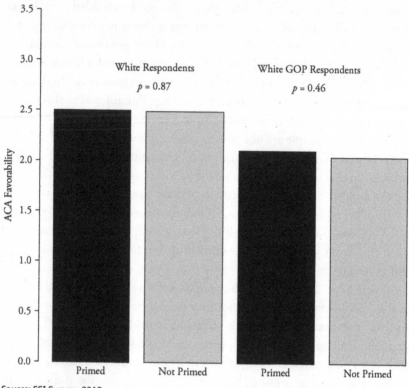

Source: SSI Survey, 2018.

the 18 million adults included "more than 7 million Black and Hispanic Americans."

We administered one variant of this experiment to a set of political activists recruited via YouGov in the fall of 2016. To qualify, these activists had to do more than simply vote for a candidate; they had to have more extensive political engagement, such as having volunteered on campaigns or even having worked as political staffers.[77] In short, these should be highly engaged respondents with well-formed political views.

What was the impact of priming these activists to think about the ACA's black and Hispanic beneficiaries just before expressing a view on the law? Among the 608 white activists, those primed to think about black and Hispanic beneficiaries were essentially no different in their self-reported

Figure 6.8 Attitudes toward Expanding the ACA among White Activists by Experimental Racial Prime and Political Party Identification, 2016

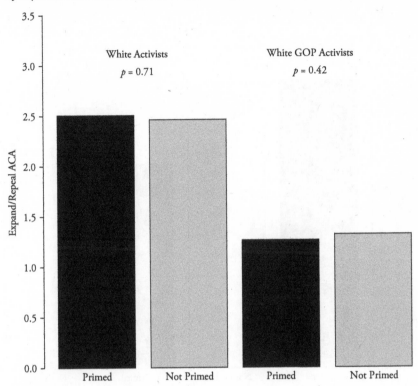

Source: YouGov activist survey, fall 2016 (Hopkins and Noel 2022).

views of what to do with the ACA (2.50 versus 2.46, p-value = 0.71), as shown in figure 6.8. Among the Republican activists, the priming reduced support for the ACA (1.26 versus 1.32, p-value = 0.42), but even that result is substantively small and statistically insignificant.

In the 2017 SSI survey, we replicated the 2016 experiment with a broader group of online, opt-in white survey respondents. We again analyze two groups, all 1,023 white respondents and the 430 white Trump supporters. As figure 6.9 illustrates, for the respondents overall, there is no evidence of an effect either way: those who read the racial prime averaged 2.45 on the 1–4 scale, roughly halfway between saying, "The 2010 health reform law should be scaled back but not repealed" (2) and "The 2010 health reform law should be left as it is" (3). Those who did not see the prime scored 2.42,

Figure 6.9 Attitudes toward Expanding the ACA among White Voters by Experimental Racial Prime and Presidential Preference, 2017

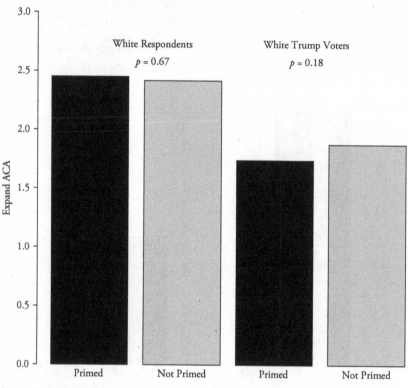

Source: SSI Survey, 2017.

which is just slightly less supportive, and certainly not significantly so ($p = 0.67$). Overall, that prime had little effect on the answers given just seconds later.

Of course, the population of white respondents includes many with high levels of racial sympathy, so it is valuable to also consider the effects only on the 430 Trump supporters. The right two bars in figure 6.9 show tentative evidence of reduced ACA support among Trump supporters who were primed—ACA support drops from 1.88 among the control group to 1.74 among the treated group—but the difference is far from significant ($p = 0.18$).

We replicated the experiment in a 2018 survey with SSI, which had 1,366 white respondents. Respondents were again asked to answer whether they wanted the ACA to be repealed, wanted it to be expanded, or took a middle position—and some were randomly selected to be primed with information about the approximate number of newly insured Americans who were black or Hispanic. Here priming does slightly reduce ACA support overall, from 2.47 to 2.39 ($p = 0.18$). But the effect is now smaller for Republicans (1.86 to 1.81; $p = 0.51$) and is insignificant in any case.

In particular experiments, there are tentative suggestions of possible effects, albeit in different directions. But across the seven different survey experiments, the overall conclusion is inescapable: in the 2016–2018 period, racial primes did not consistently move Americans' attitudes toward the ACA. There is also a methodological lesson here. Although our survey experiments returned mostly null results, we did find (conflicting) results from a few, reinforcing the critical importance of conducting multiple survey experiments in different settings or with different populations.[78]

Conclusion

The chasm of racial divisions has been a feature of the American political landscape since before the nation's founding, and its impact remains deeply inscribed in our nation's politics and public policy to this day.[79] This chapter took up the relationship between white Americans' racial attitudes and their views on the ACA. Observational data indicate a meaningful connection between racial attitudes, partisanship, and ACA attitudes. Still, across seven experiments conducted with varied samples, we find that priming racial attitudes does not consistently heighten hostility to the ACA. What's more, the policy attitudes that ACA attitudes appear most closely correlated with are not attitudes on the most clearly racialized policies, like food stamps. Instead, they are policies like student loan regulation and disability insurance that are not seen as especially benefiting racial or ethnic minorities.

In sum, the evidence that racial attitudes do not have much immediate, short-term influence on views of the ACA is strong. To the extent that racial divisions shape white Americans' ACA views, both the evidence from panel data and prior research indicate that these divisions operate at a distance, shaping ACA attitudes through their long-run influence on partisan divisions and on the narratives through which the public makes sense of social policies. Racial divisions and prejudices set the stage more than they act the parts. We will uncover similar patterns with respect to trust in government, another deep-seated political predisposition, in the next chapter.

Chapter 5 demonstrated that the ACA's complexity limited its capacity to produce consistent policy feedback effects. From the evidence presented in this chapter, it seems plausible that the ACA's complexity may also have had an upside: to some degree, it may have shielded the law from the racialized dynamics of other programs, including food stamps and welfare. Indeed, the ACA's complexity may serve to integrate more closely white Americans' views of the law with their overall partisan predispositions, which themselves are tethered to their racial attitudes yet remain distinct. One of the mysteries of the ACA's Medicaid expansion—and so of the law overall—is that it did not fall prey to the same extent to the racialized politics that characterized the issue of welfare in the 1980s and 1990s. The ACA's complexity may be part of the answer.

This chapter's findings also provide a caution to contemporary scholarship on racial divisions. In recent decades, encouraged by a newfound attention to causal inference, researchers have conducted a torrent of survey experiments to better understand racial attitudes.[80] That research has produced critical insights. But since survey experiments take existing racial attitudes and their salience as a baseline by design, they are ill positioned to address long-running causes.[81] There is good reason to think that racial attitudes have shaped the narratives through which Americans understand redistributive policies generally—and thus there is good reason to not rely exclusively on survey experiments when studying racial attitudes. At the same time, the distinction between short- and long-term causes may help explain why some social scientists can downplay the contemporary political impacts of race while others center it as the skeleton key unlocking so much of American politics. The answer depends to some extent on the time frame of the researcher's question.

Likewise, this conception of white Americans' racial prejudices as primarily an upstream influence on ACA attitudes places limits on contemporary elites' capacity to gain political advantage by priming race. Ironically, the more integrated racial attitudes and partisanship become, the fewer cross-pressured citizens there are who are available to switch sides in response to a racialized appeal.[82] Having established the stability of public opinion on the ACA in the face of racial primes, we next turn to the impacts of ACA rhetoric more generally. Whereas this chapter has focused on public opinion, the next chapter analyzes elite rhetoric as well.

CHAPTER 7

Framing's Limited Short-Term Impacts

IN THE EYES of politicians, the ability to use rhetoric to frame complex issues appears to be a central tool to shape public opinion. In 2000, a state legislator named Barack Obama premised his congressional candidacy on his capacity to communicate, arguing that he was able to "best articulate and frame the issues that are most important to voters."[1] Obama lost that congressional race but went on to a political career of some distinction.

Obama is far from unique as a politician with faith in the power of rhetoric. In the wake of the 2002 midterms, which had gone poorly for Democrats, newly installed House Democratic leader Nancy Pelosi reflected, "The party had not been clear in terms of the message it put out to the public. I said never again would the Democrats go into a campaign where the public didn't know who we were, what we stood for."[2]

In emphasizing communications, leading Democrats can (and do) point to academic backing. In 2004, linguist George Lakoff became a well-known apostle of messaging in political circles, arguing in his book *Don't Think of an Elephant*: "What you want to do is to get [the people in the middle] to use your model for politics—to activate your worldview and moral system in their political decisions. You do that by talking to people using frames based on your world view." Later, Lakoff says simply, "Democrats ignore the power of framing at their peril."[3]

It's not just Democrats either. In a 2004 interview, the Republican pollster Frank Luntz emphasized the importance of staying on message: "There's a simple rule. You say it again, and you say it again and you say it again, and then again and again and again and again, and about the time that you're absolutely sick of saying it is about the time that your target audience has heard it for the first time."[4] Although in recent years Republicans and Democrats have disagreed on almost everything, there is one political truth that seems universally acknowledged: the words that politicians use to advance their arguments matter.

Journalists, too, commonly point to political rhetoric as a key reason why some policies prove popular while others do not. In 2011, the *New York Times* stated the conventional wisdom when it wrote that "the Obama administration and Democrats . . . largely lost the health care message war in the raucous legislative process."[5] Many viewed the strength of public opposition to the ACA after the law's passage as evidence of the effectiveness of Republicans' messaging efforts (and the failure of Democrats'). Nine years after campaigning on his ability to frame issues, and six years after giving a breakout speech to the Democratic National Convention, Obama was perceived as having lost the messaging battle on his signature domestic policy initiative.

It is not surprising that journalists emphasize messaging as a source of elite influence on public opinion. The craft of journalism, after all, is an exercise in finding compelling ways to explain contemporary events, so it makes sense that claims about the power of messaging would resonate for its practitioners. It is similarly unsurprising that politicians put a lot of stock in messaging—their rhetoric is one of the few political tools under their control. Likewise, political consultants' livelihoods depend on the prospect of changing citizens' minds through messaging—often conveyed via television ads and social media—so consultants are also likely to view messaging as crucial to political success. In the words of TV producer Peter Pomerantsev, "Everything is PR."[6] But what does the evidence say?

Given the consensus among politicians and journalists about the impact of messaging, you might think that there is an extensive body of evidence backing up that claim. Certainly, political scientists have devoted significant attention to the influence of political elites' word choice, commonly calling such effects "framing" rather than "messaging." From 2010 to 2020, there were an extraordinary 213 separate articles on the topic in three leading political science journals.[7] As James Druckman, Jordan Fein, and Thomas Leeper summarize, a "generation of research shows that elites can use frames . . . to affect public opinion."[8] On the ACA specifically, some scholars have joined commentators in contending that politicians' rhetorical choices influenced public opinion. Former Alaska governor and 2008 Republican vice presidential candidate Sarah Palin's use of the phrase "death panels" in a 2009 Facebook post is cited as especially effective anti-ACA rhetoric.[9]

As we explain here, we are examining influence on public opinion in general, not on the views of activists or specific groups like copartisans.[10] And when it comes to research methods for detecting such influence, the deck has been stacked in favor of finding elite-level framing effects. To date, research on framing has been primarily experimental, with impacts on captive audiences typically measured just moments after exposure.[11] Moreover, public opinion has been measured overwhelmingly via closed-ended questions, whereas elite frames have been measured mostly through more nuanced, observational studies of rhetoric and word choice.[12] As a result of this asymmetry, prior research has been positioned to detect only elite frames and public responses; if public opinion were actually shaping elite-level frames instead of the reverse, existing methods offer no way of knowing.

Relative to experimental research, scholars know less about how framing operates in real-world conditions.[13] But despite those methodological biases, existing research provides a mixed assessment of the strength of elite framing. There is some observational evidence of framing's impacts, especially over longer time periods, but other research emphasizes the limits of framing effects.[14] Even Lynn Vavreck's book entitled *The Message Matters* contends that the broad theme of presidential campaigns can be influential, not that more specific wordsmithing wins many votes.[15]

In fact, there are a number of substantive reasons to suspect that framing's short-term influence is quite limited in real-world settings.[16] One comes from the combination of public inattention and selective information-seeking.[17] Since only a small fraction of U.S. citizens follow politics closely, the vast majority of Americans may not ever be exposed to politicians' rhetoric. A member of Congress can spend weeks honing her message, but if her words reach only the small population of regular C-SPAN watchers, that message is unlikely to leave an imprint. In one indicator of public attention, as the debate over the ACA was kicking into high gear in 2010, 41 percent of survey respondents could not name the vice president of the United States.[18]

At the same time, millions of Americans are strongly attached to one of the major political parties, including many of the citizens most engaged with politics.[19] That partisanship may serve as a filter for incoming political information.[20] Zaller's influential framework in his 1992 book *The Nature and Origins of Mass Opinion* predicted opinion change among people with middle levels of political awareness—those who paid sufficient attention to politics to register new messages but not so much attention that they had extensive preconceptions that would lead them to disregard new messages.[21] In today's polarized times, however, it may be a stretch to think that large numbers of Americans occupy this middle ground who are both persuadable *and* paying sufficient attention to politics.[22]

Politicians' power to shape public opinion through rhetoric is further limited by the news media, whose incentives lead them to transmit a very limited subset of what politicians say.[23] Journalists can convey only a fraction of the quotes they receive through press releases, tweets, and interviews. Also, journalists and politicians are familiar with and invested in existing frames, making it hard to get coverage for novel ones.[24] If everyone understands and discusses a problem in a certain light, it is virtually impossible for a lone politician to shift that collective understanding. In addition, elites craft their language using polling and focus groups.[25] This practice might make salient frames a reflection of public opinion more than an independent influence on it.[26]

We use "elite frames" to mean selective presentations of an issue from high-profile politicians. As we saw in chapter 2, the complex and multifaceted nature of health care reform gives supporters and opponents alike opportunities to frame it.[27] And frame it they did. In September 2009, President Obama gave a prime-time congressional address devoted entirely to health care. Between January 2009 and December 2010, U.S. senators sent out a total of 1,488 press releases related to the issue. If politicians can influence public opinion on any issue, the high volume of rhetoric focused on the ACA makes it a likely case.

To measure this oft-cited channel of elite influence, this chapter reports experimental and observational evidence, employing research methods old and new. It draws extensively from my earlier study of the 2009–2010 debates over the ACA's enactment, but it also integrates novel evidence alongside a survey experiment I conducted with Jonathan Mummolo and a field experiment with David Yokum and our colleagues.[28] This chapter first uses survey experiments with population-based and opt-in samples to illustrate the effects (and limits) of framing in one-sided communication environments.[29] These experimental results provide valuable context for the subsequent observational analyses that are at the heart of this chapter.

There are good reasons to pay special attention to real-world communication effects during the initial ACA debate. The KFF's monthly surveys provide researchers with more than thirty thousand respondents who had no missing data and who were asked about health care reform between February 2009 and January 2012. As we saw in chapter 3, the Pew Research Center and the KFF together asked open-ended questions about health care reform in seven surveys; to our knowledge, there is no comparable data set of open-ended questions spanning another major American policy debate. By coupling these data with tools for automated content analysis, we can observe the specific frames that both elected officials and American citizens used in describing their views of health care reform—and we can do so before and after the issue reached peak salience. This focus on word choice allows us to measure elite frames and public opinion on the same scale, as well as to identify the extent to which elite frames induce shifts in public arguments. Unlike many prior studies, this approach does not build the presumption of elite influence into its very design.[30]

To what extent are ACA-related communications impactful in real-world settings? This chapter's final empirical section turns to a large-scale field experiment that I conducted with a team of researchers and government officials to complement the observational analyses.[31] Americans who considered but then delayed purchasing insurance on the exchanges were more likely to ultimately enroll if they received a letter from a federal agency encouraging them to do so. Still, the effects came primarily from receiving the letter itself; most experimental variations in the letter's content did not demonstrably change its impact. What's more, the 0.3-percentage-point uptick in enrollments is substantively meaningful but not transformative.

A caveat is in order. Our argument here is about political elites' capacity to use messaging to influence public opinion in general—that is, the views held by citizens of all political stripes. The average of everyone's attitudes is the best yardstick by which to understand whether elites can meaningfully reshape the public opinion landscape to their side's benefit. But in a polarized era, moving average public opinion requires that elites successfully influence citizens who do not identify with their political party, or else induce shifts among copartisans that are large enough to offset any backlash from others. There is already extensive evidence that information flows can influence copartisans and sometimes citizens more generally, especially when they are one-sided.[32] In the aftermath of Donald Trump's lies about the 2020 election, many Republicans came to believe that Trump had in fact won.[33] The argument and evidence of this chapter do not dispute the possibility of such intraparty influence. But it sets a higher bar for elite-level influence by focusing on influence overall—that is, the ability to move out-partisans alongside copartisans. By that measure, politicians' ability to influence ACA attitudes through their rhetoric proves quite limited. Elites' rapid cycling through health care frames makes framing a poor explanation for public attitudes, which change only gradually.

Perhaps our strongest tests of elite influence come from comparing word usage among politicians and the public over time and testing whether elite rhetoric comes to be used by the public. There is evidence that the public incorporates the language used by political elites during the most intense phase of the debate, and that it does so roughly symmetrically.[34] However, the broad contours of the public's arguments for and against health care reform were visible as early as July 2009—and that was prior to health care reform's spike in public salience. In short, elite rhetoric appears more likely to change the rationale underpinning citizens' evaluations of the ACA than to change the evaluations themselves.[35] Messaging is not the tool of elite influence that many (including most political elites) believe it to be.

Certainly, as discussed in the prior chapter and in this chapter's conclusion, these results are compatible with the existence of framing effects that unfold over longer time horizons, those that are more pronounced for less salient issues, and those that influence only copartisans.[36] In its emphasis on the difference between short-term and long-term effects, this chapter picks up where chapter 6 left off. But these results not only reinforce the limits on the effects of elite rhetoric during a high-salience policy debate like that over the ACA but also underscore the complex, interactive nature of real-world communication effects.[37] While political observers commonly appeal to the power of messaging or framing in the short term, its real-world influence on public opinion at a given political moment is far more constrained.

Prior Research on Framing

Here we take a step back from the ACA to consider the pathways through which rhetoric might (or might not) shape public opinion. Scholars have defined framing effects in a variety of ways.[38] Our goal is not to resolve such debates but to identify a workable definition of framing before discussing its study in real-world contexts like the ACA. This section grounds the chapter's core hypothesis: for various reasons, real-world framing effects on overall public opinion are likely to be quite limited, at least in the short run.

Framing is a process through which communications influence attitudes by shifting the weights that people put on different considerations.[39] Research on framing commonly conceives of human minds as containing a jumble of potentially relevant considerations about a given topic. For example, when someone thinks about the ACA, she may think about premium spikes (a negative consideration) or a neighbor's newfound access to insurance (a positive one). After hearing a speech focusing on rising premiums, related considerations are likely to be top of mind for a citizen, and her view of the ACA might sour as a result. In this view, frames do not change people's considerations. Instead, they change the weights that people give to existing considerations.[40]

There is also a burgeoning, related body of research on interpersonal persuasion, a more general psychological process in which recipients may gain new considerations. This research finds that sometimes conversations between canvassers and individuals on their doorsteps can shape attitudes in durable ways, such as David Broockman and Joshua Kalla's experimental study of transphobia.[41] If any brief encounter is going to persuade people to shift their attitudes for weeks to come, it is likely to be an in-person encounter.[42] Someone standing on a doorstep can command their interlocutor's full attention and use the full arsenal of active listening and nonverbal communication to connect with her.[43] But it is noteworthy that even trying to persuade someone in person is a challenging enterprise, one that can sometimes fail or even produce backlash.[44] This difficulty suggests that politicians' messaging as conveyed through the news and social media is likely to be even weaker.

In observational settings, we often lack the tools to differentiate framing from related avenues of elite influence like priming or persuasion.[45] But politicians do not care much whether they move public opinion through what academics term "framing" or "persuasion"—they only care about shifting it to their advantage.

The Limits of Elite Influence through Framing

The study of framing has developed rapidly in recent years, driven by experimental survey research.[46] This research generates expectations about real-world framing, including the hypothesis that framing effects will be especially pronounced when the frames come from trusted elites within people's own party.[47]

Still, challenges remain in translating these experimental findings to real-world settings. In the typical framing experiment, the researcher chooses frames with few limitations. In real-world settings, however, politicians and political elites face significant constraints in their attempts to frame. One limitation stems from intraparty coordination problems, as lone officials are unlikely to advance frames that are at odds with their copartisans or with contemporary discourse generally.[48] Even if parties successfully agree on a frame, the news media might prove uninterested in transmitting that frame to the public.[49]

An additional limitation stems from the use of polling and focus groups in shaping contemporary elite rhetoric.[50] To the extent that political elites craft messages based on public opinion research, the causal effect in practice might be the opposite of that identified in experimental studies, with elites adopting the language and frames already used by the public rather than creating new ones. These pathways suggest the importance of measuring not simply baseline opinion but also baseline word choice in public discussions of a given issue to help pinpoint where such language originated.

Additionally, citizens with partisan loyalties are likely to discount frames offered by the other party.[51] What's more, few prospective voters closely follow political discourse. The effects of political rhetoric are also likely to decay rapidly after exposure, further limiting framing effects.[52]

Given the barriers facing political elites who seek to influence the public through framing, it is not surprising that studies of real-world framing report mixed results.[53] Studies of political advertising find that its impacts are detectable but often small, short-lived, and undercut by opposition advertising.[54] In light of these theoretical considerations and prior results, we expect that real-world framing effects will be more limited than those observed in most survey experiments—and far more limited than politicians or journalists seem to believe.

Even when political communications do reshape citizens' ultimate evaluations, such effects are not necessarily evidence of framing.[55] Framing is distinct from other communication effects in that it attempts to change the accessibility and applicability of preexisting cognitive considerations. Alternatively, it is quite plausible that citizens will adopt their overall issue positions based on their partisan loyalties or other heuristics and then turn to salient political rhetoric to justify those evaluations. Such claims are consistent with evidence from political psychology about the extent to which voters engage in motivated reasoning.[56] As Milton Lodge and Charles Taber note, "Conscious deliberation and rumination is from this perspective the *rationalization* of multiple unconscious processes that recruit reasons to justify and explain beliefs, attitudes, and actions."[57] This implies that on a salient partisan issue, such as the ACA, citizens may first adopt an overall evaluation of the law based on partisan cues, affect, or other heuristics. Only subsequently will they adopt justifications for those views, often using the same reasons given by prominent party leaders. If so, we should not expect framing but rather what we might call "parroting" or motivated reasoning— the use of copartisans' rhetoric to justify the party's position. Communications may change the relative weights given to different considerations without changing people's overall evaluations.

Survey Experiments on Distrust

In a polarized era, just how much can framing move public opinion under optimal conditions? We begin our empirical investigation by using survey experiments to benchmark the extent and limits of one-sided framing effects. In these experiments, respondents are close to a captive audience, and there is no competing frame to counterbalance the argument. Thus, these results should provide an upper bound on any framing effects. Yet even in this case, framing effects are often small or even undetectable.

Distrust and Framing Effects

Here our goal is to estimate the substantive magnitude of framing under auspicious conditions—and more narrowly to assess whether the connection between trust and ACA attitudes might be causal.[58] To do so, we ran experiments designed to frame health policy in terms that were likely to reduce ACA support. Our respondents came from three separate surveys administered in separate years. The first is drawn from a 2011 Knowledge Networks (KN) panel of American adults (n = 2,228); the second and third were conducted in the fall of 2017 and the fall of 2018 with opt-in online samples recruited by the survey firm SSI (n = 1,631 and 1,945, respectively). In all three cases, respondents were randomly assigned to either one of two treatment conditions or a control group with no frame.

To find frames that are likely to be impactful, we turn to Americans' deep-seated distrust of government. In a pioneering 2005 book, Marc Hetherington laid out the logic for how trust might influence citizens' attitudes toward social programs such as the ACA.[59] The basic logic is this: if Americans do not trust the government to enact social programs effectively, they will not be supportive of those programs, even if they do not object to them in principle. In this account, such effects are especially pronounced with redistributive programs, since most Americans are not able to verify the programs' operations through their own experiences. And as we saw in chapter 2, the ACA was certainly redistributive, making it a likely case for this hypothesis. Indeed, Bill Clinton's 1993–1994 attempt at health care reform was one of Hetherington's primary examples.[60]

Self-reported levels of trust in government are quite low. In our 2011 KN panel, for example, just 13 percent of respondents said that they trusted the national government "just about always" or "most of the time"; in other words, 87 percent of respondents gave answers expressing distrust. Given the prevalence of distrust, we developed experimental cues that would resonate with a majority of our respondents by impugning the government's trustworthiness. Specifically, the one-third of respondents assigned to the low-trust frame read the following text: "Health care is one of the most complicated issues we face. It involves 1 of every 6 dollars spent here in the United States. The health care system includes millions of doctors and nurses and thousands of hospitals and clinics. Together, they regularly make decisions that can mean life or death. The government in Washington can't even balance its own budget. We certainly can't trust it to run something as complicated as the health care system." The goal of this manipulation was to bring trust-related considerations to the forefront of respondents' minds.

In all three experiments, the outcome is a measure of respondents' attitudes toward the ACA. In the 2011 KN experiment, we assessed those attitudes via a standard question: "Given what you know about the new health reform law, do you have a generally favorable or generally unfavorable opinion of it?" In the 2017 and 2018 SSI experiments, to avoid redundancy, we instead asked respondents' support for repealing the ACA: "Some people think the 2010 health care reform law should be kept as it is. Others want to repeal the entire 2010 health care law. Still others are somewhere in between. What about you?" Respondents could indicate that they preferred to repeal the ACA in full (1), preferred to keep the ACA as is (7), or took a position somewhere in between (2 to 6). To avoid triggering a backlash among out-partisans, there was no explicit partisan cue in the question, although politically engaged respondents might well have suspected that the source of the low-trust argument was a Republican.

The experiments each employed an alternative treatment as well as a control group. Because our experimental cue pushed respondents in an anti-ACA direction, it is critical to identify whether arguments invoking distrust are effective relative to other anti-ACA arguments. Accordingly, the alternative treatment group received an anti-ACA message that was similar in length, structure, and language but was grounded in conservative ideology rather than distrust. These respondents read: "Health care is one of the most complicated issues we face. It involves 1 of every 6 dollars spent here in the United States. The health care system includes millions of doctors and nurses and thousands of hospitals and clinics. Together, they regularly make decisions that can mean life or death. Let's leave these decisions to the private actors who know best—the doctors, patients, insurers, and hospitals—rather than getting the government involved where it doesn't belong." The one-third of respondents assigned to the control group simply answered the question about their support for repealing the ACA without reading any preceding text. Their responses thus represent a neutral baseline.[61]

Figure 7.1 illustrates the results for each of the three experiments separately. In the 2011 experiment, those who were exposed to the low-trust argument were very slightly *more* supportive of the ACA relative to the control or ideology frames (2.24 versus 2.20 and 2.16), but none of the differences are substantively or statistically significant ($p > 0.19$). The same holds in 2017, when those who read the low-trust argument were again slightly *more* supportive of the ACA than those who read nothing (4.25 versus 4.13), but

Figure 7.1 Support for the ACA under Different Experimental Trust-Related Frames, 2011, 2017, and 2018

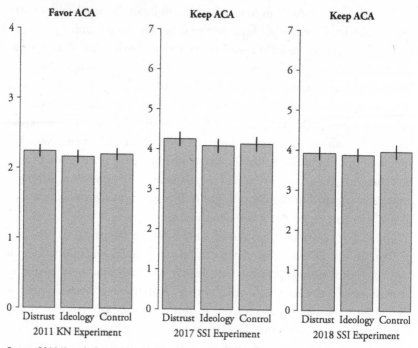

Source: 2011 Knowledge Networks (KN) Survey, 2011; SSI Surveys, 2011 and 2017.

the result is neither substantively large nor statistically significant ($p = 0.34$). In 2018, there was essentially no difference between the low-trust framing and the control who read nothing (3.93 versus 3.97, $p = 0.71$).[62]

Whether we are analyzing the full set of respondents or only the majority who expressed distrust, the experimental message on distrust did little to reshape ACA attitudes.[63] Overall ACA attitudes were surprisingly stable in the face of trust-related arguments designed specifically to move them. The stability of aggregate attitudes that we saw in chapter 2 is echoed in these results.[64]

November 2011 Framing Experiment

In another November 2011 survey—after the ACA had been signed into law, but before most of its provisions were implemented—Jonathan

Mummolo and I sought to answer a related research question about the breadth of framing effects across several issues.[65] As part of the experiment, we exposed a population-based sample of 3,318 Americans recruited via KN to one-sided messaging, including one message about health care policy. Very similar in wording to the distrustful frame described earlier, the message was again designed to tap into the deep vein of American distrust in government.[66] The fact that 67 percent of respondents found the distrustful argument convincing is evidence that our frame did resonate. However, it reduced support for health care spending by a relatively modest 2.2 percentage points (with a standard error of 1.2) relative to the control group. That effect is at once meaningful but not substantively enormous, especially given the absence of any competing frame in support of the law. Given that attitudes are already integrated with partisanship on a high-salience issue like health policy, there are limits on the extent to which these attitudes are likely to move in response to communications.[67] If framing effects under such ideal conditions are limited, they are likely to be even more constrained in real-world conditions.

Measuring ACA Frames through Automated Content Analysis

In the artificial environments of survey experiments, one-sided frames can sometimes move public opinion, but even there, the effects are minimal, or at least not substantively large. We now turn to an even harder case for framing effects: their real-world impacts in the initial debates over the ACA. This section measures prominent frames in real-world political debates through extensive analyses of textual data, including senators' press releases and open-ended survey responses.

Earlier, we defined issue frames as rhetorical structures that call attention to a subset of the considerations relevant to an issue. Frames are thus closely associated with a speaker's choices of words. Given this association, we might measure frames quantitatively by measuring the frequency of word usage within a given topic. For example, a health care frame emphasizing an expansion of governmental authority is more likely to use words like "government," "takeover," and perhaps "death" or "panel" (in light of Sarah Palin's famous comment). In such a frame, terms like "affordable" or "preexisting condition" are much less likely to be used.

In recent years, computer scientists have developed models that closely match this conception of frames as probability distributions over a vocabulary within a given topic. The most prominent of such models is latent Dirichlet allocation, or LDA.[68] Simply put, LDA is a form of cluster analysis that returns groups of words commonly found together in a collection or corpus of texts. A single document can draw from different clusters—or frames, in the applications described here. Each cluster is in turn represented by a distinctive probability distribution over the corpus's vocabulary— a distinctive set of typical words. By using an unsupervised technique such as LDA, researchers can be open to clusters of language they may not have anticipated ex ante.[69]

Open-Ended Survey Responses

The impacts of real-world frames are almost always measured using survey questions with fixed responses because they allow for easy comparisons across respondents. However, these questions have limitations. Although they are hard to categorize, open-ended survey questions can provide a better window into citizens' cognitive processes.[70] In this specific application, for instance, open-ended survey responses enable us to study changes in the rationale underlying a given attitude.

That said, automated techniques like LDA can reduce the disadvantages associated with open-ended questions, as they enable us to cluster responses based on word use. For instance, we can determine that a respondent complaining about "too much control" and another talking about a "government takeover" are voicing related concerns.[71]

Even without clustering, the ability to analyze public word choice provides leverage in understanding framing. Words are the way that we identify elite frames, but word choice has only rarely been part of scholars' strategy for measuring framing effects among the public. By comparing elites' and citizens' word use, we can measure whether the public adopted elite-level word choices—and thereby their messages—as the health care debate unfolded.

Elite Framing on the ACA: Observational Data and Results

Over the course of a campaign or debate, elite frames shift as circumstances change. Claims that health care reform was being passed through corrupt backroom deals became meaningful only as the legislative process unfolded. To observe shifting frames we need sources of political rhetoric that are available at many points in time. Since this chapter's primary goal is to assess politicians' framing capacities, we also seek at least some rhetoric not yet filtered by the media. Speeches on the House or Senate floor might prove useful, but they are available mostly when a bill is formally being debated, truncating the over-time variation. For these reasons, press releases are an unparalleled source of information, as Justin Grimmer has shown.[72] From January 2009 to July 2010, U.S. senators sent out 1,488 press releases using at least one health care–related term.[73] Often written in a form that mimics newspaper articles, press releases enable politicians to frame the issues in the ways they choose. We also analyze 218 television appearances to ensure that our results hold with content more likely to reach the public in figure E.2.[74]

Figure 7.2 depicts the distribution, by month, of U.S. senators' press releases that contained at least one health care–related term. The figure shows that new releases spiked at times when key legislative events occurred. It also illustrates the arc of the public debate: the number of press releases grew in the summer of 2009, spiked in the fall and winter of 2009, and then spiked again with the bill's passage in March 2010.[75] The figure's gray lines show select surveys and reinforce that the bulk of the public debate took place after our baseline surveys in February and July 2009. Even in early 2009, however, the issue was not wholly unfamiliar.[76]

To assess framing effects, we must first identify the elite frames employed in a given policy area. This section does so by applying LDA to 1,488 press releases from U.S. senators between January 2009 and December 2010.[77] After experimenting with various options and soliciting outside advice, we chose twelve clusters, which include the major frames we had expected ex ante.[78] For every topic, LDA provides the probability that every word appears in that topic, meaning that words can and do occur frequently in multiple topics.

With the LDA mode in hand, we can compute various quantities of interest. Here we focus on the share of a group of documents (say, Republican press releases) that fall into each of the topics and how that topic changes over time. Figure 7.3 illustrates this quantity for each of the twelve clusters.[79] In the figure, we average the shares of each press release classified into each topic for all press releases issued in the previous thirty days. The solid gray lines indicate trends in cluster usage among Democrats, while

Figure 7.2 Number of U.S. Senators' Health Care–Related Press Releases by Month, Key Legislative Events, and Select Surveys, 2009–2010

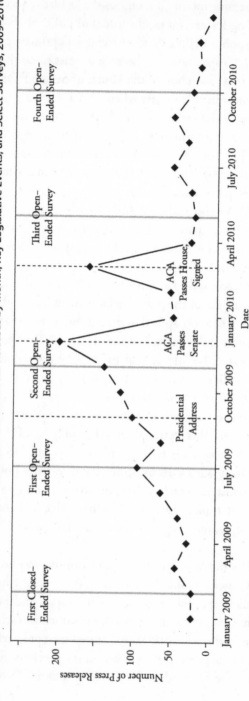

Source: KFF surveys, press releases compiled by author. Figure reprinted with permission from Springer (Hopkins 2018a).

Note: The black lines denote legislative events and the gray lines the dates of surveys.

Figure 7.3 Variation in Topics over Time in Senators' Press Releases, 2009–2010

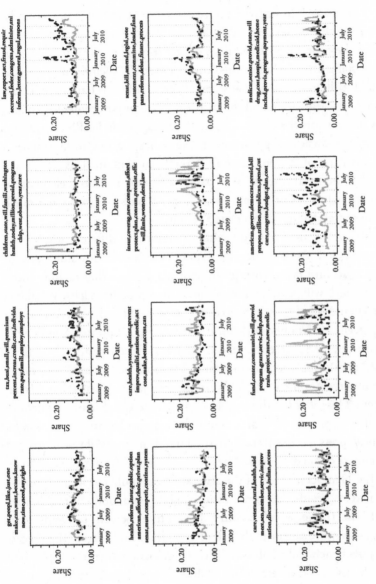

Source: Hopkins 2018a. Reprinted with permission from Springer.

Note: Model: LDA, fit to 1,488 press releases. The twelve clusters are separate topics returned by an LDA model fit to senators' press releases. The lines depict the share of all press release content that falls into each topic for Republicans (dashed black lines) and Democrats (solid gray lines). These shares have been smoothed over the prior thirty days.

the dashed black lines do the same for Republicans. Each cluster is labeled with the fifteen word stems with the largest differences in probabilities between that cluster and the corpus overall.

The LDA results in figure 7.3 have several notable features. Certainly, the returned clusters correspond in sensible ways to our expectations. For instance, one prominent Republican cluster throughout the debate draws on word stems that include "American," "govern," "Democrat," "presid," "bill," and "trillion" (bottom row, second from right). This frame emphasizes the cost of the legislation and the increasing role of government it entails, a focus that mirrors the GOP's consistent messaging on health care reform as a costly expansion of government; the corresponding topic reaches a maximum share of 32 percent of all Republican content. It is also worth noting that the words "death" and "panel" are not constitutive elements of this (or any) cluster. For the most part, other Republicans were not quick to borrow Sarah Palin's "death panels" phrasing.[80]

Republican senators framed health care reform in different ways as the debate unfolded. Another heavily Republican cluster is oriented toward business costs and taxes, with prominent word stems that include "tax," "busi," "small," "will," and "premium" (first row, second from left). This frame emerged in the fall of 2009 but was used throughout the debate, accounting for 17 percent of Republican rhetoric at its zenith. Additionally, notice the Medicare-oriented frame, defined by stems such as "medicar," "senior," "provid," and "state" (bottom row, far right). Both parties used this frame, but we observe a spike in Republican usage in January 2010 that reaches 27 percent.[81] Just after health care reform passed the U.S. Senate, Republican press releases portrayed health care reform as undermining Medicare. Republican press releases also emphasized fraud and oversight, as illustrated by the cluster defined by "law," "report," and "fraud" (top row, far right).

On the Democratic side of the aisle, we see a "public option" frame—constituted by "health," "reform," "insur," "public," and "option" (middle row, far left). This frame, which accounts for up to 21 percent of Democratic rhetoric, was more salient in the fall of 2009 than it was later. The suggestion of Julia Lynch and Sarah Gollust that Democratic rhetoric emphasized affordable insurance coverage and middle-class economic security proves accurate.[82] See, for example, the cluster defined by the stems "insur," "coverag," "new," "compani," and "afford" (middle row, second from right), which reaches a maximum share of 26 percent of Democratic content.[83]

The Democrats' focus on "children," "state," and "families" in one topic that spiked in early 2009 is indicative of the surprisingly contentious fight over reauthorizing state CHIP programs.

Not all clusters are dominated by one party. For example, senators from both parties commonly talked about rural and veterans' health care (bottom row, far left); many of these press releases were not directly about the ACA and appeared to be less consistently polarized. We also see considerable attention to legislative procedure, which spiked in late 2009, just when the ACA came up in the Senate (middle row, far right). A third cluster provides generic health care language used by both parties (middle row, second from left). When considering the difference between the 916 Democratic press releases and the 552 Republican press releases, the average absolute difference across topics is 0.04. Substantively, this means that the average difference between Republican and Democratic usage of a category is four percentage points—for example, if a given topic represents 9 percent of all GOP rhetoric, it would represent just 5 percent of Democratic rhetoric. An average difference of 0.04 is sizable given that each of the twelve categories account for an average of 0.08 of the total content. When viewed over time, the average standard error within a topic is 0.06 for Republicans and 0.08 for Democrats. These measures indicate the over-time variability in each party's usage of each topic; the fact that they are so large relative to the averages is evidence of substantial over-time variability.[84] The most salient topics differ markedly over time.[85]

Obviously, even the most engaged citizens do not typically read press releases. Instead, members of the public watch and read journalists who serve as important filters of the elite rhetoric aimed at the public. Accordingly, we also fit an LDA model using the transcripts from 218 appearances on Sunday talk shows by members of Congress and Obama administration officials between July 2009 and March 2010, when the legislation was signed into law.[86] In this data set, we use 1,999 separate word stems that appear in more than 1 percent of the observed television appearances.[87]

In television appearances, when officials speak to much broader audiences, we are able to observe exactly what attentive citizens observe (see figure E.2 for results). Despite the markedly smaller sample size, the findings of this sample corroborate the core claims made using senators' press releases. Republicans were consistently more likely to talk about "trillions," "taxes," and "government," and their discussion of "Medicare" peaked in late 2009 and early 2010. Early in the debate, Democrats were likely to draw from a cluster of words that included "public" and "option" and to highlight issues related to costs and coverage. Later in the debate, Democrats' rhetoric shifted to a focus on insurance companies and affordability. For representatives of both parties, discussions of Senate voting and procedure ramped up as the Senate's formal consideration of the ACA in December 2009 approached.[88] Although our conclusions about framing are drawn initially from senators' press releases, these conclusions are not specific to that mode of communication. Elite frames on health care show considerable over-time variability. Even if political elites did want to follow Frank Luntz's advice and hammer home a single message repeatedly, the news cycle demands novelty, and political elites seemed to oblige.

A New View of Public Opinion

To increase this study's comparability with prior research and to ensure that its results are not a product of its novel method, sections of chapter 3 followed the traditional approach of analyzing closed-ended survey questions. The stability in health care attitudes documented in that chapter stands in contrast to the variability of elite frames identified here—and thus in contrast to claims that the public is strongly responsive to the elite frames salient at particular moments in time.[89]

Still, it is plausible that frames could influence public opinion without shifting overall policy attitudes. Frames might instead operate, for example, by shifting the reasons people give to justify a policy attitude. In this section, we apply LDA to open-ended responses from seven surveys during the health care debate to examine the reasons that respondents gave for their views. This analysis affords us a more subtle understanding of public opinion than we could attain by focusing exclusively on closed-ended survey questions.

Analyzing Open-Ended Responses

We identified seven telephone surveys that asked open-ended questions about health care reform and that were conducted from July 2009 through November 2011.[90] In all, we observed 8,533 responses over a period of twenty-nine months spanning from before the salient public debate until a year after the 2010 midterm elections. To illustrate this research design, figure 7.2 depicts the first four open-ended surveys alongside the distribution of press releases by month (gray lines). As this figure shows, while attempts at framing were already underway in July 2009, the most intense efforts at framing were still to come. What's more, given the punctuated elite frames uncovered in figure 7.3, it is clear that our open-ended baseline took place before key shifts in the content of elites' frames (see table E.4 for the full results).

Our analyses focus on the 6,363 respondents who used at least one of the 225 most common words in their responses.[91] Figure 7.4 presents the results using six panels, each of which illustrates the share of responses in a particular category over the first thirty-six months of the Obama administration. As a reference point, health care reform became salient in August and September 2009, and the bill was signed into law in March 2010. The response shares among supporters (solid lines) and opponents (dashed lines) are shown separately.

The cluster of words at the top left shows one coherent set of responses dominated by concerns about the expansion of government control. Unsurprisingly, this cluster was far more likely to be used by health care reform's opponents: the cluster never accounts for more than 9 percent of supporters' words and always accounts for at least 18 percent of opponents' words. Although there is some evidence of a decline in this cluster's use in October 2010, the general trend is toward consistency. Opponents were concerned about health care reform's impact on the scope of government as early as July 2009, before the issue became salient nationally, and they remained concerned well after the polarized debate and the passage of the law. The same is generally true for a separate cluster emphasizing the legislation's cost and tax impacts (top right); although it declined in use, this cluster always accounts for at least 19 percent of opponents' explanations.

These two clusters correspond to clusters of words identified earlier in the Republicans' press releases. Note, however, that these clusters were prominent in public opinion even before health care reform became a central issue in the late summer and early fall of 2009. The timing strongly suggests that the elite-level frames did not have causal effects: the core sources of opposition to the ACA were visible well before the legislation itself took shape. There is some evidence of a shift in rhetoric among health care reform opponents, but there is also considerable stability. Opponents were consistently concerned that the ACA represented an increase in governmental

Figure 7.4 Variation in Open-Ended Responses from Health Care Reform Supporters and Opponents over Time, 2009–2010

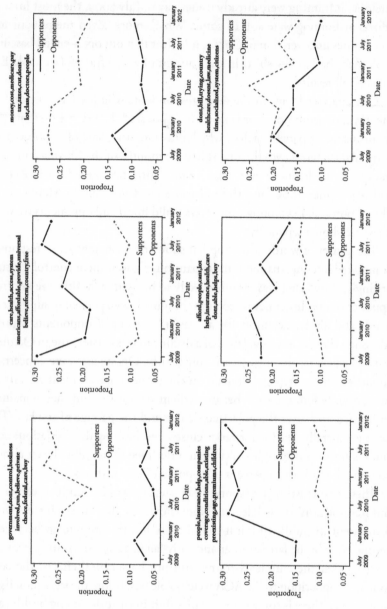

Source: Press releases compiled by author. Figure reprinted with permission from Springer (Hopkins 2018a).

Note: Model: LDA, fit to 6,355 open-ended survey responses in seven surveys.

authority that was likely to entail significant costs to taxpayers. Even the catchall sixth cluster, shown on the bottom right, reinforces this point, as "socialized" is among its prominent words. In no case do we see the words "death" or "panel," an observation that further limits the direct impact of Governor Palin's formulation. In fact, in the first survey after Palin's use of the term, not a single respondent employed the phrase.

Stability is clear among ACA supporters as well. We do see health care reform supporters shifting into the category defined by words like "people," "insurance," "help," and "companies" (bottom left), although the associated decline is from a similar cluster emphasizing the affordability of health insurance (bottom middle). What's more, even after the decline, 17 percent of all rhetoric by supporters drew on the affordability-related frame. Supporters also made heavy use of a frame emphasizing universal access and affordability (top middle), one defined by words such as "access," "affordable," "provide," and "universal." This frame always accounts for at least 19 percent of the explanations given by supporters for their views. One indication that this frame might be a default frame among supporters is that it was used somewhat more before the salient political debate (30 percent in July 2009) than afterwards (27 percent in November 2011).

Elite-level framing might explain the observed subtle shifts from focusing on universal coverage and affordability to focusing more specifically on insurance companies. Earlier we saw that Democratic senators focused on words like "insurance," "coverage," and "afford," a focus that grew more pronounced after the passage of the ACA in March 2010. Still, the overall finding is one of stability among mass-level supporters and opponents alike. There are shifts in the prominence of frames, but all of the core frames that citizens used after the salient moments of the health care debate were commonly used beforehand.

Does Language Diffuse from Elites to the Public?

Both in experimental and real-world settings, studies of framing analyze the effect of variation in frame exposure on public opinion as measured through closed-ended survey questions. That is precisely the approach we employed in the survey experiments on distrust detailed here. Yet this approach has multiple limitations. We already began to address one limitation: framing might influence the rationale behind a policy attitude without changing the attitude itself, making it plausible that the typical approach underestimates elite influence. Second, politicians might choose precisely those frames that resonate with preexisting public opinion, meaning that the frames' causal impact is unclear. This section reports the results of an approach examining the dynamic relationship between elite and mass-level word choice despite differences in these two modes of expression. At its base, this technique examines the changing similarity in word choice between elite and mass speech.[92]

We begin by identifying the word stems that appear in more than 1 percent of the 1,488 press releases and more than 0.25 percent of the open-ended survey responses. There are exactly 100 such word stems; neither "death" nor "panel" is among them. For parsimony, we focus on the open-ended responses from the three surveys that span the most salient parts of the debate. The first is in July 2009, before health care reform became highly salient with the August town hall meetings and the September presidential address. The second is in November 2009, in the thick of the legislative debate. And the third is in May 2010, more than one month after the passage of the ACA. We then identify the press releases that were issued between each of these surveys, giving us three measurements of opinion and two measurements of elite framing.

With baseline measures of public and elite language on the issue, we can then estimate how public language changed as the issue became salient and as political leaders deployed their frames. We can thus distinguish framing effects from elites' co-optation of public language. Specifically, we compare the frequency of word usage in the press releases with the frequency of the same words' usage among the public via multiple measures of association or distance.[93] If the press releases and the public use almost identical language, the distance between them will be low; if they rarely use the same words, it will be much higher. With these distance estimates, we can then calculate how the distances change at different points in time. Declines in distance indicate that when elites adopted certain language in their press releases, the members of the public subsequently shifted their vocabulary by adopting the same words.

To give some sense of the word-frequency distributions that are our core building blocks, we plot the difference in the distributions of words from four open-ended survey questions in figure 7.5. On the x-axis, we plot each word's overall frequency on the logged scale, while on the y-axis we plot the

Figure 7.5 Difference in Citizens' Word Usage for ACA Supporters and Opponents as a Function of Each Word's Frequency on the Log Scale, 2009–2010

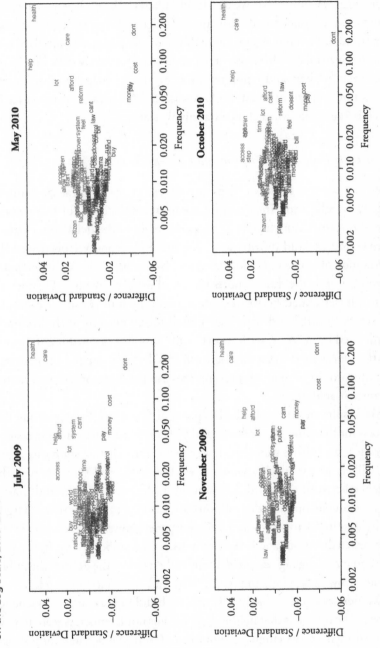

Source: Press releases compiled by author. Figure reprinted with permission from Springer (Hopkins 2018a).

Note: The y-axis has been rescaled by dividing by the word's standard deviation across responses. Words that appear more frequently in supporters' comments are above 0 on the y-axis, while those used more frequently by opponents are below 0 on the y-axis.

difference in word usage between supporters (positive numbers) and opponents (negative numbers). We divide this difference by each word's standard deviation across documents, reducing the magnitude for words whose usage is more variable. Here again, the stability of the popular vocabulary over time is on display, with opponents consistently using words like "pay," "cost," and "money" and supporters using words like "help," "health," "care," and "afford." Framing could not have changed Americans' word choice by much because that word choice was highly stable.

Connecting Politicians' Rhetoric and Citizens' Responses

How can we use these word-frequency estimates to measure framing effects? To take a specific example, we measure the effect of Democratic frames on American citizens in the early stages of the debate by creating three vectors of word distributions. The first and second vectors denote the distribution of words in the July 2009 and November 2009 Pew open-ended responses, while the third denotes the distribution of words in Democratic press releases issued between those surveys. In July 2009, for example, the stems "health" and "care" accounted for 29 percent of the common words used by citizens, with "don't" and "cost" being prominent as well. We then measure the distance between this distribution and the distribution of words in subsequent press releases using a common distance metric in content analyses.

The results are shown in the left panel of figure 7.6. By replicating this process for the same press releases and the open-ended responses measured *after* the press releases were issued, we can measure whether supporters grew more likely to use specific words after elites employed those words. The distance between the word distribution in the press releases and that in the subsequent open-ended responses measured in November is larger, as the upwards arrow in figure 7.6's left panel shows. This result is in the unexpected direction (and is also not statistically significant): the fit between elite and mass language *declined*. In the early stages of the debate, the public did not grow more likely to use the words in Democratic press releases.

We next assess how likely it is that such differences appear by chance alone.[94] The upshot is that neither Republicans nor Democrats seem to have adopted their party's language about the ACA in the debate's early stages. However, when we conduct the same analyses for the second period,

Figure 7.6 Distances or Correlations between Words Used in Senators' Press Releases and All Survey Respondents' Open-Ended Responses before and after the Issuance of Press Releases, 2009–2010

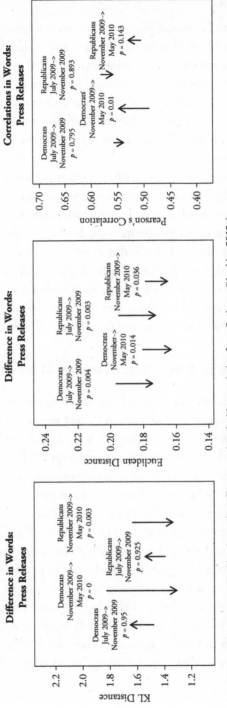

Source: Press releases compiled by the author. Figure reprinted with permission from Springer (Hopkins 2018a).

Note: Declining differences (left-hand and center panels) and increasing correlations (right-hand panel) indicate that the public is using words more similar to the words found in the press releases when surveyed after the press releases were issued. *p*-values are estimated through bootstrapping using ten thousand iterations.

between November 2009 and May 2010, we see a substantial and statistically significant decline in distance ($p < 0.001$), and it holds for the language of both Republican senators and citizens ($p = 0.003$). So we do see clear evidence of citizens adopting copartisans' language at the height of the debates over the ACA's passage.[95] We find not just that political elites and the public use similar words but that the similarity actually grew after the elites' public statements. This conclusion holds when we use alternative measures of distance.

From November 2009 to May 2010, citizens increasingly used the words commonly used by Democratic senators, and the same appears true for Republican senators' word choices. Elite rhetoric might not influence aggregate public opinion in demonstrable ways, but it does shape how citizens talk about an issue. The fact that it did so primarily after November 2009 further motivates this analysis's emphasis on the period from July 2009 to May 2010. Also, in contrast to the arguments of several commentators about Republicans' messaging advantage, there is no evidence that Republican words were more likely to be adopted than Democratic words.

Field Experiment: Government as the Messenger

At the same time, and on some of the same television stations where politicians were making appearances to deliver messages about the ACA, another public information campaign was underway: the promotion of enrollment in health insurance via the exchanges.[96] To varying degrees, many state governments and the federal government sought to encourage uninsured residents to buy insurance on the local exchanges. We saw earlier that messaging from explicitly partisan actors did not produce large-scale effects on public opinion, though it did have some influence on the words that Americans used to explain their ACA attitudes. But what about messaging on the concrete question of whether to purchase insurance via the exchanges? Were messages coming from government officials rather than politicians able to influence behavior?[97] Answers to these questions provide an opportunity to consider the effects of messaging on consequential behaviors instead of attitudes. They also enable us to integrate this chapter's prior analyses by providing causal estimates of real-world messaging.

In part, these questions are about the breadth of partisanship's influence. It is clear that citizens respond to messages from explicitly partisan actors by accounting for the messenger's partisanship.[98] But are ostensibly non-partisan government actors capable of having a wider impact? Prior research is mixed.[99] One estimate of governments' capacity to increase enrollments via messaging comes from Paul Shafer and his colleagues.[100] That study finds that the volume of state-level advertising—but not federal-level advertising—predicts marketplace enrollments.[101] It is possible that state governments are more influential because they are seen as less overtly partisan, or because their partisanship is more likely to match that of their citizens. Here we supplement existing evidence by briefly recounting a large-scale randomized field experiment on ACA enrollment conducted in 2015.[102]

During that year's open-enrollment period, I joined researchers and federal officials at the General Services Administration and the U.S. Department of Health and Human Services to administer a randomized experiment on the impact of government messaging on insurance enrollment.[103] Specifically, we identified people who had set up an account on the federal exchange website—which covered thirty-seven states at the time—but who had not yet enrolled as of mid-January 2015. Many of these people had considered their options on the exchanges but tentatively decided against buying insurance. Our total sample size was 744,510 people. After setting aside a control group, we sent citizens variants of a letter encouraging them to enroll, with each randomized feature designed to trigger different mechanisms highlighted in recent social and behavioral research. Some variants included action language, some suggested a descriptive norm of being insured, others showed a picture of the then-CEO of the marketplaces, and still others included a combination of these elements. This experiment differs from the studies described here. The letters were sent by a government actor, so they all featured broad appeals and conveyed no explicitly partisan cues. The interventions involved tweaking language, not conveying different issue frames. But the experiment provides a large-scale, real-world test of the effects of messaging on ACA-related behaviors.

Of the members of the control group who received no letter, only 4.0 percent wound up enrolling in a plan through the exchanges. Those who did receive a letter were 0.3 percentage points more likely to enroll overall. That effect is certainly meaningful but not overwhelmingly large; in all,

Figure 7.7 Respondents' Enrollment via the Exchanges after Receipt of Different Randomly Assigned Letters from the U.S. Government Encouraging Enrollment, 2015

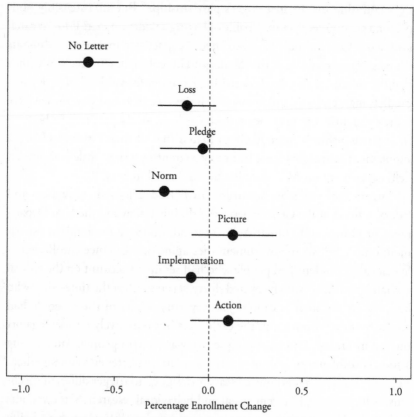

Source: Administrative data from U.S. government (Yokum et al. 2022).

it translated to an additional 1,753 enrollments. More importantly, as figure 7.7 illustrates, the primary effect on enrollment was induced by receiving any letter at all: while attempts to invoke a descriptive norm were not as effective as other elements in the letters, the differences between most of the letter variants were not substantively or statistically significant. Communication and messaging clearly play a role in shaping citizens' knowledge about public policies, yet this experiment adds to the evidence shown throughout this chapter that tweaking language on its own is not likely to have large effects on attitudes or behaviors. That was true not only for attitudes toward the ACA but also for enrollment via the newly created exchanges.

Conclusion

For mass- and elite-level opponents of the ACA, the legislation's cost and call for an increased governmental role were central reasons for opposition. Consider the following argument: "This may be your last chance to weigh the consequences of taking the first step toward establishment of socialized medicine in the United States. . . . When costs get out of line . . . there are three possible courses of action. The first is to reduce the benefits; the second is to increase taxes; the third is to impose government controls of the services."[104] Certainly, that message would have been an unsurprising addition to the press releases and TV appearances analyzed in this chapter. But that particular quotation, written by the president of the American Medical Association, actually comes from the 1965 debates over Medicare. Even across the decades, the rhetoric used to support and oppose health care reform has been notable in its consistency, a point that our mass-level results reinforce. Such consistency places a low ceiling on the extent of the influence of politicians' frames at any one moment: a variable cannot explain a constant. This observation in turn suggests the value of studying not just specific political debates but also the contours of public debate over broad swaths of time.[105] As we saw in chapter 6, framing is not a source of short-term elite influence over public opinion, but a complex, interactive process that unfolds over many years.

This chapter first reported four survey experiments, three of which found no evidence of framing effects and one of which found a detectable but not game-changing effect. (The three experiments on distrust found no meaningful impacts on ACA attitudes, while the 2011 messaging experiment found discernible effects on health spending preferences.) We then applied automated content analyses to the health care rhetoric of public officials and American citizens from 2009 to 2010. These tools enable us to summarize the central arguments for and against health care reform and to analyze shifts over the course of the debate. They provide a more granular view of public opinion than typical approaches allow. We saw, for example, that supporters at the elite and mass levels alike emphasized the expansion of insurance and increased access to health care. Yet the fact that citizens supportive of the ACA used these arguments to explain their views even before the health care reform debate came to dominate headlines suggests the limited influence of elite rhetoric on overall evaluations. Key elements of public opinion toward the ACA were in place even before political elites began their most visible attempts at framing the law to their advantage. In particular, the phrase "death panels," which many observers thought to be profoundly influential, shows little evidence of having penetrated public opinion.[106]

Analyzing the fit between elite and mass word choice enables us to measure communication effects—whether frames or not—with increased precision and subtlety. When doing so, we see that citizens grew more likely to use the same words as their elected officials over the course of the public debate over the ACA. In this case, such effects appear to be roughly symmetric: the word choices of both Democratic and Republican senators and citizens at large became increasingly correlated. Although it does not move overall evaluations by much, elite rhetoric appears to shape the rationale underpinning those evaluations.[107]

By using press releases, television appearances, and open-ended survey questions to test hypotheses about framing, this chapter has provided an example of how text and automated content analysis can provide new vantage points on old questions. And on one specific old question, the results of such analyses are unequivocal: elite influence through messaging or framing is quite limited. Yes, framing can influence how citizens describe their views, but the content of their views proves harder to move. In the case of a large-scale government communications effort to encourage ACA enrollment, the main effect stemmed simply from receiving the letter, not from the specific psychological levers triggered by the different letters. The writer and television producer Peter Pomerantsev describes the public as "just bit-part players in the political technologists' great reality show."[108] But at least with respect to Americans' health care attitudes and behaviors, that overstates the case. Political elites, and even presidents, are quite limited in their ability to reframe a political debate.

"We are a species that delights in story. We look out on reality, we grasp patterns, and we join them into narratives that can captivate, inform, startle, amuse, and thrill."[109] Those are the words of the physicist Brian Greene. There is nothing in this chapter that contradicts those ideas. Narratives and metaphors are central ways in which people organize information.[110] Studies of real-world framing indicate that the frames adopted by journalists, politicians, and academics can have long-term impacts on the shape of politics.[111] The point of this chapter is not that such frames are irrelevant, but simply that politicians alone are very limited in their capacity to shape them.

CHAPTER 8

Conclusion

IN LATE 2021 and well into 2022, the Democratic Party found itself riven by two separate debates. One was about policy and legislation: with unified control of the U.S. House of Representatives, U.S. Senate, and the presidency, Democrats were trying to pass a federal budget that would expand elements of the ACA while also tackling climate change and transforming social policy—all while winning the support of virtually every congressional Democrat given the party's razor-tight margins in both chambers. The second debate was focused on political strategy: which groups of would-be voters should the Democrats target in an attempt to preserve or expand their electoral coalition for the 2022 midterm elections and beyond?[1]

In both debates, the starting premise was that the Democrats' choices were likely to have meaningful and direct electoral consequences, whether via the policies they enacted or via the messaging they adopted. On the policy side, key proposals were evaluated partly in electoral terms. For example, some hoped that offering health insurance coverage to low-income Americans in states that had not expanded Medicaid might help Georgia Democratic senator Raphael Warnock in his 2022 reelection bid. Others touted the electoral benefits of offering dental coverage through Medicare or extending the pandemic-era child tax credit. Politicians do not tend to cite political science in justifying their actions, but in this case they could have. Extensive research on policy feedbacks finds that enacting policies *can* change political behaviors and—at least under some conditions—attitudes.

On the messaging side, the key question was about coalition-building: at whom should the party's messaging be targeted? Which policies should the party trumpet, and which should it downplay or drop? Here, too, politicians' assumptions are grounded in an extensive political science literature, this one on messaging and framing. Still, the core claim of this book is that both debates are built on a false premise—an overstatement of just how much elites can move public opinion through either policy or messaging in today's highly polarized and nationalized era. To date, researchers have framed these questions in binary ways, asking yes/no questions about the presence of elite influence. This book has asked a related but different question, one that is relevant to politicians and researchers alike: Just how large are messaging or policy feedback effects on policy attitudes? The answer, in this period, is that such effects are typically quite small.[2] Careful attention to effect sizes can bridge some of the discrepancies between theory and practice. And it can illuminate the powerful limitations on political elites' influence.

To better understand the interplay between public policy, Americans' lived experiences, and their reactions to contemporary politics, this book has sought to provide a comprehensive assessment of Americans' ACA attitudes in the period between 2009 and 2021. During the law's first tumultuous decade, it was a lightning rod for interparty conflict, as Republicans and Democrats battled over the law in Congress, statehouses, and courthouses. The stakes were high: the cost and availability of health insurance for millions nationwide, as well as the expanding scope of governmental authority. Through their messaging and policymaking, political elites from both parties tried to influence citizens' thinking and win their support.

If we are looking for a policy area that touches on citizens' daily lives and so represents a potential avenue of elite influence through personal experience, health care seems a promising starting point. When explaining Revolutionary America to his late-twentieth-century readers in *Undaunted Courage*, historian Stephen Ambrose notes that "people in the late eighteenth century were helpless in matters of health. They lived in constant dread of sudden death from disease, plague, epidemic, pneumonia, or accident. Their letters always begin and usually end with assurances of the good health of the letter writer and a query about the health of the recipient."[3] Long before the Covid-19 era, people valued their own health and the health of their families more than almost anything.

Despite the personal importance of good health, and despite health care's preeminence as an issue in the 2009–2021 period, elite attempts to shift public opinion on the ACA were largely unsuccessful. This book has shown that elite influence—through policy as well as messaging—was far more limited than suggested by either Democratic Party debates or prior scholarship. The Medicaid expansion did lead to demonstrable increases in ACA favorability among low-income Americans in affected states, but even these effects were not very large, and they were blunted not only by the incomplete implementation of the Medicaid expansion but also by this group's relatively low levels of political engagement (chapter 4). For at least some of the ACA's beneficiaries, the benefits were quite sizable and unambiguously positive, suggesting that benefit size alone is not the primary explanation for why the ACA failed to produce more of an imprint on public opinion.

The ACA bundled various policy levers and so provides insights on the extent to which different levers produce different effects. The ACA's exchanges dispensed subsidies averaging $4,000 to 6.1 million Americans in 2016 alone and were originally expected to be the main driver of increased insurance uptake.[4] But their complex, backdoor policy design—plus the rocky implementation and unpopular individual mandate—led to offsetting impacts overall (chapter 5). In a polarized and nationalized environment, the ACA's complexity let it become synonymous with its least popular element for millions of Americans.

To construe this research as producing evidence against policy feedbacks in general overstates the case. In fact, as chapter 2 detailed, within American political institutions, policy feedbacks shaped the ACA in profound ways. The law was a complex patchwork of subsidies and backdoor regulations precisely because it sought to extend health insurance without significantly disrupting the existing employer-provided system for those under sixty-five. Ironically, those very institutional policy feedbacks led to a law whose ability to generate consistent feedback effects among the mass public was circumscribed.

Messaging's impacts on public opinion are limited as well, especially over the time frames most relevant to politicians. In chapter 6, we saw that the clearest case for the influence of racial attitudes came through their long-term effects on partisanship and on policy narratives. Neither observational nor experimental evidence suggests that rhetoric that primed racial attitudes had much influence on white Americans' ACA views in the short term. Likewise, the barrage of elite messages did influence the words that supporters and opponents of the ACA used but had little impact on the underlying distribution of opinions on the law (chapter 7).

This study focuses on a single policy in a single country advanced by the Democratic Party at a specific moment in time. Given the well-documented asymmetries in the political parties and their coalitions, it is quite possible that elite influence works differently for GOP-backed policies or for issues beyond social policy. That said, the preliminary evidence suggests that politicians' influence on public opinion is limited in other arenas besides ACA attitudes.[5] In March 2020, Covid-19's arrival in the United States prompted a dramatic response from policymakers, who shuttered schools and businesses while urging the public to stay home. In the pandemic's early days, politicians' communications and stay-at-home policies proved impactful.[6] But political polarization on Covid-related policies set in rapidly, and subsequent waves of elite-level rhetoric and policy were less influential in changing the public's willingness to stay at home or engage in social distancing.[7] As the pandemic dragged on, citizens' behaviors remained responsive to local levels of Covid-19, but less so to politicians' policies or rhetoric. Like the ACA's first decade, the experience of the Covid-19 pandemic and America's political response demonstrate the profound limits that politicians face when trying to change citizens' minds.

The federal aid offered in response to the pandemic also provided added (though preliminary) evidence about the limits of policy feedbacks on public opinion. Early in 2021, President Biden and congressional Democrats expanded the Child Tax Credit (CTC) to between $3,000 and $3,600 per child for all families, a policy that significantly reduced the number of American children in poverty. But despite the policy's popularity and the size of the benefit, Congress opted not to extend the expanded CTC, and it lapsed with little fanfare at the end of 2021.[8] The CTC was but one element of the mammoth 2021 American Rescue Plan (ARP), which dramatically increased U.S. government spending and surely merits more detailed study as a potential source of policy feedbacks and elite influence. But the initial evidence certainly does not suggest much of a pro-Democratic impact, as the party downplayed the law in 2022 campaigns despite payments to citizens that were unconditional as well as unprecedented. Certainly, the passage of the law didn't prevent the Democrats from losing the House of Representatives in 2022 after a meaningful pro-GOP shift in House voting. And of course, the ARP wasn't the only new legislation in 2021–2022: Congress also passed an infrastructure bill and the Inflation Reduction Act, which made broad changes to taxes, climate policy, and health care.

Still, if the politics of the Covid-19 pandemic reinforces this book's core argument, the more general experience of America's president during the pandemic's early days might seem to contradict it. That is because Donald Trump is thought to be able to persuade at least the sizable fraction of American citizens who view him favorably. In the wake of the 2020 election, for instance, Trump falsely claimed that he had won several key states; in a survey of Republican activists that Hans Noel and I conducted in April 2021, a striking 77 percent of them agreed, saying that Trump "probably won" or "definitely won" the election.[9] Surely Trump's ability to generate such doubts about the legitimacy of the election despite all the evidence to the contrary shows the impacts of elite-level rhetoric? Well, yes, intraparty rhetorical influence is very real, and it undoubtedly deserves more study. Still, even such influence has its limits. In challenging the legitimacy of the 2020 election, Trump drew on long-standing racially inflected narratives about voter fraud that some supporters had little reason to disbelieve. In August 2021, however, after Trump told an audience, "I recommend taking the vaccines," the boos that followed were audible.[10] Trump's apparent influence with his supporters may stem not only from his invocation of familiar narratives (chapters 6 and 7) but also from his avoidance of positions they are likely to disagree with.

More to the point, this book has analyzed the influence of elite rhetoric on the public generally, not on politicians' supporters—and not during the height of political campaigns. By this book's metric, the evidence is clear that even Donald Trump was not especially persuasive. We saw in chapter 3 that soon after Trump's 2016 election, just as his bully pulpit was growing, public support for the ACA grew as well. Although not our focus here, similar dynamics were at work on immigration attitudes and prejudice.[11] As Trump became increasingly prominent politically, opinion among the broader public shifted *against* his core messages. Like Obama, Trump appeared unable to move the opinion of those who were not his supporters— at least not in the direction he wanted. He could polarize more than he could persuade. Still, the example of Trump is a useful reminder that this book is focused on persuasion overall—that is, on attempts to persuade those not already predisposed to agree.

The question of *why* contemporary elite influence is so circumscribed is beyond our scope here. That said, this book has repeatedly proposed political polarization and nationalization as engines stabilizing public opinion in the face of elite actions.[12] A highly polarized and nationalized polity may be one in which citizens are moved more by national symbols than by personal experiences. Other related social changes merit scrutiny too, from the decline of organized mass-membership organizations to the fragmentation of the media landscape.[13] In tandem, these transformations may have led to a complex, atomized social and political world in which the proliferation of organizations and information sources limits the influence of any one.[14] In such a complex and fragmented political landscape, it is difficult for politicians to focus sustained public attention on any one problem or policy, and maybe we shouldn't expect uniform effects across broad swaths of the population.

The Impact and Limits of Public Opinion

This book has focused on explaining public opinion toward the ACA and documenting its remarkable stability. Of course, the dynamics of public opinion are not necessarily the central explanation for why the elite-level politics of the ACA played out as they did. Indeed, one of the book's themes has been the enduring disconnect between elite actions and public opinion. Many of the policy decisions that shaped the ACA—even decisions that affected millions of people—took place well outside the public's view and often with little direct public input.[15] Instead, these decisions were typically the products of bargaining and contestation between politicians, interest groups, bureaucrats, lobbyists, lawyers, and judges.[16] As we saw in chapters 2 and 3, dramatic shifts in the elite-level politics of the ACA were often invisible in citizens' aggregate evaluations of the law. Elites have a hard time moving public opinion, but they still have substantial leeway to act in its blind spots.[17]

The Trump administration's executive actions on the ACA are a useful example. After the failure of congressional attempts to repeal the ACA in 2017, the Trump administration faced a choice about how to administer the law. Would it oversee the law in a way that would encourage enrollment and try to limit premiums? As we saw in chapter 2, the Trump administration chose to do the opposite, seeking to undermine the ACA through a set of legal, administrative, marketing, budgetary, and regulatory avenues. But that was not what the public wanted. In October and November 2018, the ISCAP panel included a question about how the administration should handle the ACA. Specifically, it asked: should "President Trump and his administration . . . do what they can to make the current health care law work, or should they do what they can to make the current health care law fail so they can replace it later?" Overall, 57 percent of respondents said that the Trump administration should make the current health care law work, while just 17 percent said that it should work to sabotage the law. Among Republicans, the split was almost even, with 32 percent opting for making the law work and 30 percent saying that it should undermine the law. The fact that 24 percent of all respondents said that they did not know or were not sure indicates that there was considerable uncertainty among the public. Even if the ACA overall was highly visible, specific questions about its implementation were not, and so Trump, like Obama before him, had significant latitude within which to maneuver.

Still, the imprint of public opinion is clearly visible in the ACA's evolution during its first decade. In some cases, the role of the public was quite direct and supportive of the law. Some states—for example, Idaho, Kansas, Maine, Missouri, South Dakota, Utah, and Oklahoma—were prodded to expand their Medicaid programs by voter-passed initiatives mandating that they do so. Chapter 4 told the stories of Maine and Oklahoma in some detail. And chapter 6, by discussing the role of racial prejudice in ACA attitudes, made clear that the politics of the Medicaid expansion differed from the politics of welfare reform in the 1980s and 1990s. Race provided one lens that shaped white Americans' views of the ACA, but it was not the only lens, and it was not an especially immediate one.

In other cases, public opinion's influence worked to circumscribe the law. A January 2010 poll found that the individual mandate was opposed by 62 percent of respondents, even as other ACA elements garnered majority support.[18] The mandate's unpopularity also showed up in election returns: Ohio voters passed a symbolic 2011 initiative exempting state residents from the ACA's mandate to purchase health insurance by more than thirty percentage points. As a candidate, Barack Obama himself had opposed the individual mandate, although he then came to embrace it as a tool to avoid adverse selection and keep premiums down. But it is critical to note that the individual mandate was the one element of the ACA that the Republicans were able to repeal, as they did by setting the penalty at $0 in a late-2017 tax bill. (Ironically, the mandate also proved an ineffective policy, as Molly Frean, Jonathan Gruber, and Benjamin Sommers show.)[19]

As we have seen, the public's views of the ACA did not closely track elite-level debates or machinations. Even so, by 2022 the ACA had evolved in line with the popularity of its constituent elements: the individual mandate had been eliminated, but an increasing number of states had expanded Medicaid. In their study of state-level policies and public opinion, Devin Caughey and Christopher Warshaw find strong evidence that American states update their policies in the direction of public opinion over long periods of time.[20] Likewise, we have seen compatible evidence from health care reform: in its broad outlines, the ACA evolved in precisely the directions the public wanted. The public's influence on policymaking hinges on the policy's salience—the public is better positioned to get what it wants on big-ticket questions than on narrower, less visible policy issues.

In still other cases, the role of public opinion was less direct but none-theless formidable. The Republican Party made the ACA a centerpiece of its congressional campaigns in 2010 and 2014 in part because public opinion toward the law was generally negative. In the 2010 national exit polls, for example, 48 percent of respondents advocated repealing the law, while 31 percent thought it should be expanded and just 16 percent thought it should be left as is.[21] In such an environment, it is not surprising that Republicans came to prioritize ACA repeal. Potentially more surprising is how committed the GOP was to the goal of repeal in later years, after overall public opinion began to shift in the law's favor. Having campaigned extensively on ACA repeal when it was popular, Republicans found them-selves boxed in when it became less so. It is instructive as well that GOP repeal attempts managed to do what the ACA's implementation could not: make the law popular with a majority of Americans. Post-enactment, the one major shift in ACA attitudes moved *against* the direction of elite policy-making. So much for elite influence.

Certainly, the salience of the ACA over more than a decade may have crowded out other items on the political agenda. In that way, the ACA may have jeopardized the connection between public opinion and subsequent public policymaking on other issues, hindering the capacity of policymakers to respond to citizens' wishes. But in broad strokes, the ACA of 2022 matched public opinion more closely than did the ACA of 2010.

Distilling the ACA's Lessons for Policy Advocates

One goal of this book is to distill the key lessons of public opinion on the ACA for future fights over other policy areas. Most of the lessons emerge principally from the research reported here, while some synthesize long-standing arguments and evidence in political science:

1. When the public evaluates a complex, multifaceted policy, *the whole is not equal to the sum of its parts.* Some aspects of the policy may be highly visible to the public, while others may be all but invisible. And the public may not see any integral connection between a policy's more and less popular features. When it comes to policy, a spoonful of sugar may not help the medicine go down.
2. After enactment, *the design of a policy can influence which of its aspects trigger self-interest, thus shaping attitudes toward the policy.* But self-interest's effects are limited in size, and they have a negative skew: policies that impose costs are more likely to trigger reactions than policies that provide benefits.
3. Because they are likely to generate heterogeneous experiences among citizens, *complex policies are unlikely to foster consistently positive policy feedback effects in aggregate.*
4. *Surveys offer only a partial glimpse of political reality.* Citizens' reactions to positions described in a survey are not always reliable guides to how they will react when a concrete proposal is on the table and subject to partisan attacks.
5. Public opinion reliably moves away from the direction being advanced by the president. It commonly acts like a thermostat, shifting to counterbalance the direction in which the president and Congress move policy.[22] Here we have seen that *even the threat of a major policy change can be enough to move public opinion.*
6. In an era of intense political polarization, *one side's indication that a policy is among its top priorities may push the opposing party into all-out opposition.* Frances Lee terms this "reflexive partisanship."[23]
7. A key decision that opposition parties make is whether or not to stridently oppose a policy. Outspoken opposition is likely to bring voters who share their partisanship into alignment. However, *more*

tactical decisions about the specific messages to use do not do much to move public opinion.

8. Even a policy that is seemingly novel to its architects is not likely to be thought of as such by most citizens. Instead, *citizens typically view new policies through the lens of long-standing narratives about the role of government and the deservingness of visible social and racial groups.*

9. Considered jointly, *these observations demonstrate a critical disconnect between the public's views on policy and those of policymakers.* In a democracy, there is a presumption that public opinion should decide issues that divide elites. But this evidence indicates that aggregate public opinion, though coherent, is nevertheless not positioned to be the ultimate arbiter on more technical, low-salience policy questions. When deciding many midlevel policy issues, political leaders are often operating within the public's "electoral blind spot."[24] And to the extent that contemporary political polarization and gridlock keep Congress from addressing big-ticket issues, that electoral blind spot may include a growing share of the policies that Congress is able to pass.

Implications for Studying Politics

These results point to an important distinction that gets little emphasis in political science research—the distinction between the *statistical* and *substantive* significance of effects. As this book makes clear, the public does respond to policies and elite-level rhetoric to some degree. At the same time, these effects are quite modest relative to broader swings in public opinion.[25] From a researcher's vantage point, are there policy feedback effects on public opinion in the near term? Definitely. Such effects are detectable. But from a politician's point of view, are such effects large enough to meaningfully change the balance of political support? No. Enacting any one new policy may provide an edge in the tightest of races, but it is unlikely to build a durable political coalition or to be the difference between victory and defeat.

In a highly competitive era, politicians often justify policies in electoral terms.[26] But the evidence here shows that politicians should not expect policy to build coalitions, especially if the policy is incremental or complex and the political environment remains polarized. The implication, in turn, is that the public will neither reward nor punish politicians for many of their policy choices—and thus that elected officials have significant latitude to enact policies without worrying about their political impacts. After all, as long as those policies do not lead to significant losses for citizens, their political effects are likely to be limited. In theory, this latitude could allow policymakers to focus on designing and implementing effective policies, safe in the knowledge that they are probably not missing an opportunity to foster constituent support directly. In practice, however, policymakers are certain to face competing considerations. (Among those considerations are activists—key political actors whose demands may be obscured by an exclusive focus on elites and the mass public.)[27]

Beyond its emphasis on substantive significance, this book has challenged contemporary practice in political science in another way. In recent decades, the study of public opinion and political behavior has come to rely heavily on experiments, a valuable development that has led to marked improvements in causal inference.[28] But as we saw in chapters 6 and 7, there are critical sources of influence that do not act contemporaneously and so are not as easily tested via survey experiments.[29] In particular, chapter 6 emphasizes the historical role of racial divisions in sorting white Americans into political parties and also in reinforcing narratives about social policy, redistribution, and fairness. Born partly of racial animus and reinforced over decades, such narratives can retain some power even in situations that are not themselves explicitly racialized. Understanding the hold of such narratives is thus critical. But in contemporary political science, there is an enduring tension between the research questions we ask and the methods we use to answer those questions.[30] That tension has limited our knowledge of the influence of such narratives, as well as our knowledge of other factors whose effects unfold over long periods of time. Still, the claim that narratives matter does not mean that they are easily influenced by any one political actor.

The Contours of Future Health Policy Battles

Even in 2022, thirteen years after the ACA was first debated in Congress, health care policymaking remains unsettled. The parties are deeply divided, certainly, but there are divisions within the parties as well. During the early stages of the 2020 presidential campaign, Democratic candidates split on the path forward: candidates Joe Biden and Pete Buttigieg backed an expansion of the ACA, while Bernie Sanders and Elizabeth Warren argued for expansive single-payer health care plans. Such proposals were clearly grounded in dissatisfaction with the ACA and the patchwork health insurance system of which it is a part. But any attempt to further reform health care or insurance is likely to trigger many of the same public opinion dynamics observed with the ACA. In fact, the ACA has already picked much of the low-hanging political fruit, as it increased insurance enrollment without substantially disrupting employer-sponsored health care. Health care reforms that go significantly beyond the ACA are likely to pose a more direct threat to citizens' existing interests and thus to provoke a sharper short-term backlash. We saw in chapter 5 that the cancellation of noncompliant health care plans alongside the individual mandate worked to suppress any positive impacts of the ACA's exchanges on other citizens. Now imagine scaling up such disruptions by a factor of ten or more if Congress sought to curtail or end private health insurance.

Meanwhile, on the right, we noted that in December 2017 congressional Republicans and President Trump successfully repealed the ACA's mandate that most people have health insurance. And Trump's administration took a variety of executive actions to undercut the ACA between 2017 and 2021, from reducing ACA outreach efforts to extending short-term plans that do not meet the ACA's requirements for comprehensive insurance.[31] By the end of 2018, the rate of uninsured Americans had climbed to 13.7 percent, from a low of 10.9 percent two years prior.[32]

At the same time, other conservative health policy ideas advanced during Trump's 2017–2021 term. For example, as of June 2019, sixteen states had formally proposed modifying their Medicaid programs to mandate work requirements.[33] The Biden administration subsequently rejected these proposals, but they signal one possible policy direction for future Republican administrations.[34] The ACA's first decade provides hints and warnings about how the public is likely to respond to these opposing policy choices.

On a given day, much of the punditry about American politics starts from the assumption that Americans are paying close attention to political events and that any elite-level event needs to be viewed partly through the lens of public opinion. Politicians, the story goes, pass policies to gain advantages with voters. This book has demonstrated why I disagree, and that disagreement has implications for policymaking. The immediate electoral rewards for enacting most policies in today's polarized environment are likely to be low. There is an asymmetry, however, that the ACA makes clear: both parties were penalized for pursuing unpopular policies. Voters seem better positioned to punish than to reward.

This book has highlighted the stark disconnect between the frenetic and relentless elite-level maneuvering over the ACA and the public's steady attitudes. At a high level, public opinion toward the ACA was largely stable and coherent: it was shaped by similar factors and stabilized by common narratives over long periods of time. The public acts like something of an absentee parent, with authority it rarely uses. For that reason, explanations for shifts in American political behavior are not likely to emerge from sudden changes in what the public thinks about a given issue. Instead, such changes are likely to come from changes in the attitudes mobilized into politics at a particular political moment. Public opinion does not change on a dime, but the aspects of it that are politically relevant sometimes do.[35] In the medium run, a primary challenge facing political organizers and elites is not shifting opinions, but fostering collective action among the already like-minded.

APPENDIX A (CHAPTER 3)

ISCAP Panel Details

Table A.1 summarizes the dates and sample sizes of the ISCAP panels.

Table A.2 details the demographics of the ISCAP panel. Our respondents were older than the U.S. population, but that is to be expected: they had to be eighteen in late 2007 to participate. On a variety of other metrics, even those who participated in the final waves are a reasonable approximation of the target population of U.S. adults over twenty-five. For example, our sample's mean income in 2016 was $58,400, which is not far from the 2015 U.S. median household income of $54,900. Of particular importance is the fact that there is no evidence of heightened attrition rates among those who were less politically engaged. We merged our data with validated vote histories provided by the data vendor Catalist and found that voter turnout was essentially indistinguishable among those who remained in the panel between 2012 and 2016 and those who did not. Specifically, 2008 turnout was 69.4 percent among the 2,471 respondents to the post-election 2012 wave and 69.0 percent among the 1,075 respondents who participated in the post-election 2016 wave.

Table A.1 ISCAP Panel Waves and Sample Sizes

Wave	Start Date	End Date	N
Wave 1	October 2, 2007	December 31, 2007	19,190
Wave 2	January 1, 2008	March 31, 2008	17,747
Wave 3	April 2, 2008	August 28, 2008	20,052
Wave 4	August 29, 2008	November 4, 2008	19,241
Wave 5	November 5, 2008	January 20, 2009	19,234
Wave 6	October 19, 2012	October 29, 2012	2,606
Wave 7	November 14, 2012	January 29, 2013	2,471
Wave 8	October 17, 2014	October 31, 2014	1,693
Wave 9	November 19, 2014	January 14, 2015	1,493
Wave 10	January 22, 2016	February 8, 2016	1,562
Wave 11	October 14, 2016	October 24, 2016	1,227
Wave 12	November 28, 2016	December 7, 2016	1,075
Wave 13	October 23, 2018	November 5, 2018	1,024

Source: ISCAP panel, 2007–2018 (Hopkins and Mutz 2022).

Coding Open-Ended Health Care Responses

Codebook Version 1.3

BASIC INSTRUCTIONS

In the spreadsheet, please create twelve new columns, labeling them "ARGUMENT," "SELF," "GROUP," "GROUPNAME," "POLITICIAN," "POLITICIANNAME," "POLICY," "POLICYNAME", "PLACE," "PLACENAME," "METAPHOR," and "FIT." Also, please rename the spreadsheet to add your initials (for example, "openendjul09DJH.csv").

Then, please read each open-ended response carefully. Please (1) *correct any spelling errors* you see, so as to enable the automated procedures to recognize the word in question, but *do not worry about grammar* or punctuation. It may be more efficient to simply *use spell-check* on all responses first. Then, for each response, please (2) *enter the appropriate numeric codes* in the spreadsheet as described below. If more than one code is appropriate, please code the first segment of the open-ended response.

Table A.2 Demographics of Respondents across Surveys

	Minimum	Maximum	Wave 4 2008		Wave 7 2012		Wave 16 2016		ACS 2015
			Mean	Missing[a]	Mean	Missing[a]	Mean	Missing[a]	Mean
Income, 2008[b]	2.50	250.00	61.38	0.31	57.72	0.07	58.40	0.00	54.89
Years of education, 2008	4.00	19.00	14.33	0.00	13.76	0.00	13.68	0.00	
High school degree, 2008	0.00	1.00	0.96	0.00	0.94	0.00	0.94	0.00	0.87
Bachelor's degree, 2008	0.00	1.00	0.40	0.00	0.31	0.00	0.30	0.00	0.30
Party identification, 2008	1.00	7.00	3.87	0.15	3.82	0.17	3.87	0.14	
Union household, 2008	0.00	1.00	0.09	0.00	0.12	0.00	0.13	0.00	
Catholic, 2008	0.00	1.00	0.16	0.00	0.21	0.00	0.20	0.00	
Protestant, 2008	0.00	1.00	0.27	0.00	0.31	0.00	0.33	0.00	
Female, 2008	0.00	1.00	0.56	0.00	0.53	0.00	0.50	0.00	0.51
Age, 2008	18.00	110.00	50.13	0.00	47.12	0.00	48.84	0.00	
Over sixty-five, 2008	0.00	1.00	0.17	0.00	0.14	0.00	0.15	0.00	0.15
Black, 2008	0.00	1.00	0.09	0.00	0.13	0.00	0.12	0.00	0.13
Hispanic, 2008	0.00	1.00	0.06	0.00	0.10	0.00	0.10	0.00	0.17
White, 2008	0.00	1.00	0.80	0.00	0.71	0.00	0.71	0.00	0.77
Voted, 2012					0.69	.21	0.69	0.21	
N			19,241		2,471		1,075		

Source: American Community Survey, 2015 (U.S. Census Bureau 2020; ISCAP panel (Hopkins and Mutz 2022).

Note: The American Community Survey benchmarks come from July 1, 2015, estimates for the full U.S. population.

[a] "Missing" refers to the share of that variable which is missing for respondents to the designated panel wave.

[b] The U.S. census reports median household income, not mean income.

1. **Argument:** What is the main reason this person supports or opposes health care reform?

Arguments in Support

    11. *Access:* "People will be able to get care more easily"; "people will be able to see a doctor"; "people won't go without care"; "gives people with preexisting conditions health care."

    12. *Fairness/equality/right to health care:* "Everyone should have health care." Note that this category is a normative claim about what people should have or deserve to have.

    13. *Affordability/personal costs:* "It will make health insurance more affordable."

    14. *Governmental costs/deficit/lower taxes:* "It will help us reduce the deficit"; "get control over runaway entitlement spending."

    15. *Quality of health care:* "It will improve the quality of care."

    16. *Consumer protection/distrust insurance companies:* "Insurance companies shouldn't discriminate or take advantage"; "insurance companies can no longer discriminate by preexisting conditions."

    17. *Step in right direction:* "While I wanted a public option, this is better than the current system."

    18. *Process/timing/overdue:* "It's about time"; "we've waited so long"; "need to move on and worry about other things."

    23. *Abortion:* "The law will not directly fund abortion."

    24. *Economic/other systemic benefits:* "People will be able to find new jobs more easily"; "this bill will help fix the economy"; "healthy people are more productive."

    25. *Positive opinion leadership:* "Jesse Jackson supports this law."

    26. *Positive for specific social group/program:* "This will help children"; "this will strengthen Medicare."

    27. *Positive international comparison:* "This will make our system more like Canada's."

    28. *General positive:* "The country needs this."

Arguments in Opposition

    31. *Access/constrain choice/rationing care:* "I won't be able to pick my doctor"; "I'll have to wait for care"; "I won't be able to get the care I need"; "it will bring about death panels."

32. *Fairness/deservingness/opposition to paying for others:* "I shouldn't have to pay if someone doesn't get health insurance"; "health care is not a right."

33. *Affordability/personal costs:* "It will make it impossible for people to afford health insurance/drive up costs for consumers."

34. *Government cost/deficit/raise taxes:* "It will cost too much and drive taxes/the deficit up."

35. *Quality of health care:* "It will hurt the quality of health care in the U.S."

36. *Governmental inefficiency:* "We can't trust the government to run the health care system"; "the government won't be able to provide health care well at all."

37. *Single payer/public option:* "This bill doesn't create a single-payer system"; "this bill doesn't include a public option."

38. *Legislative/policymaking process:* "This bill wasn't bipartisan, it was rammed down the throat of Congress/rushed through/wasn't read by legislators."

39. *Rights/Constitution/mandate:* "It infringes on my rights to have to buy health care"; "bill is unconstitutional"; opposition to individual mandate; "don't like being forced to buy something."

40. *Proper role of government/government control/government take-over:* "Government shouldn't run health care"; "bill is socialism/communism"; "we should leave this to the free market." [Notice that these are statements of principle rather than empirical claims about what the bill's impact will be.]

41. *Complexity/lack of information about the bill:* "The law is too complicated and I don't understand it"; "it is over two thousand pages long."

42. *Immigration:* "The law will allow undocumented/illegal immigrants to get health care."

43. *Abortion:* "The law will fund abortions."

44. *Economic/other systemic costs:* "It will drive small companies out of business."

45. *Negative opinion leadership:* "Glenn Beck opposes the law."

46. *Negative for specific social group/program:* "This will hurt seniors"; "this will undermine Medicare."

47. *Negative international comparison:* "This will make our system more like France's."

48. *General negative:* "It's going to break the country"; "prefer current system"; "this bill doesn't solve the problem."

2. **Self:** Default is "0." Please code this as a "1" if the response invokes the person's self-interest (for example, "this will help me get health care," "my wife had cancer and this would have limited her care"). Both mentions of individual interest and those of family members are considered self-interest. Mentions of taxpayers in general do *not* count as mentions of self-interest.

3. **Group:** Default is "0." Please code this as a "1" if the response makes reference to a specific group in a positive way, such as "this will help seniors," "this will help children get healthy," "young adults can stay on their parents' insurance," etc. Please code this as a "2" if the response makes reference to a specific group in a negative way, for example, "illegal immigrants shouldn't get free health care," "people on welfare don't need this," etc. Note that *positive references to a group can be in opposition to the legislation or vice versa.* For example, "this bill will hurt rural Americans" is a positive reference to rural Americans (because hurting them is a bad thing); it is not a negative reference to the bill. It would thus receive a "1." Please code this as a "3" if the group is not mentioned with a positive or negative valence. Then, in the **GROUPNAME** column, type in the group's name.

4. **Politician:** Default is "0." Please code this as a "1" if the response makes reference to a specific politician (such as then–Minority Leader Boehner, President Obama, etc.) in a positive way. Please code this as a "2" if the response makes reference to the politician in a negative way. Please code this as a "3" if the politician is not mentioned in a positive or negative way. Then, in **POLITICIANNAME**, please enter the politician's name. Please include clear references to a politician that do not use a name (for example, "he had to start somewhere" as a reference to the president), but not ambiguous references.

5. **Policy:** Default is "0." Please code this as a "1" if the response makes reference to a specific policy element or area in a positive way (for example, "the bill will eliminate discrimination based on preexisting conditions"). Please code this as a "2" if the response makes reference to a specific policy element or area in a negative way (for example, "this bill will

undermine Medicare"). Please code this as a "3" if the response makes reference to a specific policy in a neutral way. Then, in **POLICYNAME**, please indicate the specific policy. References count even if they don't formally name the policy—for example, "my prescription drugs will cost less"; "my son can stay on my insurance."

6. **Place:** Default is "o." Please code as a "1" if the response makes a specific reference to a place (for example, "rural America," "East Coast," "heartland," "Nebraska," etc.). Please code as a "o" otherwise. Please exclude references to Washington, D.C. Then, in **PLACENAME**, please indicate the specific place.

7. **Metaphor:** Default is "o." Please code as a "1" if the response uses any metaphor or simile to express a view and/or make sense of the law. For example, "you would not insure a house that is currently on fire," or "this is just a band-aid."

8. **Fit:** Default is blank. Please indicate a "1" if the argument does not fit neatly into the **Argument** categories. Then, please do your best to choose among the available categories.

APPENDIX B (CHAPTER 4)

Table B.1 OLS Models Predicting Town-Level Support for the Medicaid Expansion in Maine, 2017

	Dependent Variable					
	Share Voting for Medicaid Expansion					
	(1)	(2)	(3)	(4)	(5)	(6)
Share with public assistance income	0.255* (0.108)			0.264* (0.108)		0.091 (0.120)
Median income (logarithmic)		−0.049 (0.037)				−0.014 (0.043)
Share with income under the poverty level			0.134* (0.049)			0.085 (0.058)
Rural hospital municipality				−0.011 (0.017)		
Share employed in health care					0.076 (0.084)	
Share voted for LePage in 2014	−0.421* (0.052)	−0.469* (0.053)	−0.401* (0.052)	−0.424* (0.052)	−0.456* (0.051)	−0.458* (0.053)
Share voted for Trump in 2016	−0.539* (0.056)	−0.487* (0.056)	−0.543* (0.056)	−0.539* (0.056)	−0.503* (0.056)	−0.491* (0.056)
Share with a bachelor's degree	0.088* (0.039)	0.119* (0.041)	0.102* (0.040)	0.087* (0.039)	0.099* (0.039)	0.135* (0.042)
Share non-Hispanic white	0.202* (0.101)	0.224* (0.100)	0.253* (0.103)	0.199 (0.101)	0.170 (0.101)	0.247* (0.101)
Population (logarithmic)	−0.002 (0.006)	0.011 (0.006)	0.001 (0.006)	−0.001 (0.006)	0.004 (0.006)	0.009 (0.006)
Population density (thousand people per square mile)	0.008 (0.017)	−0.003 (0.016)	0.006 (0.017)	0.007 (0.017)	0.001 (0.017)	−0.004 (0.016)
Constant	0.787* (0.103)	0.942* (0.176)	0.706* (0.108)	0.789* (0.103)	0.796* (0.104)	0.748* (0.210)
N	485	478	485	485	480	478
R^2	0.699	0.721	0.700	0.700	0.712	0.723

Source: ACS, Maine Secretary of State (U.S. Census Bureau 2020).

Note: $p < 0.05$.

Table B.2 OLS Models Predicting County-Level Support for the Medicaid Expansion in Oklahoma, 2020

	Dependent Variable				
	Share Voting for Medicaid Expansion				
	(1)	(2)	(3)	(4)	(5)
Share with public assistance income	0.579			0.572	0.207
	(0.353)			(0.357)	(0.362)
Median income (logarithmic)		−0.142*			−0.092
		(0.045)			(0.063)
Share with income under the poverty level			0.380*		0.170
			(0.132)		(0.183)
Share employed in health care support				0.555	
				(0.555)	
Share voted for Trump in 2016	−1.143*	−1.066*	−1.077*	−1.120*	−1.060*
	(0.117)	(0.114)	(0.115)	(0.118)	(0.115)
Share with a bachelor's degree	−0.263*	−0.194	−0.251*	−0.247	−0.184
	(0.119)	(0.115)	(0.112)	(0.126)	(0.118)
Share non-Hispanic white	0.002*	0.003*	0.003*	0.002*	0.003*
	(0.001)	(0.001)	(0.001)	(0.001)	(0.001)
Share American Indian	0.001	0.001	0.001		0.001
	(0.001)	(0.001)	(0.001)		(0.001)
Population (logarithmic)	−0.012	−0.005	−0.005	−0.011	−0.004
	(0.007)	(0.007)	(0.007)	(0.007)	(0.007)
Population density (thousand people per square mile)	0.064	0.075*	0.061	0.053	0.068
	(0.036)	(0.034)	(0.035)	(0.036)	(0.035)
Constant	1.229*	2.515*	1.031*	1.229*	1.961*
	(0.128)	(0.414)	(0.146)	(0.132)	(0.653)
N	77	77	77	77	77
R^2	0.793	0.812	0.808	0.790	0.815

Source: ACS, Oklahoma State Election Board (U.S. Census Bureau 2020).

Note: * $p < 0.05$.

Table B.3 OLS Regression Estimates from Models Predicting a 1–4 Measure of ACA Favorability among Respondents under Sixty-Five

	Dependent Variable		
	Among All Respondents under Sixty-Five (1)	Among Low-Income Respondents under Sixty-Five (2)	Among High-Income Respondents under Sixty-Five (3)
Intercept	2.557* (0.058)	2.717* (0.087)	2.373* (0.077)
Male	−0.057* (0.008)	−0.026* (0.012)	−0.068* (0.010)
Republican	−1.459* (0.010)	−1.157* (0.017)	−1.650* (0.013)
Independent	−0.801* (0.009)	−0.620* (0.014)	−0.962* (0.012)
Age (in years)^2/100	−0.406* (0.029)	−0.358* (0.043)	−0.443* (0.040)
Black	0.437* (0.012)	0.408* (0.017)	0.523* (0.018)
Hispanic	0.280* (0.012)	0.387* (0.017)	0.074* (0.019)
Asian American	0.270* (0.023)	0.307* (0.041)	0.235* (0.028)
Other ethnic-racial identification	0.051* (0.017)	0.032 (0.023)	0.061* (0.026)
Education	0.028* (0.002)	0.019* (0.002)	0.040* (0.002)
Income	−0.000* (0.000)	−0.003* (0.000)	0.000* (0.000)
Expansion state	−0.061 (0.054)	−0.009 (0.078)	−0.151* (0.075)
Post-expansion	−0.017 (0.039)	−0.088 (0.057)	0.033 (0.049)
Expansion state x post-expansion	0.041* (0.016)	0.101* (0.024)	−0.002 (0.020)
N	68,757	30,153	38,604
R^2	0.318	0.247	0.385

Source: KFF Health Tracking Poll (Kaiser Family Foundation 2022).

Note: * $p < 0.05$.

Table B.4 Multilevel Models Predicting ACA Favorability (1–4) Using the HTP for 2014–2016 and 2017–2019

	Dependent Variable	
	ACA Favorability	
	2014–2016	2017–2019
	(1)	(2)
Intercept	4.926*** (0.133)	4.047*** (0.136)
Medicaid	0.162*** (0.030)	0.168*** (0.030)
Insured through exchanges	0.421*** (0.041)	0.293*** (0.044)
Medicare	−0.009 (0.023)	0.095*** (0.024)
Employer insurance	−0.031 (0.020)	0.069** (0.021)
Insurance coverage	0.190*** (0.027)	0.099*** (0.028)
Asian	0.297*** (0.038)	0.174*** (0.041)
Hispanic	0.324*** (0.021)	0.171*** (0.021)
Black	0.433*** (0.020)	0.227*** (0.021)
Income = $25,000	−0.058* (0.024)	−0.052* (0.026)
Income = $35,000	−0.052* (0.025)	−0.071** (0.027)
Income = $45,000	−0.127*** (0.026)	−0.062* (0.028)
Income = $62,500	−0.081*** (0.024)	−0.070** (0.026)
Income = $82,500	−0.107*** (0.027)	−0.043 (0.029)
Income = $95,000	−0.040 (0.033)	−0.056 (0.035)
Income = $200,000	−0.049* (0.024)	−0.072** (0.026)
Male	−0.037** (0.012)	−0.044*** (0.013)
Age	−0.060*** (0.008)	−0.031*** (0.008)
Age^2	0.001*** (0.000)	0.000** (0.000)
Age^3	−0.000** (0.000)	−0.000 (0.000)
Education = ten years	−0.405*** (0.052)	−0.363*** (0.055)
Education = twelve years	−0.475*** (0.046)	−0.363*** (0.046)
Education = thirteen years	−0.412*** (0.047)	−0.391*** (0.047)
Education = fourteen years	−0.417*** (0.048)	−0.351*** (0.048)
Education = sixteen years	−0.266*** (0.047)	−0.242*** (0.047)
Education = seventeen years	−0.187** (0.066)	−0.213*** (0.061)
Education = nineteen years	−0.092 (0.048)	−0.149** (0.048)
Party identification = weak Democrat	−0.835*** (0.019)	−0.156*** (0.019)
Party identification = independent	−0.936*** (0.020)	−0.821*** (0.023)
Party identification = weak Republican	−0.810*** (0.019)	−1.504*** (0.020)
Party identification = strong Republican	−1.499*** (0.017)	−1.627*** (0.017)
N	26,980	22,569
Number of months	26	19
Month-level variance	0.004	0.001
Residual variance	0.959	0.880

Source: KFF Health Tracking Poll (Kaiser Family Foundation 2022).

Note: $* p < 0.05$; $** p < 0.01$; $*** p < 0.001$.

Table C.1 Key Variables and Their Associations with Insurance Sources among Respondents to Surveys after December 2013

	Income	Education	Age	Male	Black	Hispanic	Republican Party Identification	N
Used exchanges	59.8	14.7	47	0.50	0.12	0.13	2.5	1,074
Medicaid	26.8	12.7	46	0.42	0.23	0.21	2.5	3,469
Self-purchased	76.6	14.6	53	0.51	0.09	0.09	3.0	4,708
Uninsured	37.1	12.5	41	0.58	0.17	0.33	2.8	5,069
Employer-insured	106.6	15.3	48	0.53	0.10	0.09	2.9	22,624
Medicare	58.5	14.3	70	0.44	0.09	0.05	2.9	12,379
Other	57.5	13.4	44	0.54	0.00	0.45	2.6	2,499
All	77.9	14.4	52	0.51	0.11	0.12	2.9	52,424

Source: KFF Health Tracking Poll (Kaiser Family Foundation 2022).

Note: "Used exchanges" is a subset of "self-purchased." Republican party identification is a five-point scale. All summary values are means.

Trends in Self-Reported Harm or Benefit from the ACA

In addition to questions about ACA favorability and insurance status, the HTP also asked respondents, "So far, would you say you and your family have (personally benefited from/been negatively affected by) the health reform law, or not?"[1] Although such self-reported perceptions of impacts

Figure C.1 Personal Benefit or Harm Attributed to the ACA, 2010

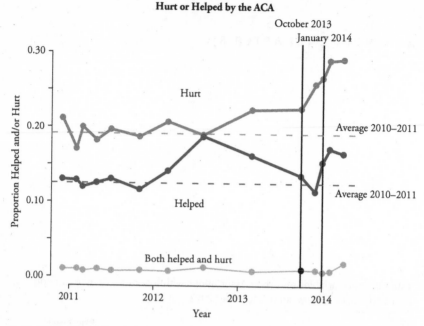

Hurt or Helped by the ACA

Source: KFF Health Tracking Poll (Kaiser Family Foundation 2022). Figure reprinted with permission from Hobbs and Hopkins 2021.

Note: This figure shows responses to the HTP question, "So far, would you say you and your family have (personally benefited from/been negatively affected by) the health reform law, or not?" The y-axis is the monthly proportion reporting "personally benefited from" or "negatively affected by ACA."

are prone to obvious perceptual biases from partisanship and other factors, the over-time trends can nonetheless be instructive. For example, figure C.1 illustrates that the share of people reporting either being helped or harmed by the ACA did increase markedly right as the exchanges were opening in late 2013 and early 2014. Such results are certainly consistent with the claim that the exchanges' rollout had heterogeneous effects.

Tables C.2 and C.3 help give meaning to these results by showing the words that uninsured or self-purchasing respondents used most commonly in post-2014 open-ended responses to a follow-up question about how the ACA helped or hurt them. The use by uninsured respondents of words like "forced," "canceled," and "penalized" and the use by those who were self-insured of terms like "didn't," "affordable," and "insurance" suggest that these groups' attitudes were based to some extent on personal experiences.

Text Analysis of Uninsured Respondents Reporting Harm and Respondents with Self-Purchased Insurance Reporting Benefit

In the section on self-reported help and harm, we analyzed yes/no responses to the question, "So far, would you say you and your family have (personally benefited from/been negatively affected by) the health reform law, or not?" If a respondent answered "yes," the question was followed by an open-ended question: "In what ways would you say you have (benefited from/been negatively affected by) the health reform law?" The interviewer would record the response verbatim.

As a descriptive analysis to better understand the experiences of the uninsured and those who self-purchased insurance after January 2014, we also identify keywords that can distinguish whether an open-ended response was written before or after the ACA's implementation. To do this, we use mutual information to identify words with the most information for classifying a document—in this case an open-ended response—into a class, which is an indicator of being pre- or post-implementation.[2] In this setup, we use the pre-implementation responses as controls, since these are more likely to be misattributions of benefit or harm than the post-implementation responses. Note that this analysis is subject to the same selection concerns as other descriptive analyses, and that the specific words used might be driven by changes in rhetoric.

In table C.2, the keywords identified in the uninsured sample suggest that the individual mandate was common in the post-implementation complaints by uninsured respondents, in addition to responses mentioning "price," "choice," and "canceled"/"dropped" (insurance). In the sample of those with self-purchased insurance shown in table C.3, we see mentions of both lower cost ("lower," "affordable") and words suggesting increased access ("coverage"), but some of this shift might be due to changes in tense.

As chapter 5 details, table C.4 reports linear regression models in which I analyze ACA favorability (measured on a 1–4 scale) as a function of a variety of standard demographic questions as well as respondents' sources of insurance for respondents to the late-2015 Kentucky survey. For the

Table C.2 Open-Ended Keywords Used by Uninsured Respondents to Denote Harm by the ACA Pre- and Post-Implementation

Harmed before January 2014	Harmed in or after January 2014
financially	forced
care	penalized
Medicaid	lost
going	hospital
doctors	insurance
family	get
Law	couldn't
Bill	price
company	able
gone	like
harder	enough
increase	cost
affected	fine
doctor	one
right	take
getting	choice
husband	good
know	information
health	longer
amount	back
anything	canceled
Got	dropped
need	medication
needs	said
costs	covered
$N = 346$	$N = 171$

Source: KFF Health Tracking Poll, 2010–2014, subset of uninsured respondents (Kaiser Family Foundation 2022).

Table C.3 Open-Ended Keywords Used by Respondents with Self-Purchased Insurance to Denote Benefit from the ACA Based on Mutual Information, Pre- and Post-Implementation

Helped before January 2014	Helped in or after January 2014
condition	now
don't	didn't
existing	insurance
lot	affordable
people	time
pre-	got
will	month
can't	preexisting
costs	lower
help	cost
helps	good
keep	money
received	companies
without	insured
get	premium
law	really
pay	spend
can	afford
benefits	plan
well	coverage
doctor	less
kids	policy
plans	cover
prescriptions	free
able	better
$N = 119$	$N = 79$

Source: KFF Health Tracking Poll, 2010–2014, subset of self-insured respondents (Kaiser Family Foundation 2022).

Table C.4 Select Coefficients from Fitted Models of Kentucky Respondents' Support for the ACA, Including Indicators for Those Who Received Subsidies and Used Kynect

| | Dependent Variable | | | |
| | ACA Favorability | | | |
	(1)	(2)	(3)	(4)
Intercept	3.60* (0.33)	3.32* (0.36)	3.58* (0.33)	3.31* (0.36)
Received Medicaid	0.30* (0.14)	0.21 (0.15)	0.35* (0.15)	0.27 (0.15)
Self-purchased insurance	0.11 (0.18)	−0.06 (0.20)	0.12 (0.18)	−0.07 (0.20)
Employer-provided insurance	0.03 (0.13)	−0.09 (0.15)	0.005 (0.14)	−0.12 (0.15)
Received subsidy		0.32 (0.40)		0.46 (0.41)
Insured		0.41* (0.20)		0.41* (0.20)
Used Kynect			−0.20 (0.15)	−0.24 (0.15)
N	567	567	567	567

Source: KFF Kentucky survey, 2015 (Kaiser Family Foundation 2022).

Note: Models also include basic demographics such as gender, income, education, age, partisan identification, and ethnic-racial self-classification. $* p < 0.05$.

ISCAP panel, table C.5 shows the effect of including or excluding demographic covariates when modeling 2018 ACA repeal support. Table C.6 uses the ISCAP panel to illustrate the changes in support for repealing the ACA in 2018 that are associated with changes in insurance status between 2016 and 2018.

Additional Panel Analyses

In chapter 5, we employ a difference-in-differences or change score estimation strategy to analyze the panel data. Here we instead use an "analysis of covariance" strategy in which the first measure of the outcome goes on the right-hand side of the regression equation. Specifically, we model 2018 respondents' views of the ACA as a function of their fall 2018 insurance status, their January 2016 insurance status, their attitudes toward the ACA in 2012 and 2016, their 2012 partisan identification, and a series of basic demographics such as gender, education, and income.

Such models are well suited to isolating the extent to which *changes* in insurance status predict subsequent shifts in ACA attitudes, although their leverage comes from the forty respondents whose status as uninsured changed

Table C.5 OLS Models of Anti-ACA Attitudes, Measured on a 1–7 Scale, as a Function of Various Variables, Fall 2018

	Dependent Variable	
	Support for ACA Repeal (1–7)	
	(1)	(2)
Intercept	3.83* (0.26)	3.78* (0.29)
January 2016: Medicare	0.04 (0.28)	−0.14 (0.29)
January 2016: Plan through parent	−0.78 (1.09)	−0.73 (1.10)
January 2016: Plan through employer	0.08 (0.27)	0.04 (0.27)
January 2016: Self-purchased plan	−0.31 (0.33)	−0.33 (0.33)
January 2016: Insurance refused	−0.98 (0.99)	−1.02 (0.99)
January 2016: Other government program	0.19 (0.41)	0.10 (0.41)
January 2016: Other insurance	0.34 (0.42)	0.19 (0.43)
January 2016: Uninsured	0.53 (0.35)	0.54 (0.35)
October 2012: ACA attitudes	0.61* (0.10)	0.59* (0.11)
November 2012–January 2013: ACA attitudes	0.03 (0.10)	0.03 (0.10)
October 2016: ACA attitudes	0.75* (0.08)	0.76* (0.08)
October 2012: Republican partisan identification	0.35* (0.07)	0.32* (0.07)
October 2012: Years of education		0.09 (0.06)
October 2012: White		0.17 (0.14)
October 2012: Black		−0.20 (0.22)
Fall 2007: Income		0.00 (0.05)
October 2012: Female		0.04 (0.11)
October 2012: Age		0.18* (0.08)
Fall 2007: Union household		0.12 (0.17)
Fall 2007: Catholic		−0.09 (0.15)
Fall 2007: Protestant		0.19 (0.13)
R^2	0.62	0.63
N	573	573

Source: ISCAP panel, 2007–2016 (Hopkins and Mutz 2022).

Note: Fully observed respondents completing fall 2016 and fall 2018 ISCAP waves. Excluded baseline categories include insurance through Medicaid. * $p < 0.05$.

Table C.6 Select Coefficients from a Change Score Model of the Change in Respondents' Support for Repealing the ACA, Measured on a 1–7 Scale, Fall 2016 to Fall 2018

	Dependent Variable	
	Support for ACA Repeal (1–7)	
	(1)	(2)
Intercept	−1.878* (0.602)	−1.099* (0.450)
Uninsured status	0.641 (0.357)	
Self-purchased insurance status	0.312 (0.277)	0.302 (0.278)
Medicaid status	0.360 (0.349)	0.435 (0.352)
Became uninsured, 2018		0.935* (0.447)
Became insured, 2018		−0.156 (0.617)
Weak Democratic identification, October 2016	−0.012 (0.222)	−0.032 (0.222)
Lean Democratic, October 2016	−0.284 (0.214)	−0.266 (0.214)
Pure independent, October 2016	−0.394 (0.404)	−0.382 (0.405)
Lean Republican, October 2016	−0.304 (0.247)	−0.314 (0.248)
Weak Republican identification, October 2016	−0.588* (0.270)	−0.606* (0.271)
Strong Republican identification, October 2016	−0.462 (0.258)	−0.445 (0.259)
2016 ACA repeal = 2	−0.021 (0.210)	0.016 (0.210)
2016 ACA repeal = 3	0.167 (0.297)	0.157 (0.298)
2016 ACA repeal = 4	0.131 (0.217)	0.125 (0.218)
2016 ACA repeal = 5	−0.120 (0.352)	−0.141 (0.353)
2016 ACA repeal = 6	0.496 (0.306)	0.535 (0.306)
2016 ACA repeal = 7	0.461 (0.249)	0.474 (0.249)
Education (in years)	0.057 (0.030)	0.035 (0.028)
Female	−0.022 (0.126)	−0.007 (0.126)
Black	−0.394 (0.214)	−0.299 (0.210)
Hispanic	0.038 (0.197)	0.104 (0.195)
Age (in years)	0.010* (0.005)	
R^2	0.042	0.037
N	593	593

Source: ISCAP panel, 2016–2018 (Hopkins and Mutz 2022).

Note: * $p < 0.05$.

Figure C.2 Coefficients for Being Uninsured in 2016 and 2018 (Included in the Same Model) When Predicting 2018 Support for ACA Repeal

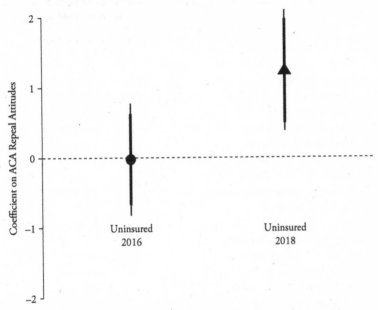

Source: ISCAP panel, 2016 and 2018. Figure reprinted with permission from Hobbs and Hopkins 2021.
Note: The thick lines indicate 90 percent confidence intervals, while the thin lines indicate 95 percent confidence intervals.

between 2016 and 2018.[3] However, these models are again a conservative test, as we are isolating people who became uninsured only after 2016, nearly three years after the ACA's implementation. As a result, those who were uninsured in the first few years after the ACA's 2014 implementation will not influence our estimate.

The core results are presented graphically in figure C.2, while table C.7 provides the full fitted model. Most of the indicators of different insurance statuses are not predictive of 2018 ACA attitudes. Importantly, those who self-purchased insurance plans in 2018 were not much more or less supportive of the ACA. Figure C.2 illustrates only the coefficients for being uninsured in 2016 and 2018, alongside the associated 90 percent (thick lines) and 95 percent (thin lines) confidence intervals. As it shows, respondents who were uninsured in 2018 were dramatically less supportive of the ACA, even accounting for 2016 insurance status. The coefficient is 1.23 (SE = 0.43),

Table C.7 OLS Model of Anti-ACA Attitudes, Measured on a 1–7 Scale, as a Function of Various Variables, Fall 2018

	Dependent Variable
	Support for ACA Repeal (1–7)
Intercept	3.56* (0.35)
Uninsured, fall 2018	1.23* (0.43)
Uninsured, January 2016	−0.03 (0.40)
January 2016: Medicare	−0.13 (0.33)
January 2016: Plan through parent	−0.91 (1.10)
January 2016: Plan through employer	−0.15 (0.34)
January 2016: Self-purchased plan	−0.62 (0.40)
January 2016: Refused insurance	−1.04 (0.99)
January 2016: Other government insurance	−0.30 (0.47)
January 2016: Insured (other)	0.38 (0.45)
October 2018: Medicare	0.07 (0.37)
October 2018: Plan through parent	2.80 (1.66)
October 2018: Plan through employer	0.45 (0.39)
October 2018: Self-purchased plan	0.56 (0.46)
October 2018: Refused insurance	1.03 (1.76)
October 2018: Other government insurance	0.75 (0.53)
October 2018: Other insurance	−0.68 (0.51)
October 2012: Repeal ACA	0.60* (0.11)
November 2012–January 2013: Repeal ACA	−0.02 (0.10)
October 2016: Repeal ACA	0.76* (0.08)
October 2012: Republican partisan identification	0.34* (0.07)
October 2012: Years of education	0.10 (0.06)
October 2012: White	0.19 (0.14)
October 2012: Black	−0.27 (0.22)
Fall 2007: Income	0.01 (0.05)
October 2012: Female	0.02 (0.11)
October 2012: Age	0.24* (0.08)
Fall 2007: Union household	0.13 (0.17)
Fall 2007: Catholic	−0.05 (0.15)
Fall 2007: Protestant	0.21 (0.13)
R^2	0.65
N	567

Source: ISCAP panel, 2007–2018 (Hopkins and Mutz 2022).

Note: * $p < 0.05$.

meaning that those who became uninsured between 2016 and 2018 also downgraded their opinion of the ACA by a pronounced 1.23 on a 1–7 scale. That effect is 61 percent of a standard deviation. The figure also shows that being uninsured in 2016 has little association with ACA attitudes, which is a valuable placebo test: these results appear to be driven by the experience of being uninsured in 2018, not by other factors that are consistently associated with being uninsured.

Most Likely Case 1: Geographic Variability in Exchange-Based Insurance Prices

Table C.8 Full Multilevel Models with Insurance Market Conditions (and Other Independent Variables) Predicting ACA Favorability, Measured on a 1–4 Scale and Fit to KFF Respondents, 2015, 2016, and 2017

	Dependent Variable			
	ACA Favorability			
	Among Nonmarket- Insured (1)	Among Market-Insured (2)	Among Uninsured (3)	Among Market-Insured (4)
Weak Democratic identification	−0.63*	−0.19	−.42*	−0.19
	(0.02)	(0.15)	(0.07)	(0.15)
Independent	−0.87*	−0.60*	−0.63*	−0.59*
	(0.03)	(0.16)	(0.07)	(0.17)
Weak Republican identification	−1.01*	−0.94*	−0.50*	−0.94*
	(0.03)	(0.15)	(0.07)	(0.15)
Strong Republican identification	−1.51*	−1.27*	−0.91*	−1.25*
	(0.02)	(0.14)	(0.08)	(0.15)
Education	0.03*	−0.01	−0.03*	−0.01
	(0.003)	(0.02)	(0.01)	(0.02)
Income	−0.0003*	−0.001	−0.002*	−0.001
	(0.0001)	(0.001)	(0.001)	(0.001)
Black	0.37*	0.40*	0.36*	0.41*
	(0.03)	(0.16)	(0.07)	(0.16)
Hispanic	0.28*	0.01	0.46*	0.03
	(0.03)	(0.16)	(0.07)	(0.17)
Asian	0.20*	0.74*	0.19	0.73*
	(0.05)	(0.35)	(0.19)	(0.35)

(*Table continues on p. 216*)

Table C.8 (*Continued*)

	Dependent Variable			
	ACA Favorability			
	Among Nonmarket-Insured (1)	Among Market-Insured (2)	Among Uninsured (3)	Among Market-Insured (4)
Age	−0.001	0.001	−0.01*	0.001
	(0.0005)	(0.004)	(0.002)	(0.004)
County: percent Black, 2010	−0.20*	0.54	0.38	0.52
	(0.08)	(0.53)	(0.23)	(0.53)
County: percent Hispanic, 2010	0.03	0.23	0.38*	0.23
	(0.06)	(0.36)	(0.17)	(0.37)
County: median household income 2010	−0.0000	0.0000	−0.0000	0.0000
	(0.0000)	(0.0000)	(0.0000)	(0.0000)
County: percent poor, 2010	0.003	1.01	−0.16	0.99
	(0.30)	(1.81)	(0.92)	(1.82)
County: percent unemployed, 2010	5.15*	−6.40	2.24	−6.19
	(0.90)	(6.14)	(2.62)	(6.18)
County: percent unemployed, 2010–2016	3.56*	−2.43	4.30	−2.35
	(1.15)	(7.88)	(3.51)	(7.92)
County: percent with bachelor's degree, 2010	0.97*	1.24	0.48	1.24
	(0.13)	(0.79)	(0.40)	(0.80)
Number of plans (logged, in standard deviations)	0.001	−0.07	−0.004	−0.08
	(0.01)	(0.06)	(0.03)	(0.07)
Mean premium (in standard deviations)	0.004	0.04	0.05	0.04
	(0.01)	(0.07)	(0.03)	(0.07)
Mean change in premium (in standard deviations)	0.001	−0.19*	−0.02	−0.17*
	(0.01)	(0.07)	(0.04)	(0.08)
Mean change in benchmark premiums (in standard deviations)				−0.0003
				(0.002)
Constant	2.17*	2.87*	2.65*	2.84*
	(0.11)	(0.70)	(0.34)	(0.71)
N	15,987	442	1,772	438
Month Fixed Effects	Y	Y	Y	Y
County-level demographics	Y	Y	Y	Y
Clusters (year)	3	3	3	3

Source: KFF Health Tracking Poll, 2015–2017 (Kaiser Family Foundation 2022); Robert Wood Johnson Foundation's National Narrow Network Project (Polsky and Weiner 2015).

Note: Data taken from KFF's Health Tracking Poll, merged with Health Exchange. * $p < 0.05$.

Most Likely Case 2: Individuals in Their Early Sixties

Table C.9 presents checks of the key assumption underpinning the regression discontinuity design (RDD) analyses, which is that potentially confounding variables are distributed smoothly at the point of the discontinuity. Using the same specification as in the RDD models in table C.10, table C.9 presents the coefficient (Beta), standard error, and *t*-value from models in which the listed variable is the dependent variable predicted by being sixty-five or older. As the table makes clear, none of these variables are significantly different for those just over sixty-five years old, save for being Asian American, which is slightly more common among those just over sixty-five.

Although we do not control for partisanship in other causal models—to avoid post-treatment bias—we include it here. Removing partisanship from these models does not meaningfully change the RDD coefficient.

Table C.9 Regression Coefficients, Standard Errors, and *t*-values for Potentially Confounding Dependent Variables Predicted by Being Sixty-Five or Older

	Beta	**Standard Error**	***t*-value**
Education	−0.108	0.133	−0.813
Black	0.015	0.013	1.158
Hispanic	0.008	0.011	0.698
Asian American	0.012	0.005	2.285
Male	−0.000	0.022	−0.020
Republican	−0.024	0.080	−0.296
Income	−1.250	2.912	−0.429

Source: KFF Health Tracking Poll (Kaiser Family Foundation 2022).

Table C.10 RDD Models Fit to Respondents between Sixty-Two and Sixty-Eight before and after the ACA's Implementation

	Dependent Variable	
	Pre-ACA (1)	Post-ACA (2)
Intercept	3.57* (1.24)	1.91 (1.37)
Older than sixty-five	−0.12 (0.06)	0.01 (0.06)
Age	−0.02 (0.02)	−0.00 (0.02)
Survey month	1.92* (0.92)	1.43 (1.65)
Survey month^2	−2.18 (1.14)	−0.60 (1.00)
Education	0.05* (0.01)	0.03* (0.01)
Black	0.49* (0.06)	0.44* (0.05)
Hispanic	0.37* (0.07)	0.40* (0.06)
Asian American	0.29* (0.13)	0.28* (0.13)
Male	−0.04 (0.03)	−0.01 (0.03)
Income	0.20 (0.29)	0.09 (0.26)
Weak Democratic identification	−0.24* (0.05)	−0.85* (0.05)
Pure independent	−0.96* (0.06)	−0.82* (0.05)
Weak Republican identification	−1.60* (0.05)	−0.94* (0.05)
Strong Republican identification	−1.60* (0.04)	−1.56* (0.04)
R^2	0.42	0.32
N	3,843	4,791

Source: Kaiser Family Foundation Health Tracking Poll (Kaiser Family Foundation 2022).

Note: * $p < 0.05$.

APPENDIX D (CHAPTER 6)

Table D.1 Regression Results Predicting ACA Attitudes over Time

				Dependent Variable			
				Support for ACA Repeal			
	December, 2012	October, 2014	October, 2016	December, 2016	October, 2018	January, 2020	October, 2020
	(1)	(2)	(3)	(4)	(5)	(6)	(7)
Intercept	2.996* (0.700)	4.182* (0.748)	5.323* (0.739)	4.209* (0.765)	3.053* (0.809)	4.030* (0.891)	4.429* (0.717)
Anti-black prejudice	0.666 (0.444)	1.132* (0.470)	1.045* (0.417)	1.545* (0.427)	0.651 (0.522)	1.027 (0.548)	1.005* (0.429)
Years of education	-0.054 (0.034)	-0.117* (0.037)	-0.134* (0.036)	-0.099* (0.038)	-0.068 (0.040)	-0.098* (0.043)	-0.122* (0.035)
Female	0.244 (0.132)	0.336* (0.143)	0.050 (0.136)	0.173 (0.141)	0.094 (0.155)	0.161 (0.163)	-0.029 (0.133)
Protestant	-0.194 (0.153)	0.053 (0.166)	-0.143 (0.154)	-0.067 (0.161)	-0.064 (0.182)	-0.071 (0.188)	-0.001 (0.154)
Catholic	-0.206 (0.173)	-0.301 (0.188)	-0.338 (0.179)	-0.125 (0.186)	-0.236 (0.205)	-0.082 (0.211)	-0.097 (0.174)
Union	0.191 (0.195)	0.282 (0.212)	0.145 (0.205)	0.295 (0.204)	0.263 (0.232)	0.506* (0.240)	0.351 (0.199)
Age	-0.005 (0.006)	-0.009 (0.006)	-0.008 (0.006)	-0.004 (0.006)	0.007 (0.007)	-0.011 (0.007)	-0.012* (0.006)
Partisan identification = 2	1.155* (0.249)	1.176* (0.286)	0.634* (0.257)	0.917* (0.263)	0.701* (0.287)	0.900* (0.308)	0.658* (0.248)
Partisan identification = 3	1.135* (0.224)	1.120* (0.241)	0.947* (0.225)	1.109* (0.232)	0.813* (0.258)	1.126* (0.273)	1.018* (0.228)
Partisan identification = 4	3.081* (0.666)	2.690* (0.566)	2.846* (0.745)	1.560* (0.669)	1.112 (0.676)	1.865* (0.704)	2.433* (0.511)
Partisan identification = 5	3.228* (0.218)	3.305* (0.235)	2.604* (0.224)	2.483* (0.229)	2.676* (0.261)	2.686* (0.268)	2.554* (0.223)
Partisan identification = 6	3.284* (0.222)	3.450* (0.239)	2.710* (0.231)	2.389* (0.247)	2.510* (0.266)	2.462* (0.276)	2.652* (0.226)
Partisan identification = 7	4.081* (0.222)	3.632* (0.240)	3.095* (0.223)	2.963* (0.233)	3.086* (0.256)	3.174* (0.267)	3.248* (0.228)
N	607	541	495	453	445	515	667
R^2	0.482	0.475	0.448	0.404	0.400	0.320	0.370
Adjusted R^2	0.471	0.462	0.433	0.386	0.382	0.302	0.357

Source: ISCAP panel, 2012–2020 (Hopkins and Mutz 2022).

Note: * $p < 0.05$.

Figure D.1 Word Clouds of Open-Ended Responses by SSI Respondents

1. Words Used to Explain Favorable Attitudes on the ACA

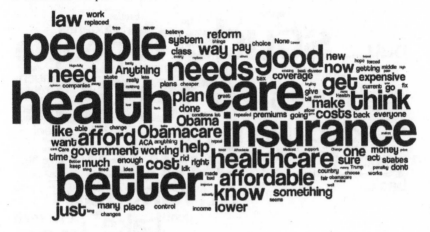

2. Words Used to Explain Unfavorable Attitudes on the ACA

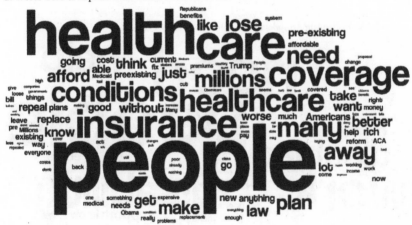

(*Figure continues on p. 222*)

Figure D.1 (*Continued*)

3. Words Used to Explain Attitudes on Student Loan Spending

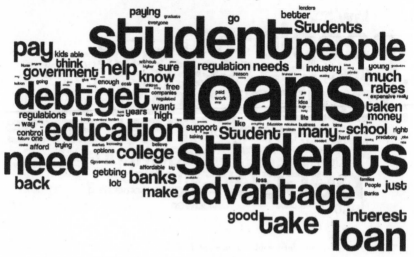

4. Words Used to Explain Attitudes on Disability Insurance Spending

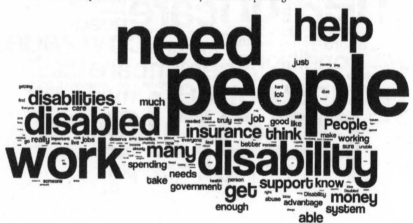

Figure D.1 (*Continued*)

5. Words Used to Explain Attitudes on Food Stamp Spending

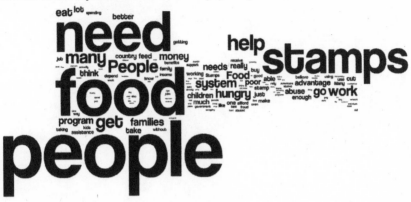

6. Words Used to Explain Attitudes on Unemployment Spending

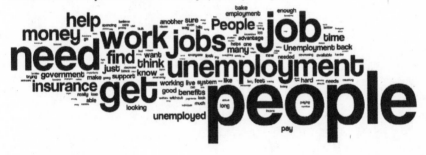

Source: SSI Survey, 2017.

APPENDIX E (CHAPTER 7)

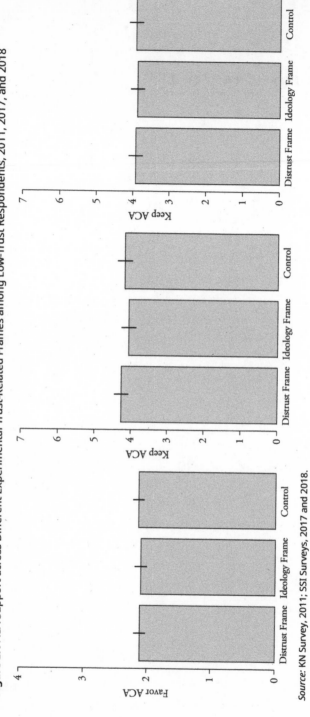

Figure E.1 ACA Support across Different Experimental Trust-Related Frames among Low-Trust Respondents, 2011, 2017, and 2018

Source: KN Survey, 2011; SSI Surveys, 2017 and 2018.

Figure E.2 Variation in Topics, April 2009 to February 2010, with Topic Probabilities Smoothed over the Prior Twenty-Eight Days

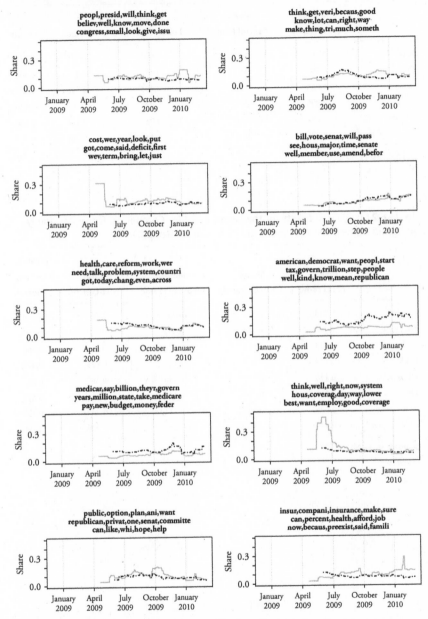

Source: Media appearances by administration officials and congressional leaders.

Note: Model: LDA, fit to 218 transcripts from television appearances by administration officials and congressional leaders. The dashed black lines indicate Republican press releases, and the straight gray lines indicate Democratic press releases.

Table E.1 Means and *t*-tests for the Listed Variables Comparing Those Randomly Assigned to the Trust Argument with the Control Group, 2011

	Mean, Trust Frame	Mean, Control Frame	Mean, Ideological Frame	*p*-value	*p*-value
Republican	0.482	0.455	0.507	0.345	0.390
Democrat	0.498	0.519	0.472	0.475	0.468
White	0.764	0.748	0.783	0.516	0.434
Black	0.095	0.100	0.071	0.780	0.136
Hispanic	0.082	0.106	0.089	0.144	0.686
Over sixty-five	0.226	0.178	0.236	0.038	0.687

Source: KN Survey, 2011.

Note: N = 2,228.

Table E.2 Means and *t*-tests for the Listed Variables Comparing Those Randomly Assigned to the Trust Argument with the Control Group, 2017

	Mean, Trust Frame	Mean, Control Frame	Mean, Ideology Frame	*p*-value, Trust-Control	*p*-value, Ideology-Control
Republican	0.243	0.255	0.259	0.663	0.543
Democrat	0.402	0.383	0.392	0.527	0.728
White	0.633	0.662	0.614	0.324	0.506
Black	0.134	0.132	0.151	0.929	0.429
Hispanic	0.138	0.127	0.140	0.587	0.924
Over sixty-five	0.154	0.186	0.149	0.165	0.818
Trump voter	0.326	0.334	0.311	0.784	0.597
Clinton voter	0.445	0.409	0.453	0.236	0.790

Source: SSI Survey, 2017.

Note: N = 1,631.

Table E.3 Means and *t*-tests for the Listed Variables Comparing Those Randomly Assigned to the Trust Argument with the Control Group, 2018

	Mean, Trust Frame	Mean, Control Frame	Mean, Ideology Frame	*p*-value Trust-Control	*p*-value, Ideology-Control
Republican	0.431	0.440	0.405	0.753	0.361
Democrat	0.421	0.444	0.457	0.437	0.213
White	0.773	0.760	0.780	0.608	0.771
Black	0.099	0.100	0.095	0.932	0.829
Hispanic	0.067	0.072	0.067	0.782	0.958
Over sixty-five	0.202	0.190	0.205	0.596	0.896
Trump voter	0.424	0.429	0.402	0.863	0.424
Clinton voter	0.387	0.413	0.388	0.352	0.948

Source: SSI Survey, 2019.

Note: N = 1,945.

Open-Ended Responses Identified through LDA

Table E.4 Most Commonly Occurring Words in Each of the Six Clusters of Open-Ended Responses Identified through LDA, 2009–2012

	Cluster					
	1	2	3	4	5	6
1	government	people	care	afford	money	don't
2	don't	insurance	health	people	cost	bill
3	control	help	access	can't	Medicare	trying
4	business	companies	system	lot	pay	country
5	involved	coverage	Americans	help	tax	health care
6	run	conditions	affordable	insurance	taxes	doesn't
7	believe	able	provide	health	cut	law
8	private	existing	universal	care	don't	medicine
9	choice	preexisting	believe	don't	lot	time
10	federal	age	reform	able	class	socialized
11	care	premiums	country	helps	doctors	system
12	buy	children	free	buy	people	citizens
13	purchase	que	costs	pay	paying	public
14	forced	income	Canada	benefit	middle	change
15	individual	covered	coverage	time	health care	passed
16	program	covers	countries	health care	costs	senior
17	tell	pre-	quality	expensive	social	read
18	freedom	low	American	sick	dollars	didn't
19	socialism	helps	change	elderly	debt	feel
20	choose	health	world	issues	Medicaid	that's

Source: Various open-ended surveys, 2009–2012.

NOTES

Chapter 1: Introduction

1. Kristol 1993.
2. Ibid.
3. Bachrach and Baratz 1962; Gaventa 1980.
4. Brunner, Ross, and Washington 2011; Campbell 2003, 2012; Hacker and Pierson 2019; Lerman and Weaver 2014; Mettler 2005, 2011; Nall 2018; Pierson 1994; Soss 1999; Soss and Schram 2007; and Svallfors 2007. "Policy feedback" refers to the influence of a government policy on subsequent political behavior or public opinion.
5. Broder and Johnson 1996; Hacker 1999; Skocpol 1997.
6. Cohn 2021; Jacobs and Skocpol 2015.
7. Kaiser Family Foundation, "State Health Facts: Medicaid Expansion Enrollment," https://www.kff.org/health-reform/state-indicator/medicaid-expansion-enrollment/.
8. Internal Revenue Service 2019.
9. Campbell and Shore-Sheppard 2020; Dorn, Garrett, and Holahan 2014.
10. Anzia, Jares, and Malhotra 2021; Gordon 2011; Keech and Pak 1989; Kogan 2020; Kriner and Reeves 2012, 2015; Tufte 1978; see also Béland, Campbell, and Weaver 2022; Campbell 2012.
11. Wesleyan Media Project 2018.
12. Nyhan et al. 2012.
13. Edwards 2012.
14. Political elites are defined here as a small group of politicians, journalists, and others who are able to play a direct role in the formulation of public policy as well as to make their positions on public policy widely known. I use "messaging," a term common in political circles, as a synonym of "framing." We follow Chong and

Druckman (2010, 665) by focusing on issue framing, which occurs "when a communication changes people's attitudes toward an object by changing the relative weights they give to competing considerations about an object."

15. Steinhauer and Pear 2011.

16. Lawrence and Schafer 2012; Scherer 2010; Shapiro and Jacobs 2010; see also Berinsky 2017; Fowler et al. 2017; Gollust et al. 2014; Jacobs and Shapiro 2000; Karaca-Mandic et al. 2017; Kriner and Reeves 2014; Nyhan 2010; Skocpol and Williamson 2016.

17. Hiltzik 2014. Similarly, in an assessment of why Vermont's 2011–2014 push for single-payer health care failed, the health policy expert John McDonough (2015, 1584) contends that the gubernatorial administration that backed the effort "had neglected to launch a serious and sustained effort to educate the public—a crucial missed opportunity."

18. Kam 2012; Zaller 1992. See also Berinsky 2009; Broockman and Butler 2017; Zaller 2012.

19. For example, Arceneaux and Vander Wielen 2017; Baumgartner, De Boef, and Boydstun 2008; Boudreau and MacKenzie 2014; Boydstun et al. 2014; Broockman and Butler 2017; Broockman and Kalla 2016; Chong and Druckman 2010; de Vreese 2003; Druckman 2001; Edwards 2009; Entman 2004; Garz and Martin 2021; Hopkins, Kim, and Kim 2017; Iyengar and Kinder 1987; Jacobs and Shapiro 2000; Kalla and Broockman 2018; Kellstedt 2003; Lenz 2012; Sides, Vavreck, and Warshaw 2022; Smith 2007; Vavreck 2009.

20. Kaiser Family Foundation 2010.

21. Blendon and Benson 2014.

22. Kaiser Family Foundation 2022.

23. See also Galvin and Thurston 2017; Hacker and Pierson 2018; Jacobs and Mettler 2016, 2018; Patashnik and Oberlander 2018; Patashnik and Zelizer 2013.

24. Fukuyama 2018a, 2018b; Gest 2016; Lilla 2018; see also Gidron 2020; Grossmann and Thaler 2018; Sides, Tesler, and Vavreck 2019.

25. Bartels 2008, 2018; Gidron 2020.

26. Jacobs, Mettler, and Zhu 2019.

27. DeBonis 2019.

28. For example, Banks 2014a, 2014b; Béland, Rocco, and Waddan 2016; Blendon and Benson 2017; Brodie, Hamel, and Kirzinger 2019; Clinton and Sances 2018; Fowler et al. 2017; Grande, Gollust, and Asch 2011; Henderson and Hillygus 2011; Jacobs and Mettler 2016, 2020; Jacobs, Mettler, and Zhu 2019; Kriner and Reeves 2014; Lerman, Sadin, and Trachtman 2017; Lerman and Trachtman 2021; McCabe 2016, 2019; Reny and Sears 2020; Sances and Clinton 2020; Shapiro and Jacobs 2010.

29. Wlezien 1995.

30. Following Hafner-Burton, Hughes, and Victor (2013, 369), we define elites as "the small number of decision makers who occupy the top positions in social and political structures." Political elites are those whose actions and stated positions in the political arena are likely to be widely known and reported on.

31. Miller 2018; Schumpeter 1943.

32. Druckman and Jacobs 2015; Ginsberg 1986; Jacobs and Shapiro 2000.

33. Bachrach and Baratz 1962; Constant 1988; Gaventa 1980.

34. Azari 2018; Grumbach 2022; Hopkins, forthcoming; Howell and Moe 2020; Levitsky and Ziblatt 2018; Lieberman et al. 2019.

35. Kam 2012.

36. Achen and Bartels 2016; Converse 1964; Kinder and Kalmoe 2017.

37. Ellis and Stimson 2012; Page and Shapiro 1992; Stimson 2004; Wlezien 1995.

38. Hacker and Pierson 2019; Mettler 2019; Pacheco, Haselswerdt, and Michener 2020.

39. Angrist and Pischke 2010; King, Tomz, and Wittenberg 2000; Sekhon 2009.

40. Zaller 2012, 571.

41. Berinsky 2009; Druckman 2001; Lenz 2012; Levendusky 2009, 2010; Zaller 2012.

42. Zaller 1992; Berinsky 2009.

43. Zingher 2022.

44. Abramowitz 2013; Lee 2016; McCarty 2019; McCarty, Poole, and Rosenthal 2006; Zingher 2022. On the ACA in particular, see Pacheco, Haselswerdt, and Michener 2020; Putnam and Garrett 2020.

45. Lerman and Trachtman 2021.

46. Roy 2014.

47. See also Broockman and Skovron 2018.

48. Centers for Medicare & Medicaid Services 2021.

49. Kaiser Family Foundation, "State Health Facts: Marketplace Enrollment, 2014–2022," https://www.kff.org/health-reform/state-indicator/marketplace-enrollment.

50. Finkelstein et al. 2012; McKenna et al. 2018; Sommers, Gawande, and Baicker 2017. Health insurance can also influence political participation, potentially through its effects on people's resources (Baicker and Finkelstein 2019; Clinton and Sances 2018; Haselswerdt and Michener 2019; Michener 2017, 2019a).

51. Cohn 2008; Michener 2018.

52. Campbell 2014.

53. Kirzinger et al. 2020.

54. Clinton and Sances 2018; McCabe 2016.

55. Rosenthal 2012.

56. Hopkins and Barry-Jester 2017.

57. Associated Press 2013.

58. *Politifact* 2020.

59. See also Haselswerdt and Michener 2019; Patashnik 2019.

60. Achen and Bartels 2016; Ahler and Sood 2018; Conover and Feldman 1984; Converse 1964; Mason 2018.

61. On racial attitudes, see Banks 2014b; McCabe 2019; Michener 2020; Tesler 2012. On political partisanship, see Brodie, Hamel, and Kirzinger 2019; Kriner and Reeves 2014.

62. Hetherington 2005; Lerman 2019.

63. For example, Sears and Funk 1991; Haselswerdt 2020; Kumlin 2004.

64. Sears and Citrin 1982.

65. For example, Achen and Bartels 2016; Converse 1964; Delli Carpini and Keeter 1996; Krupnikov and Ryan 2022; Lippmann 1922; Lupia 2016; Popkin 1994; see also Zingher 2022.

66. Lerman and Trachtman 2021.

67. Chattopadhyay 2018; Hosek 2019; Mettler 2011, 2018; Morgan and Campbell 2011.

68. Michener 2017, 2018.

69. Blendon and Benson 2017; Brodie, Hamel, and Kirzinger 2019.

70. On "thermostatic response," see Stimson 2004; Wlezien 1995. On common behaviors in political psychology, see Kahneman and Tversky 1979; Samuelson and Zeckhauser 1988. On loss aversion and the ACA, see Mettler, Jacobs, and Zhu 2022.

71. Malhotra, Margalit, and Mo 2013.

72. See also Michener 2017, 2018.

73. Kahneman and Tversky 1979; Tversky and Kahneman 1991.

74. See Benedictis-Kessner and Hankinson 2019; Hankinson 2018; Haselswerdt 2020; Hersh and Nall 2016; Malhotra, Margalit, and Mo 2013; Marble and Nall 2018; Margalit 2013; Michener 2019b; Soss and Weaver 2016. But see Mansfield and Mutz 2009; Mutz 1992, 1994.

75. See especially Jacobs and Shapiro 2000; see also Kalla and Broockman 2018.

76. Cramer 2016; Hochschild 1995, 2018; Jones-Correa 1998; Lee 2002; Michener 2018. For the latter accounts, see Achen and Bartels 2016; Converse 1964.

77. Berinsky 2009; Zaller 1992.

78. On political divisions generally, see Carmines and Stimson 1989; Enos 2017; Gillion 2016; Hutchings and Jardina 2009; Hutchings and Valentino 2004; Kinder and Kam 2009; Kinder and Sanders 1996; Michener 2019b; Mutz 2018; Parker and Barreto 2014; Schickler 2016; Sides, Tesler, and Vavreck 2019; Sniderman and Piazza 1993; Stephens-Dougan 2020; Tesler 2016. On particular social policy attitudes, see Gilens 1999; Goren 2003; Hancock 2004; Kellstedt 2003; Kluegel and Smith 1986; Krimmel and Rader 2017; Quadagno 1994; Sears and Citrin 1982; Sniderman and Carmines 1997; Winter 2008.

79. Gilens 1999; Goren 2003.

80. Tesler 2012; Banks 2014b.

81. Michener 2020; see also Lantz and Rosenbaum 2020.

82. Michener 2018, 10.

83. See also Acharya, Blackwell, and Sen 2018; Michener 2020.

84. Chan, Kim, and Leung 2021; Hutchings and Jardina 2009; Kinder and Sanders 1996; Mendelberg 2001; Stephens-Dougan 2020; Valentino 1999.

85. McCabe 2019; Metzl 2019.

86. Gilens 1999.

87. See also Sen and Wasow 2016.

88. Bode et al. 2020; Broockman and Butler 2017; Broockman and Skovron 2018; Canes-Wrone, Brady, and Cogan 2002; Druckman and Jacobs 2015; Edwards 2009; Garz and Martin 2021; Grimmer, Messing, and Westwood 2012, 2014; Hopkins, Kim, and Kim 2017; Lenz 2012; Page and Shapiro 1992.

89. Béland, Rocco, and Waddan 2016, 2020; Cohn 2021; Hacker and Pierson 2018; Hertel-Fernandez 2019b; Jones 2017; Patashnik and Oberlander 2018; Rocco and Haeder 2018; Skocpol and Williamson 2016.
90. Patashnik 2008; Rocco and Haeder 2018; Stokes 2020.
91. Béland, Rocco, and Waddan 2019; Jones 2017.
92. Grumbach 2018; Hertel-Fernandez 2019b; Hopkins 2018a.
93. Hacker 2019.
94. Anderson, Marinescu, and Shor 2019; Mildenberger 2020; Rabe 2018; Skocpol 2013; Stokes 2020.
95. Béland, Rocco, and Waddan 2016; Mildenberger 2020; Steinmo and Watts 1995.
96. Leonhardt 2019. Similarly, in July 2019, the pro-ACA journalist Ezra Klein (2019) argued that the health law's market-based features were its Achilles' heel politically: "The private-public construction of Obamacare has given opportunistic Republicans their most effective attacks on the bill. Those attacks have been legal, like this assault on the regulations governing private insurance purchase; and political, like the ads slamming high deductibles and complex shopping schemes and Medicare."
97. DePillis 2022.
98. But see Aklin and Mildenberger 2020.
99. Collier and Brady 2004.
100. This approach defines causal effects as the differences in two or more potential outcomes under different conditions (Imbens and Rubin 2015).
101. Pearl 2000; Collier and Brady 2004.
102. See also Jacobs and Mettler 2020; Mettler, Jacobs, and Zhu 2022.
103. Achen and Bartels 2016; Cohen 2003. See also Hobbs 2019; Krimmel and Rader 2020.
104. Michener 2018; Tallevi 2018.
105. Banks 2014b; McCabe 2019; Tesler 2012.
106. Lee 2016.

Chapter 2: The Elite-Level Politics and Policymaking of the ACA

1. Jost 2017. The employer mandate required that businesses with more than fifty employees offer health coverage meeting certain standards to full-time employees.
2. Berman 2017.
3. Hacker and Pierson 2018.
4. Congressional Research Service 2021; Tikkanen and Abrams 2020.
5. Congressional Research Service 2021; Emanuel 2020.
6. Kluender et al. 2021.
7. Congressional Research Service 2021.
8. Campbell 2014; Cohn 2008, 2021; Dawes 2016; Hacker 2002; Starr 1982.
9. Michener 2018.
10. Marmor 1973, as cited in Patashnik and Oberlander 2018, 666; see also Michener 2019b; Oberlander 2003; Zelizer 2000.

11. Hacker 1999, 3.
12. Starr 1997, 150.
13. Skocpol 1996, 15.
14. Johnson and Broder 1997; Skocpol 1997.
15. Skocpol 1997, xiii.
16. Starr 1995.
17. Steinmo and Watts 1995.
18. Volden 2006.
19. Clerk of the U.S. House of Representatives 2003.
20. Morgan and Campbell 2011.
21. Lizza 2011.
22. Holan 2009.
23. Hundt 2019.
24. Brill 2015; Dawes 2016.
25. Skocpol and Williamson 2016.
26. Holan 2009.
27. Hargrove 2009.
28. Hacker 2002.
29. Jones 2017.
30. Michener 2018.
31. Galewitz 2013.
32. Elmendorf 2010.
33. Abraham 2020; Campbell and Shore-Sheppard 2020; Hall 2020.
34. Guth, Garfield, and Rudowitz 2020.
35. See also Beauregard and Miller 2020; Rocco and Kelly 2020.
36. Weisman and Pear 2013.
37. Internal Revenue Service, "Affordable Care Act Items," https://www.irs.gov/businesses/corporations/affordable-care-act-items.
38. Weisman and Pear 2013.
39. Internal Revenue Service, "Affordable Care Act Items," https://www.irs.gov/businesses/corporations/affordable-care-act-items.
40. Béland, Rocco, and Waddan 2016; Jones 2017.
41. Jones 2017; Patashnik and Oberlander 2018.
42. See especially Abraham 2020; Campbell 2014; Michener 2018.
43. Hopkins and Barry-Jester 2017.
44. Ibid.
45. Campbell and Shore-Sheppard 2020; Rocco and Kelly 2020.
46. Tolkien 1991.
47. Hundt 2019.
48. Béland, Rocco, and Waddan 2016; Jones 2017; Levy, Ying, and Bagley 2020.
49. Levy, Ying, and Bagley 2020.
50. Gleckman 2012; Levy, Ying, and Bagley 2020; Saldin 2017.
51. Norris 2021.

52. Berry, Burden, and Howell 2010; Patashnik 2008.

53. Béland, Rocco, and Waddan 2016; Hall 2020; Jones 2017.

54. Byers 2012.

55. Stelter 2012.

56. Biskupic 2019.

57. Ibid.

58. National Public Radio 2012.

59. Biskupic 2019.

60. Ibid.

61. Simmons-Duffin 2021.

62. Brill 2015.

63. *Politifact* 2020.

64. Kliff 2013.

65. Abraham 2020; Hall 2020.

66. Levy, Ying, and Bagley 2020.

67. Barrilleaux and Rainey 2014; Hertel-Fernandez, Skocpol, and Lynch 2016; Jacobs and Callaghan 2013; Pacheco, Haselswerdt, and Michener 2020; Rose 2015.

68. Jones 2017; see also Lee et al. 2017; Mayer, Kenter, and Morris 2015; Rigby and Haselswerdt 2013.

69. Pear 2015.

70. O'Keefe 2014.

71. Levy, Ying, and Bagley 2020.

72. Supreme Court of the United States 2015.

73. Barnes 2015.

74. Cillizza 2017.

75. Conway 2017.

76. Kaplan and Pear 2017.

77. Kliff 2017c.

78. Kaplan and Pear 2017.

79. Haberkorn, Everett, and Kim 2017.

80. Stanek 2017.

81. Frean, Gruber, and Sommers 2017.

82. Levy, Ying, and Bagley 2020.

83. Kliff 2017a; Pollitz, Tolbert, and Diaz 2019.

84. Bagley 2017; Keith 2019.

85. Froelich 2019.

86. Witters 2019.

87. White House 2021; see also Fording and Patton 2020.

88. Keith 2021.

89. Liptak 2021.

90. Campbell and Shore-Sheppard 2020.

91. Lizza 2011.

92. Holan 2009.

Chapter 3: The Stability of Public Opinion

1. Elster 1989.
2. Howard 1999; Mettler 2018.
3. Achen and Bartels 2016; Ashworth 2012; Converse 1964; Delli Carpini and Keeter 1996; Healy and Malhotra 2013; Huber, Hill, and Lenz 2012; Judis 2000; Kinder and Kalmoe 2017; Lane 1962; Lippmann 1922; Miller 2018; Lupia 2016; Popkin 1994; Schumpeter 1943.
4. Achen and Bartels 2016, 10–11.
5. Ibid., 11.
6. Social Security Administration, "Social Security History: Life Expectancy for Social Security," https://www.ssa.gov/history/lifeexpect.html; see also Munger 2022.
7. Schuyler 2014. Although sickness funds did exist (Murray 2007) and may have covered as many as 20 percent of workers in some occupations, they were far from the health insurance products available today (Morrisey 2013).
8. Committee for a Responsible Federal Budget 2018.
9. The information environment has also been transformed, with a proliferation of new options as well as heightened incentives for media outlets to avoid news coverage or to cover it in conflictual, attention-grabbing ways (Baum 2011; Hindman 2008; Kim 2022; Ladd 2012; Mutz 2015; Peck 2019; Prior 2007; Stroud 2011).
10. Duggan, Gupta, and Jackson 2019; Frean, Gruber, and Sommers 2017; Fry, McGuire, and Frank 2020; Gruber and Sommers 2019; Saltzman 2019.
11. Frean, Gruber, and Sommers 2017.
12. The task of attributing the health law's varied impacts to specific politicians—some of whom were out of office by the time key provisions took effect—was more challenging still (Arnold 1992).
13. Lupia 2016, 3; see also Delli Carpini and Keeter 1996.
14. Kimmel 2013.
15. Achen and Bartels 2016; Converse 1964; Popkin 1994.
16. Kimmel 2013.
17. Kliff 2016; see also Skocpol and Williamson 2016, 54.
18. Achen and Bartels 2016; Bartels 2002; Cohen 2003; Hersh 2020; Huddy, Mason, and Aarøe 2015; Lenz 2012.
19. Bullock et al. 2015; Druckman and Levendusky 2019; Fowler 2020; Klar, Krupnikov, and Ryan 2018; Orr and Huber 2020.
20. Bursztyn et al. 2022; Lerman, Sadin, and Trachtman 2017; Sances and Clinton 2019; see also Lerman and Trachtman 2021.
21. Druckman and Bolsen 2011; Zaller 1992; but see Miller and Krosnick 2000.
22. See especially Cohn 2021.
23. As reported by Daniel Hopkins and Samantha Washington (2020), the panel tracks benchmarks for the population closely. For example, in 2012, 31 percent of respondents had a bachelor's degree (compared to 30 percent in the American Community Survey, or ACS), 53 percent were female (51 percent in the ACS), 14 percent were over

sixty-five (15 percent in the ACS), and 13 percent were black (13 percent in the ACS). The survey was conducted only in English, which partially explains why Hispanics/ Latinos represented 17 percent of the 2012 population in the ACS but only 10 percent in the panel.

The panel has thirteen waves: five in 2007–2008, two in 2012 (which included the first questions about the ACA specifically), two in 2014, three in 2016, and one in 2018. Note that this panel does not provide insurance status measures until 2016, two years *after* the implementation of the ACA's principal provisions. Even so, panel data can provide critical leverage on the possibly different attitudinal trajectories of respondents with different types of insurance (see especially Jacobs and Mettler 2016, 2018). For more details on panel administration, see table A.1. For panel demographics, see table A.2.

24. Wlezien 1995; Stimson 2004; see also Page and Shapiro 1992.
25. Nadash et al. 2018; see also Gose and Skocpol 2019.
26. It is noteworthy that immigration attitudes showed a similar pattern of movement soon after Trump's election (Hopkins 2017).
27. Hacker and Pierson 2019; Jacobs and Mettler 2011; Pacheco, Haselswerdt, and Michener 2020; Richardson and Konisky 2013.
28. The question read, "As you may know, a health reform bill was signed into law in 2010. Given what you know about the health reform law, do you have a generally favorable or generally unfavorable opinion of it?"
29. Klein 2021b.
30. Achen and Bartels 2016;Converse 1964; Delli Carpini and Keeter 1996; Kinder and Kalmoe 2017; Lupia 2016; but see Arceneaux and Vander Wielen 2017.
31. Cramer 2016; Cramer Walsh 2007; Hochschild 1981, 2018; Jones-Correa 1998; Michener 2018.
32. The firms include the Kaiser Family Foundation, the Pew Research Center, Survey Sampling International, Knowledge Networks, and YouGov.
33. Notice, too, that supporters' mentions of "access" grew in 2016, even before the Democrats sought to mobilize opinions against GOP repeal efforts in 2017. A closely related argument, one about Americans' right to health care, was mentioned by 6 percent of respondents on average and was the third most common supportive argument offered. One July 2009 respondent declared, "Health care is our right."
34. James Lynch 2020.
35. Golos et al. 2022.
36. Hartz 1955; Hetherington 2005.
37. Hopkins and Barry-Jester 2017.
38. See also Richardson and Konisky 2013.
39. See also Jacobs and Mettler 2011.
40. See Fording and Patton 2020.
41. Kaiser Family Foundation 2010.
42. MacGuill 2017. I made a similar argument in a *Washington Post* op-ed (Hacker and Hopkins 2010); see also Jacobs and Mettler 2011.

43. See, for example, Hacker 2002, 2004; Pierson 1994; Steinmo and Watts 1995.
44. Cowley and Ford 2019.
45. Fernandez and Rodrik 1991; Kahneman, Knetsch, and Thaler 1991.
46. Bowler and Donovan 1998; Kriesi and Trechsel 2008.
47. Page and Shapiro 1992; Stimson 2004; Wlezien 1995.
48. Wlezien 1995.

Chapter 4: Public Opinion and the Medicaid Expansion

1. Kersey 2014.
2. Kaiser Family Foundation 2017.
3. Baicker et al. 2013; Finkelstein et al. 2012; Kluender et al. 2021.
4. Baldwin et al. 1998; Currie and Gruber 1996. For Medicaid's effect on children's educational levels, see Cohodes et al. 2016; Levine and Schanzenbach 2009; see also Fry, McGuire, and Frank 2020; Sommers, Maylone, et al. 2017; Wherry and Miller 2016.
5. Kaiser Family Foundation 2022.
6. For example, Campbell 2012; Kumlin 2004; Svallfors 2007.
7. Medicaid and CHIP Access and Payment Commission, "Medicaid Enrollment Changes Following the ACA," https://www.macpac.gov/subtopic/medicaid-enrollment-changes-following-the-aca/.
8. Rosenthal 2022.
9. Clinton and Sances 2018; Haselswerdt and Michener 2019; Michener 2018, 2019a; Pacheco and Maltby 2017; Sances and Clinton 2020.
10. Campbell 2003; Lerman 2019; Mettler 2005; but see Tallevi 2018.
11. Sears and Funk 1991; see also Bartels 2008; Benedictis-Kessner and Hankinson 2019; Brunner, Ross, and Washington 2011; Haselswerdt 2020; Hopkins 2012; Marble and Nall 2018; Margalit 2013; Mettler 2005; Pierson 1993, 1994; Soss 1999; Soss and Schram 2007.
12. See also Clinton and Sances 2018.
13. For example, Hacker and Pierson 2019; Hopkins 2018b; Iyengar et al. 2019; Levendusky 2009; Mason 2018; McCarty 2019.
14. For example, Campbell 2012; see also Hertel-Fernandez 2019a.
15. Lerman and Weaver 2014; Lerman 2019.
16. Even in 2021, there were an estimated 2 million people who would have benefited from the Medicaid expansion in the twelve states that had not expanded their programs (Simmons-Duffin 2021).
17. Anderson, Marinescu, and Shor 2019; see also Jacobs and Shapiro 2000. In Ohio in 2011, for example, voters backed a symbolic measure to invalidate the individual mandate by a margin of nearly two-to-one. This result lends credibility to survey-based evidence of the mandate's unpopularity.
18. Kahneman, Knetsch, and Thaler 1991.
19. Kaiser Family Foundation 2019.

20. Michener 2018; Verba, Schlozman, and Brady 1995; see also Michener 2019b; Soss 1999.
21. Hopkins and Mummolo 2017.
22. Cohn 2016; Frank 2016; Fukuyama 2018a, 2018b; Klein 2021a; Lilla 2018.
23. Sayers 2021.
24. See, for example, Hacker and Pierson 2020.
25. Bartels 2018; Gidron 2020; Sides, Tesler, and Vavreck 2019.
26. Kliff 2017b.
27. Goodnough 2017. As Jonathan Rodden (2022) notes, in several states the health care sector was the only sector to produce job growth in rural areas in the period from 2008 to 2020.
28. LaCasse 2017.
29. Kilgore 2017.
30. Kirzinger et al. 2017.
31. State of Maine, Bureau of Corporations, Elections & Commissions, Department of the Secretary of State, "Tabulations for Elections Held in 2017," https://www.maine .gov/sos/cec/elec/results/results16-17.html#nov17.
32. Achen and Shively 1995; King 1997.
33. In addition, we manually labeled municipalities containing hospitals that qualify for the Maine Center for Disease Control and Prevention's Flex Grants or Small Rural Hospital Improvement Grant Program (nineteen in total) as rural hospital municipalities.
34. The political measures include the share backing Governor LePage in 2014 and the share backing President Trump in 2016, while the demographics include the share with at least a bachelor's degree, the share non-Hispanic white, the logged population, and the population density.
35. These measures are drawn from the American Community Survey's five-year estimates from 2013 to 2017. We also use two alternative measures for the share of a town's population who are likely to benefit directly: the percentage below the poverty line and logged median income.
36. Although the relationship is not substantively or statistically significant when using logged income as the key measure (model 2), it is when we instead use the share below the poverty line (model 3). Model 6 illustrates that when we include all three measures of local economic deprivation jointly, all three coefficients are in the expected directions, although their strong correlations prevent any from being statistically significant in this joint model.
37. One of the arguments made in favor of Proposition 2 was that rural hospitals in particular would benefit. Robert Peterson (2017), the CEO of the Millinocket Regional Hospital, contended that "these funds will have a profound effect on the health of many Mainers and preserve our state's rural hospitals for years to come. No public policy proposal is perfect or without challenges. However, Medicaid expansion is on balance, very good for needy Maine people and for the Maine healthcare providers who care for them." Given those claims in support of Proposition 2, we also estimate

models that include measures of local dependence on hospitals or health care. In model 4, for example, we incorporate an additional indicator variable identifying cities or towns with rural hospitals that stood to benefit from the Medicaid expansion. But it is noteworthy that the coefficient is *negative* at −0.011 and insignificant (SE = 0.017). This means that these municipalities were not more likely to back the expansion despite standing to significantly gain from it. And although the coefficient for the town's share employed in health care is 0.076, as model 5 shows, the standard error of 0.084 demonstrates that this result is not especially strong, either. That said, the benefits may stretch beyond municipal boundaries and so may mean that these estimates are a lower bound.

38. Roubein 2020.
39. Jacobs and Mettler 2016.
40. McCabe 2016; see also Lerman and McCabe 2017. There is also evidence that the Medicaid expansion increased voter turnout (Clinton and Sances 2018; Haselswerdt 2017; see also Baicker and Finkelstein 2019; but see Courtemanche, Marton, and Yelowitz 2020).
41. Campbell 2012; Gingrich and Watson 2016; Mettler 2011; Morgan and Campbell 2011; Soss and Schram 2007.
42. Campbell 2012; Lerman and Weaver 2014; Soss 1999; Weaver and Lerman 2010.
43. Campbell 2014; Michener 2018.
44. Mettler 2011; Tallevi 2018.
45. Riffkin 2015.
46. Levendusky 2009. On the GI Bill, see Mettler 2005; on Social Security, see Campbell 2003.
47. Kriner and Reeves 2014; Fowler et al. 2017; Lerman, Sadin, and Trachtman 2017.
48. Druckman, Peterson, and Slothuus 2013; Lodge and Taber 2013; Patashnik and Zelizer 2013; Hopkins 2018a.
49. For general effects, see Campbell 2011, 2012; Gingrich and Watson 2016; Morgan and Campbell 2011; Soss and Schram 2007. For effects on Medicaid expansion, see Campbell 2012; Clinton and Sances 2018; Haselswerdt 2017; see also Baicker and Finkelstein 2019; but see Courtemanche, Marton, and Yelowitz 2020.
50. Hopkins and Parish 2019.
51. The average response rate across these surveys was 13 percent, with a low of 6 percent in March 2017 and a high of 25 percent in January 2010.
52. Medicaid does make substantial payments for seniors' nursing home care, but our goal is to outline the effects of the expansion of primary insurance coverage.
53. Washington, D.C., participated in the Medicaid expansion.
54. Antonisse et al. 2016.
55. We measure Medicaid receipt via a self-reported question about respondents' primary source of health insurance, making it valuable to assess this measure's validity (see especially Tallevi 2018). Despite the difficulty of measuring income in telephone surveys, the respondents receiving Medicaid were concentrated in the lower end of the income distribution. Of our non-elderly respondents, 6.3 percent reported being

on Medicaid. However, 92 percent of those who did report being on Medicaid reported incomes less than $45,001.

56. Given that the current income cap for Medicaid eligibility is $37,825 for a family of five in states that opted for the expansion with a cap at 138 percent of the federal poverty line (Baicker and Finkelstein 2019; Campbell 2012; Clinton and Sances 2018; Haselswerdt 2017), a $45,001 cutoff is substantively appropriate.

57. The survey question asks: "As you may know, a health reform bill was signed into law in 2010. Given what you know about the health reform law, do you have a generally favorable or generally unfavorable opinion of it? Is that a very favorable/unfavorable or somewhat favorable/unfavorable opinion?" For more on the impact of question wording on reported ACA attitudes, see Grande, Gollust, and Asch 2011; Holl, Niederdeppe, and Schuldt 2018.

58. See also Sances and Clinton 2020.

59. Bertrand, Duflo, and Mullainathan 2004.

60. Democrats constitute the omitted baseline. Some KFF surveys used a single question about partisan identity that separated self-reported Democrats, Republicans, and independents without a follow-up question identifying closet partisans.

61. There are a total of fifty-one states, including Washington, D.C., but we must exclude two states: one as a generic baseline and a second in order to include a separate indicator variable for states that expanded Medicaid at any time during this period. Note that the estimated effects are substantively identical in models that do not include state fixed effects.

62. Hopkins and Parish 2019. These results prove highly robust to changes in model specification or defensible changes in estimation strategy. For example, when we respecify the outcome as a binary measure of favorability, the coefficient becomes 0.038 with a standard error of 0.011. Importantly, our results are also not highly sensitive to omitting any particular states.

63. Recent research has pointed to concerns about difference-in-difference estimators when applied to treatments whose implementation is staggered over time (for example, Goodman-Bacon 2021). It is reassuring that our estimates are virtually identical (coefficient of 0.104, standard error of 0.025) when removing the six states that implemented the Medicaid expansion during the period we study but after January 1, 2014.

64. Levendusky 2009, 2010; Zaller 1992.

65. Patashnik and Oberlander 2018.

66. There is also some evidence that the public became even more polarized, with the favorability gap between Republicans and Democrats growing after the GOP's 2017 repeal attempts.

67. Haselswerdt and Michener 2019; Sances and Clinton 2020; but see Courtemanche, Marton, and Yelowitz 2020.

68. Verba, Schlozman, and Brady 1995; Fraga 2018.

69. Haselswerdt and Michener 2019; Michener 2017, 2018; see also Clinton and Sances 2018; Hagan 2016.

70. Hamel, Norton, and Brodie 2015.

71. But see Hollingsworth et al. 2019.
72. But see ibid.

Chapter 5: The Offsetting Effects of the Exchanges

1. Brill 2015.
2. Ibid.
3. Hopkins 2018b; Lerman, Sadin, and Trachtman 2017.
4. Morgan and Campbell 2011; see also Hacker 2002.
5. Elmendorf 2010.
6. Biskupic 2019.
7. Kaiser Family Foundation, "Medicaid Expansion Enrollment," https://www.kff.org /health-reform/state-indicator/medicaid-expansion-enrollment/; Kaiser Family Foundation, "State Health Facts: Marketplace Enrollment, 2014–2022," https:// www.kff.org/health-reform/state-indicator/marketplace-enrollment/.
8. See instead Courtemanche, Marton, and Yelowitz 2020; Lerman, Sadin, and Trachtman 2017; Sances and Clinton 2019; Trachtman 2018.
9. Chattopadhyay 2018.
10. Campbell 2012; Patashnik 2008; Pierson 1994; Schattschneider 1935.
11. Campbell 2003; Lerman and Weaver 2014; Mettler 2005; Soss 1999.
12. Campbell 2011; Gingrich and Watson 2016; Mettler 2018; Morgan and Campbell 2011; see also Howard 1999; Mettler 2011, 2018. Separate research bolsters these claims, concluding that citizens' attitudes are often sociotropic—influenced by the nation's economic conditions rather than their own standing—and that self-interest typically has limited effects on public opinion (Mutz 1992; Reny and Sears 2020; Sears and Funk 1991).
13. Patashnik and Oberlander 2018.
14. Jacobs and Weaver 2015; Béland, Rocco, and Waddan 2019.
15. Clemans-Cope and Anderson 2015.
16. Congressional Research Service 2021.
17. Brill 2015, 397.
18. Lee et al. 2017; Hall 2020; Abraham 2020.
19. Clinton and Sances 2018; Haselswerdt 2017; Hopkins and Parish 2019. On the ACA's overall impact, see Courtemanche, Marton, and Yelowitz 2020; Hollingsworth et al. 2019; Jacobs and Mettler 2016, 2018; McCabe 2016.
20. But see Hosek 2019; Pacheco and Maltby 2019; see also Rigby and Haselswerdt 2013.
21. Howard 1999; Mettler 2011, 2018; Morgan and Campbell 2011; Rosen 2020. Although a topic as broad and contested as neoliberalism is beyond our scope here—see instead McKean (2020), Gerstle (2022), and Cebul (2023)—the emphasis on implementing public policy through private, market-based actors fits well within some definitions of a "neoliberal" framework.
22. Hobbs and Hopkins 2021.
23. Jones 2017; Michener 2018.

24. Lerman, Sadin, and Trachtman 2017; Sances and Clinton 2019; Trachtman 2018.

25. Jacobs and Mettler 2016.

26. The Medical Expenditure Panel Survey suggests that many older adults considered the exchanges' offerings: adults ages fifty to sixty-three disproportionately switched from employer-based or COBRA plans to the exchanges after the ACA's implementation (Glied and Jackson 2017).

27. Chattopadhyay 2017.

28. Morgan and Campbell 2011.

29. It is critical to assess the impacts of the exchanges and related policies on the law's broader targeted populations, but doing so is challenging because of rampant endogenous selection. In Hobbs and Hopkins (2021), we developed a method for assessing the effects of the new exchanges on the populations most likely to be affected, such as those whose demographics made them likely to self-purchase insurance or to be uninsured. In other words, we focused on people without group-based insurance for whom the exchanges were most likely to bring meaningful change to their health insurance options. The results of that specific analysis are consistent with the broader findings reported throughout this chapter. We find little change in political attitudes among those more likely to be self-insured. Those more likely to be uninsured, however, were significantly *less* favorable toward the ACA after its implementation. Here, too, we see favorability decline during the late-2013 enrollment period, suggesting that the rocky rollout and/or cancellation of noncompliant plans—and not just experiences after 2014—may have contributed to the backlash.

30. See also Patashnik 2019.

31. For example, Hacker and Pierson 2019; Mettler 2018; Morgan and Campbell 2011.

32. Internal Revenue Service, "Affordable Care Act Items," https://www.irs.gov/businesses /corporations/affordable-care-act-items.

33. In 2017, nearly 4 million customers automatically re-enrolled with the same insurer.

34. Internal Revenue Service, "Affordable Care Act Items," https://www.irs.gov/businesses /corporations/affordable-care-act-items.

35. Abraham 2020.

36. Goldstein 2016.

37. Abraham 2020.

38. Morgan and Campbell 2011.

39. Ibid.

40. Arnold 1992; Campbell 2012; Mettler 2011, 2018.

41. See Kogan and Wood 2018. In the words of Campbell and Shore-Sheppard (2020, 2), "Although these regulatory effects were broad and important, they were in many ways more difficult for individuals to recognize."

42. The mandate was intended to increase insurance uptake through various pathways, including employer-sponsored insurance as well as self-purchased insurance.

43. Baicker and Finkelstein 2019; Larsen 2019.

44. Fowler et al. 2017; Gollust et al. 2014.

45. Hacker and Pierson 2019.

46. Finkelstein et al. 2012.
47. Campbell 2012.
48. Chattopadhyay 2018.
49. O'Donnell 2014.
50. Campbell 2012.
51. Campbell 2003.
52. Campbell 2011.
53. Jacobs and Mettler 2018.
54. Arceneaux 2012. This tendency has been observed specifically with regard to health care politics (Eckles and Schaffner 2010).
55. This survey has been conducted in most months between 2009 and 2020; here we report results for 117,234 respondents surveyed between February 2009 and September 2017.
56. Figure 5.1 also demonstrates the uptick in Medicaid receipt that followed the expansion of Medicaid in some states, from 3.7 percent to 6.6 percent.
57. How does the small share of Americans who purchased insurance via the exchanges compare to other groups? Table C.1 summarizes the means of several key variables by insurance source for post-January 2014 respondents. Consistent with Lerman, Sadin, and Trachtman (2017) and Sances and Clinton (2019), those who bought insurance through the exchanges leaned Democratic. Partisanship was similar among Medicaid recipients and those who used the exchanges, even though those using the exchanges had higher incomes and were more likely to be white. This trend indicates that any causal analyses will have to be wary of selection biases, especially given the stability of partisan identification (Green, Palmquist, and Schickler 2002; but see Hajnal and Lee 2011). Table C.1 also shows that exchange enrollees had lower incomes and were younger than the population overall but were older than the uninsured.
58. McCabe 2016.
59. Hobbs and Hopkins 2021.
60. The poll included 692 respondents under sixty-five.
61. Asking about people who purchase their own insurance is notoriously difficult. However, KFF data indicate that in 2015 Kentucky marketplace enrollment was 106,330 individuals, which amounts to 2.4 percent of Kentucky's total 2015 population. That is virtually identical to the 2 percent in the survey.
62. We restrict our analyses to those under sixty-five given that the exchanges target that population.
63. Specifically, using the four-category measure of ACA favorability as our outcome, we estimate linear models that predict ACA attitudes as a function of basic demographics, including age, education, five-category partisan identification, and identification as male, Asian American, black, and Hispanic/Latinx.
64. But conditional on income, partisanship, and other background characteristics, respondents who received Medicaid were somewhat more favorable toward the ACA than others, with coefficients varying from 0.21 (SE = 0.15) to 0.35 (SE = 0.15) depending on the specification.

65. This estimate for Kentucky residents with subsidies matches the estimate from the analyses of all adults with nongroup insurance in 2014 nationwide reported closely in Hobbs and Hopkins (2021).

66. Morgan and Winship 2007.

67. Witters 2019.

68. Specifically, those without insurance in January 2016 shifted positively toward the ACA by 0.30, while those with insurance underwent a pro-ACA shift of 0.53.

69. Morgan and Winship 2007. All three variables are coded as respondents' 2018 status minus 2016 status, so, for example, a 1 indicates someone who loses insurance while a −1 indicates someone who gains insurance. To improve the model's precision, we also include fall 2016 partisanship as well as fall 2012 ACA attitudes and several basic demographic measures, including respondents' age, education, and identification as black or Latino. See also table C.5 for the effect of including or excluding demographic covariates when modeling 2018 ACA repeal support.

70. When interpreting these coefficients, it is valuable to keep in mind that those who reported self-purchasing insurance or being on Medicaid in 2018 had varied prior insurance statuses in 2016, so these models recover the effect of switching to or away from Medicaid from various baselines. Separately, by including indicator variables for each level of 2016 ACA repeal support, we can relax the assumption that the relationship between 2016 ACA repeal support and 2018 ACA repeal support is linear.

71. Eckles and Schaffner 2010; Jacobs and Mettler 2016. On asymmetries, see Arceneaux 2012; Soroka 2006.

72. We reach highly similar conclusions by instead employing an "analysis of covariance" modeling strategy, which conditions on 2016 ACA attitudes while predicting 2018 attitudes (Morgan and Winship 2007).

73. O'Donnell 2014.

74. Kaiser Family Foundation, "State Health Facts: Total Marketplace Enrollment," https://www.kff.org/health-reform/state-indicator/ (accessed May 4, 2020).

75. Specifically, we obtained administrative data on plan pricing and offerings by geography for 2014–2017 from the Robert Wood Johnson Foundation's National Narrow Network Project.

76. Exchange customers are divided into geographic rating areas; in 2017, there were 504 such rating areas across the country. We acquired data on the insurance options and their prices for each rating area and year between 2014 and 2017. We then matched HTP respondents based on their zip code and/or county of residence to their rating area and the corresponding options and prices available to them. In addition, we also used respondents' zip codes or county of residence to merge in basic county-level census demographic information.

77. Note that our interest in premium changes from the prior year requires excluding 2014. The APTC is tied to the second-cheapest silver plan, so it is important to note that our principal measure is of each market's *mean* premium, which has the potential to influence even subsidized exchange customers, as discussed later. Mean premiums are a coarse measure of the premium increases faced by specific customers.

However, the 2015–2016 market-level correlation between all mean premium changes and those only for silver plans is 0.95; when examining only silver plans with above-benchmark premiums, the correlation is 0.92. Thus, premium shifts are highly correlated across plans within markets, and our measure of mean premium shifts broadly captures premium shocks.

78. Hobbs and Hopkins 2021.

79. Our respondents were distributed across many counties—in 2015, the 359 respondents using the markets were in 208 counties—and thus we cannot employ county fixed effects.

80. Kaiser Family Foundation, "State Health Facts: Total Marketplace Enrollment," https://www.kff.org/health-reform/state-indicator/ (accessed May 4, 2020).

81. Hobbs and Hopkins 2021.

82. Internal Revenue Service 2015.

83. Lerman and McCabe 2017.

84. These analyses assume that people do not perfectly anticipate their reactions to becoming sixty-five; to the extent that attitudes shift in anticipation of turning sixty-five and becoming Medicare-eligible, these results are underestimates. In addition, for those in their late sixties to serve as a comparison group, it is critical that this group did *not* have other group-specific experiences that might have made their ACA attitudes more negative at roughly the same time. For example, the ACA did include policies targeting those sixty-five and older, as well as a reduction in Medicare Advantage payments beginning in 2011, the gradual closing of the "doughnut hole" in prescription drug coverage between 2010 and 2020, and newly free preventative care services as of 2011. Yet none of these policies were implemented in or around 2014. This time line suggests that our use of those sixty-five and older as a point of comparison is reasonable.

85. Multiple mechanisms are evident in the figure. For example, we see a suggestive rise and then dip among sixty-four-year-old attitudes in late 2013, when the exchanges opened and some noncompliant plans were canceled. But given the core finding that ACA favorability increased post-implementation among sixty-four-year-olds, either the ACA's positive effects outweighed those negative effects or the negative effects receded.

86. Focusing on just one discontinuity also helps preserve statistical power, given the limitations and assumptions required to estimate regression discontinuities both in general and especially across multiple dimensions simultaneously (Cattaneo, Idrobo, and Titiunik 2017).

87. Lerman and McCabe 2017.

88. One caveat: either increased positive experiences or decreased negative experiences could drive any observed post-implementation changes.

89. Imbens and Kalyanaraman 2012. The HTP includes 7,738 respondents ages sixty-two to sixty-four and 9,862 sixty-five- to sixty-eight-year-olds.

90. Lerman and McCabe 2017.

91. Notably, the findings are also consistent with those near sixty-five having especially negative health care experiences prior to 2014—experiences that became less negative post-ACA.
92. See also Chattopadhyay 2017.
93. Lassman et al. 2014.
94. We estimate the Imbens and Kalyanaraman (2012) bandwidth to be just under three years. Using this bandwidth, we then fit a parametric polynomial regression using the rddtools package in R.
95. Kiefer 2016.
96. Hobbs and Hopkins (2021) report more evidence of negative reactions to the ACA: those Americans most likely to become uninsured after the ACA's implementation were also more likely to shift their opinion against the ACA.
97. Hacker and Pierson 2018; Jones 2017; Patashnik and Oberlander 2018.
98. Kriner and Reeves 2012.
99. Rae et al. 2021.
100. Gustafsson and Collins 2022.
101. Mettler 2018; Rosen 2020.
102. Stokes 2020.

Chapter 6: The Indirect Role of White Americans' Racial Attitudes

1. Metzl 2019, 1, 2; see also Mutz 2018; but see Putnam 2007.
2. Stephens-Dougan 2020; White 2007.
3. See especially Gillion 2013, 2020; McCabe 2019; Michener 2018, 2020.
4. Gilens 1999; Hancock 2004; Kinder and Sanders 1996; Kluegel and Smith 1986; Quadagno 1994; Sniderman and Carmines 1997; Winter 2006.
5. Acharya, Blackwell, and Sen 2018; Goldman and Hopkins 2019; Sen and Wasow 2016.
6. Huber and Lapinski 2006; Hutchings and Jardina 2009; Hutchings, Walton, and Benjamin 2010; Lapinski and Huber 2008; Mendelberg 2001, 2008; Sniderman and Carmines 1997; Stephens-Dougan 2020; Tesler 2012; Valentino 1999; Valentino, Hutchings, and White 2002; Valentino, Neuner, and Vandenbroek 2017.
7. But see Broockman and Kalla 2016; Chong and Druckman 2010; Coppock 2017, 25.
8. Acharya, Blackwell, and Sen 2018; Einhorn 2006; Lieberman 1998; Michener 2019b; Smith 1997; Soss and Weaver 2016, 20.
9. Grogan and Park 2017; Michener 2020.
10. Metzl 2019.
11. Tesler 2012.
12. Michener 2020; see also Beauregard and Miller 2020.
13. Julia Lynch 2020.
14. Gilens 1999; Hancock 2004; Hutchings 2009; Kinder and Sanders 1996; Kinder and Winter 2001; Peffley, Hurwitz, and Sniderman 1997; Winter 2008; see also Huber and Paris 2013.
15. Goren 2008; see also Goren 2003.

16. Lanford and Quadagno 2016; Michener 2018, 2019b; Snowden and Graaf 2019.
17. Sides, Tesler, and Vavreck 2019.
18. Edsall 1991; Gilens 1999; Hancock 2004.
19. Carmines and Stimson 1989; Kinder and Sanders 1996.
20. Perlstein 2012; see also Gillion 2016; Hutchings, Walton, and Benjamin 2010; Mendelberg 2001; Stephens-Dougan 2020. Nixon aide John Ehrlichman connected GOP policies on drugs to the same racist political strategy: "We knew we couldn't make it illegal to be either against the war or black, but by getting the public to associate the hippies with marijuana and blacks with heroin, and then criminalizing both heavily, we could disrupt those communities. We could arrest their leaders, raid their homes, break up their meetings, and vilify them night after night on the evening news" (Hodge 2021).
21. Jacobs and Shapiro 2000.
22. Chattopadhyay 2018.
23. In chapters 4 and 5, we focused on the impacts of a policy's design on those who experience the policy firsthand. Recent research finds that policy design can also have an independent influence on other citizens' views about the policy. For instance, programs coordinated through the tax code generate more support than those involving direct transfers (Ashok and Huber 2020; Ellis and Faricy 2020). Americans also reason from policy design to a policy's likely beneficiaries: Jake Haselswerdt (2020) finds that when a policy lacks a work requirement, it is perceived as more likely to benefit black Americans and immigrants.
24. Fording and Patton 2020.
25. Kirzinger et al. 2017.
26. Carmines and Stimson 1989; Gillion 2016; Kinder and Dale-Riddle 2012; Kinder and Sanders 1996; Ogorzalek 2018; Putnam and Garrett 2020; Schickler 2016; Sniderman and Carmines 1997; Tesler and Sears 2010.
27. Engelhardt 2020.
28. Engelhardt 2019; Hajnal 2020; Hopkins 2021; Knowles, Lowery, and Schaumberg 2010; Lundberg et al. 2017; Parker and Barreto 2014; Schaffner, Macwilliams, and Nteta 2018; Sides, Tesler, and Vavreck 2019; Tesler 2012, 2016; Westwood and Peterson 2020; but see Enns 2018; Grimmer and Marble 2019.
29. Kinder and Kalmoe 2017; Kinder and Sanders 1996; Sniderman and Piazza 1993; Tesler 2016.
30. Winter 2008.
31. Stephens-Dougan 2020; Tesler 2016.
32. Edsall 1991; Kinder and Sanders 1996; Mendelberg 2001; Sniderman and Carmines 1997.
33. Hopkins 2021; see also Valentino, Neuner, and Vandenbroek 2017.
34. Sen and Wasow 2016.
35. See especially Acharya, Blackwell, and Sen 2018.
36. Hochschild 1981.
37. Hamel, Norton, and Brodie 2015.

38. Gilens 1999; Goldman and Hopkins 2019; Kluegel and Smith 1986; McGhee 2021; Mendelberg 2001; see also Soss, Fording, and Schram 2011.
39. Lieberman 1998; Michener 2019b.
40. Pratto et al. 1994.
41. Cramer 2016; Hochschild 2018.
42. See especially Valentino, Neuner, and Vandenbroek 2017.
43. Carmines and Stimson 1989.
44. For example, Hurwitz and Peffley 2005; Hutchings and Jardina 2009; Mendelberg 2001; Tesler 2012, 2016; Valentino 1999; White 2007.
45. Hopkins 2021; Hurwitz and Peffley 2005; Tesler 2012; Winter 2008.
46. Banks 2014a, 2014b.
47. Wetts and Willer 2018; see also Jardina 2019.
48. Cuddy et al. 2009; Gilens 1999; Hancock 2004; Haselswerdt 2020; Kluegel and Smith 1986; Quadagno 1994; Winter 2008.
49. A Pearson's correlation reports a fraction that varies from −1 to 1 and that indicates the strength of the linear association between two variables: 0 indicates that the two variables have no linear relationship, whereas 1 indicates that they move up together in lockstep.
50. Winter 2006, 2008.
51. Tesler 2012.
52. Hopkins 2021; Huber and Lapinski 2006; Hurwitz and Peffley 2005; Hutchings and Jardina 2009; Stephens-Dougan 2020; Valentino 1999; Valentino, Hutchings, and White 2002; Valentino, Neuner, and Vandenbroek 2017; White 2007.
53. Feldman and Huddy 2005; Carmines, Sniderman, and Easter 2011; Peyton and Huber 2020.
54. Blinder, Ford, and Ivarsflaten 2013; Ivarsflaten, Blinder, and Ford 2010; Mendelberg 2001.
55. Lenz 2012.
56. Tesler 2012.
57. Carmines and Stimson 1989; Kinder and Dale-Riddle 2012; Kinder and Sanders 1996; Sniderman and Carmines 1997; Stephens-Dougan 2020; Tesler 2016.
58. Engelhardt 2019, 2020; Grimmer and Marble 2019.
59. Huber and Lapinski 2006; Mendelberg 2001; Stephens-Dougan 2020; Tesler 2015, 2016; Valentino 1999; Valentino, Hutchings, and White 2002; Valentino, Neuner, and Vandenbroek 2017.
60. Conover and Feldman 1984; Huddy 2018.
61. Carmines and Stimson 1989; Kinder and Dale-Riddle 2012; Kinder and Sanders 1996; Schickler 2016; Sniderman and Carmines 1997; Tesler 2016; Tesler and Sears 2010.
62. Acharya, Blackwell, and Sen 2018; Billings, Chyn, and Haggag 2020; Goldman and Hopkins 2019.
63. Goodnough 2018.
64. Skocpol and Williamson 2016, 35.
65. Cunha 2019.

66. Kinder and Sanders 1996; Kinder and Winter 2001; Kluegel and Smith 1986; Quadagno 1994; Soss, Fording, and Schram 2011.
67. Banks 2014a; Gilens 1999.
68. By contrast, the correlations between views on unemployment insurance and food stamps are quite high, at 0.67 (white respondents) and 0.68 (overall).
69. We can reinforce such claims by looking at the correlations in word usage when respondents are asked to justify their views. The correlations are higher between ACA attitudes and student loan regulation attitudes than with any other policy save unemployment insurance. In word usage as well as in their stated positions, Americans' ACA attitudes do not have much in common with their attitudes on food stamps.
70. Barabas and Jerit 2010.
71. Hopkins and Gorton 2022.
72. But see Akesson et al. 2022.
73. The choice of seven separate experiments was also encouraged by a mistake. I had made a coding error in analyzing one of the initial survey experiments and so planned additional experiments in light of a misunderstanding of the preliminary results. I thank Will Hobbs for catching the error, which was corrected after I had embarked on several follow-up experiments.
74. Krupnikov and Ryan 2022.
75. Hopkins and Gorton 2022.
76. Other groups included "you and your family," "senior citizens," "people who live in cities," "people who live in rural areas," "women," "unemployed people," "Democrats," "Republicans," and "the community where you live."
77. Hopkins and Noel 2022.
78. Hopkins, Sides, and Citrin 2019.
79. Acharya, Blackwell, and Sen 2018; Dawson 1994; Du Bois 1903; Fredrickson 1982; Glaser and Ryan 2013; Kendi 2019; Kinder and Dale-Riddle 2012; McGhee 2021; McWhorter 2021; Michener 2019b; Soss and Weaver 2016; Tocqueville 1863; Weaver and Lerman 2010; Wilkerson 2020.
80. For reviews, see Hutchings and Jardina 2009; Stephens-Dougan 2020.
81. Druckman and Leeper 2012; see also Acharya, Blackwell, and Sen 2018; Goldman and Hopkins 2019.
82. Engelhardt 2020; Tesler 2016.

Chapter 7: Framing's Limited Short-Term Impacts

1. *Frontline* 2009.
2. Ruffin 2003. Meanwhile, a Democratic campaign staffer's 2013 book was subtitled: *How a Compelling Narrative Will Make Your Organization Succeed* (Friend 2013). Similarly, the podcast of the prominent Democratic campaign adviser Anat Shenker-Osorio is called *Words to Win By*.
3. Lakoff 2004, 21, 45.

4. *Frontline* 2004. Likewise, in 2021 Republican House leader Kevin McCarthy pointed to the centrality of messaging in winning elections: "Remember, majorities are not given, they are earned. And that's about the message going forward" (Segers 2021).

5. Steinhauer and Pear 2011.

6. Pomerantsev 2015, 73.

7. The three journals were the *American Journal of Political Science, American Political Science Review*, and *Journal of Politics*.

8. Druckman, Fein, and Leeper 2012, 430.

9. Jacobs and Mettler 2011; Kriner and Reeves 2014; Nyhan 2010.

10. See also Brooke, Chouhoud, and Hoffman, forthcoming.

11. But see Arceneaux and Johnson 2013; Coppock 2021.

12. But see Broockman and Skovron 2018.

13. Chong and Druckman 2011.

14. Barberá et al. 2019; Baumgartner, De Boef, and Boydstun 2008; de Vreese 2003; Edwards 2009; Entman 2004; Hopkins, Kim, and Kim 2017; Jacobs et al. 2003; Kellstedt 2003; Smith 2007.

15. Vavreck 2009.

16. Barabas and Jerit 2010; see also Broockman and Kalla, forthcoming.

17. On public attention, see Arceneaux, Johnson, and Murphy 2012; Prior 2007. For a discussion of selective information-seeking, see Druckman, Fein, and Leeper 2012.

18. Pew Research Center 2010.

19. Bartels 2002; Guess 2021; Guess et al. 2021; Krupnikov and Ryan 2022.

20. Bail 2021; Bail et al. 2018; Berinsky 2009; Druckman 2001; but see Porter and Wood 2019.

21. Zaller 1992.

22. Hersh 2020; Krupnikov and Ryan 2022; Levendusky 2009.

23. Entman 2004; Hayes 2008.

24. Baumgartner et al. 2009.

25. Druckman and Jacobs 2015; Jacobs and Burns 2004; Jacobs and Shapiro 2000; Trussler and Soroka 2014.

26. More technically, studying messaging or framing in real-world contexts also foregrounds a significant measurement problem. Framing is thought to influence public opinion by changing the relative accessibility and applicability of different considerations in citizens' minds. Yet when politicians emphasize a certain aspect of an issue, they also provide different information and employ different persuasive strategies (Leeper and Slothuus 2018; Scheufele and Iyengar 2012; see also Lenz 2012). Framing effects take place when certain aspects of a broader issue become cognitively accessible, but not when citizens learn new facts or are persuaded to evaluate existing facts differently. Thus, it is difficult in most real-world studies to distinguish framing from learning or other types of persuasion.

27. Jacobs and Shapiro 2000.

28. Hopkins 2018a; Hopkins and Mummolo 2017; Yokum et al. 2022.

29. See also Kalla and Broockman 2018.

30. This focus on natural language also provides a way of identifying whether elite frames do in fact change the aspects of a political issue that are cognitively accessible to

citizens. "Cognitively accessible" refers to mental considerations that are easily recalled or brought into memory by an individual.

31. Yokum et al. 2022.
32. For example, Berinsky 2009; Broockman and Kalla 2022; Hopkins and Ladd 2014; Zaller 1992. On the ACA specifically, see Pacheco, Haselswerdt, and Michener 2020.
33. Hopkins 2021.
34. See Berinsky 2007; Jacobs and Mettler 2011.
35. See Hopkins, Sides, and Citrin 2019; Porter and Wood 2019.
36. For framing effects over time horizons, see Smith 2007.
37. See also Jacobs and Shapiro 2000.
38. Nelson 2011; Scheufele and Iyengar 2012.
39. Chong and Druckman 2010, 665.
40. Framing effects are distinct from learning or persuasion, as the underlying mechanism of framing is cognitive accessibility (Huber and Paris 2013). Framing effects are expected to be stronger among those with more knowledge of or experience with a given subject, as they will have a wider variety of considerations to connect to that issue (Chong and Druckman 2007b; Mutz 1994; but see Lecheler, de Vreese, and Slothuus 2009).
41. Broockman and Kalla 2016.
42. Gerber and Green 2000; Putnam 2000.
43. Kalla and Broockman 2020; Kalla, Levine, and Broockman 2021.
44. Bailey, Hopkins, and Rogers 2016; Kalla and Broockman 2018.
45. Druckman and Leeper 2012; Scheufele and Iyengar 2012.
46. For example, Chong and Druckman 2007a; Iyengar and Kinder 1987; Leeper and Slothuus 2018; Nelson, Clawson, and Oxley 1997.
47. Druckman 2001; Slothuus and de Vreese 2010; but see Bullock 2011. Attentive to concerns about external validity, scholars of framing have increasingly adopted research designs that more closely approximate real-world settings, whether by allowing for competing frames (Chong and Druckman 2007a; Sniderman and Theriault 2004) or providing choices about exposure to frames (Arceneaux, Johnson, and Murphy 2012; Druckman, Fein, and Leeper 2012).
48. Baumgartner et al. 2009.
49. For example, Entman 2004; Hayes 2008.
50. Jacobs and Burns 2004.
51. Slothuus and de Vreese 2010; Taber and Lodge 2006.
52. Hill et al. 2013.
53. For example, Jacobs et al. 2003; Kellstedt 2003; Smith 2007; but see Edwards 2009.
54. Gerber et al. 2011; Hill et al. 2013; Johnston, Hagen, and Jamieson 2004; Ridout and Franz 2011; Sides, Vavreck, and Warshaw 2022.
55. See especially Leeper and Slothuus 2018; Scheufele and Iyengar 2012.
56. Lenz 2012; Lodge and Taber 2013.
57. Lodge and Taber 2013, 22.
58. See Peyton 2020.

59. Hetherington 2005; see also Mettler 2019.

60. There is some observational evidence in keeping with this account. In November and December 2011, I included questions on a two-wave panel survey using KN, a firm that provided a population-based sample of American adults. In the first wave, I measured trust in government by asking respondents: "How much of the time do you think you can trust the national government to do what is right?" Even accounting for a variety of other factors, including education, ideology, partisanship, and presidential approval, respondents' answers to that question were predictive of their ACA assessments: those who answered "just about always," on average, rated the ACA 0.30 (SE = 0.15) higher on a 1–4 favorability scale than those who answered "hardly ever." That is roughly the same effect as a shift in approval from "strongly disapproving" to "disapproving." In keeping with Hetherington's hypothesis, the more respondents trusted government, the more favorable they were toward the ACA.

61. After collecting the data, we first conducted balance tests to examine whether key variables were evenly distributed across the experimental conditions. As detailed in tables E.1 to E.3, there is no evidence of notable imbalances across any of the three experiments.

62. It is plausible that the low-trust argument might be especially compelling to those with lower levels of trust to begin with. Given that, we used the question about trust in the national government to identify low-trust respondents. We then reanalyzed the experiments after reducing the data sets to the 87 percent of 2011 respondents, 77 percent of 2017 respondents, and 71 percent of 2018 respondents who answered that they trusted the government "some of the time" or "hardly ever." But as figure E.1 demonstrates, this untrusting subset did not substantially revise their attitudes after hearing the argument tapping distrust. In 2011, low-trust respondents who saw the low-trust argument scored at 2.11 on the 1–4 favorability scale, a figure that is almost indistinguishable from the 2.14 average score observed among the control group ($p = 0.70$).

63. Using the 2011 data, which were collected through a two-wave panel, I also examined whether exposure to the distrustful argument in the second panel wave primed respondents' levels of trust measured in the first wave. It did. Among respondents assigned to the control group, the coefficient mapping trust in government to ACA assessments is 0.098 (SE = 0.049), indicating a moderate-size effect. But among those who were exposed to the low-trust argument, that coefficient almost doubles, to 0.177 (SE = 0.045). The difference between these coefficients does not reach conventional levels of statistical significance ($p = 0.12$, one-sided), but this result suggests that trust levels may be subject to priming.

64. The absence of an overall difference between the treatment and control groups— a so-called null result—is always subject to multiple explanations. In the case of the SSI surveys, for instance, the experiment took place after respondents had already answered other ACA-related questions; perhaps already having been primed to think about the ACA reduced their responsiveness to any manipulation. But the same cannot be said about the KN experiment, which asked a population-based sample about a wide range of other issues as well. In addition, because the KN respondents

were drawn from a broader sample, they were less likely to be highly knowledgeable. Moreover, with a combined total of more than 5,100 respondents, the three experiments were well powered to detect even moderately sized effects.

65. Hopkins and Mummolo 2017; see also Coppock and Green 2022.

66. Specifically, respondents assigned to treatment read that "health care is one of the most complicated issues that we face. It involves 1 of every 6 dollars spent here in the United States. The health care system includes millions of doctors and nurses and thousands of hospitals and clinics. Together, they regularly make decisions that can mean life or death. The government in Washington can't even balance its own budget. How can we trust it to run something as complicated as the health care system?"

67. Pacheco, Haselswerdt, and Michener 2020.

68. Blei, Ng, and Jordan 2003.

69. Grimmer and King 2011. To understand LDA, it is valuable to state the model using the notation from Blei, Ng, and Jordan (2003). Let K be a predefined number of clusters in a set of documents, with $\mathbf{w}$ a vector representing a document and V representing the number of unique words in the vocabulary. LDA models a collection of documents as emerging through the following process. First, the length of the document N is chosen from a Poisson distribution with a prior parameter. Then the distribution of topics in that document θ is chosen from a Dirichlet distribution with a separate prior parameter often denoted "alpha." From there, for each of the N words w_n, we first draw a word-specific topic z_n from a multinomial distribution and then choose a word w_n from $p(w_n|z_n, \beta)$ $(w_n \sim p(w_n|z_n, \beta))$, where β is a $V \times K$ matrix indicating the probability that each of the K topics associates with each of the V words. Of the estimated parameters, a few are of particular interest. One is the β (hat) matrix, which allows us to identify the words that are associated with each topic. The second parameter is the document-specific θ (hat) vector, which provides the share of each document that falls into each topic. As with similar models in political science (Quinn et al. 2010; Roberts et al. 2014), this approach can be highly valuable in reducing the dimension of a textual data set and partitioning a set of documents into meaningful subtopics (Grimmer and Stewart 2013).

70. Payne 1951, 54.

71. Even so, within the field of political science to date, LDA and similar techniques have been primarily applied to lengthier documents of at least a few hundred words (for example, Grimmer 2010; Lauderdale and Clark 2014; Quinn et al. 2010). Empirically, it remains unclear whether brief open-ended responses of several words provide sufficient density for such techniques to return meaningful clusters (Eisenstein et al. 2010; Roberts et al. 2014).

72. Grimmer 2010.

73. The search terms were "healthcare," "health care," "obamacare," "health reform," and "health insurance reform."

74. Although exposure to news through other sources is indisputably important (see Baum 2011) and such "soft news" coverage can surely convey frames, this research focuses on direct channels of influence by political elites.

75. Other measures of salience depict a similar trajectory: while public and elite attention to health care reform began growing as early as the summer of 2009, it drew far more attention in the fall and winter of 2009–2010. For example, Lexis-Nexis (now Nexis Uni) keyword searches of CNN and *Fox News* transcripts indicate that attention to health care reform rose to a peak of 603 stories in August 2009, remained high through the following fall and winter, and reached a maximum of 667 stories in March 2010. According to the Gallup "Most Important Problem" series, the share of the public citing health care as the nation's most important problem rose from 7 percent in the second quarter of 2009 to 16 percent in the third quarter, and it remained above 13 percent in the first quarter of 2010 (Eissler and Jones 2019).

76. To prepare the press releases and television appearances for model-fitting, we first pre-processed them using common techniques (for example, Hopkins and King 2010). All words were reduced to common stems such as "senat" for "Senate," "Senator," and so on (Porter 1980), and those word stems that appeared in fewer than 1 percent of the documents were removed. In addition, we removed proper nouns that were likely to be specific to certain documents, such as senators' names, states' names, and party designations (for example, "R-WY"). Preprocessing left us with 2,309 word stems for the press releases and 2,057 for the television appearances.

77. LDA returns a θ vector of length $K - 1$, indicating the topic probabilities as well as a β matrix. The β matrix has dimension $K * V$, with each cell indicating the probability that each word would be used conditional on each topic.

78. See Boyd-Graber et al. 2009; Hopkins and King 2010. The results from models fit with K set to 10 and 14 are available in the appendix of Hopkins 2018a.

79. Specifically, we allowed K to vary over the range from 5 to 15, and then we chose the value of K that maximized the share of clusters that were clearly interpretable as coherent frames. The core conclusions are not sensitive to this choice, and several results presented here attest to the utility of the particular model employed (Grimmer and Stewart 2013).

80. Some elected Republicans did play up these concerns, though they did not use the same language (Rutenberg and Calmes 2009).

81. See also Jacobs and Mettler 2011.

82. Lynch and Gollust 2010.

83. Another cluster seems to focus on the Children's Health Insurance Program, which got attention primarily from Democrats before the ACA debate started in earnest (top row, second from right). In periods when the ACA was less salient, Democrats' health care–related press releases focused more on funding for community health programs (bottom row, second from left). The twelve states include South Dakota, which voted in November 2022 to expand Medicaid.

84. While most of these clusters are legitimate frames, some are procedural clusters without significant framing value. The cluster labeled with the stems "law," "report," "act," and "fraud" (top row, far right) appears to be one such cluster.

85. We also analyzed the standard deviation across frames for each party separately in 2009 and 2010. For Democrats the standard deviation declines slightly, while for Republicans it increases slightly. Neither case constitutes strong evidence of consolidation around specific frames.

86. These analyses include television appearances by senators and representatives from both parties and members of the Obama administration who dealt with health care reform. Such press appearances are widely seen as attempts at agenda-setting and offer prime opportunities to push health care–related frames. We collected such press appearances from five media outlets: *Fox News*, CNN, ABC, NBC, and CBS.

87. We exclude a small number of names—typically those of the shows' hosts—as well as common English-language stop words.

88. As with the press releases, we also observe a few catchall clusters without substantive interpretations.

89. See also Druckman, Fein, and Leeper 2012.

90. The first two surveys were conducted by the Pew Research Center in July 2009 ($n = 1,506$) and November 2009 ($n = 1,003$), and the remaining five were conducted by the Kaiser Family Foundation in May 2010 ($n = 1,210$), October 2010 ($n = 1,202$), March 2011 ($n = 1,202$), June 2011 ($n = 1,201$), and November 2011 ($n = 1,209$). The Kaiser question was: "Can you tell me in your own words what is the main reason you have a favorable/an unfavorable opinion of the health care reform law?" Pew asked respondents, "What would you say is the main reason you favor/oppose the health care proposals being discussed in Congress?"

91. In reviewing open-ended responses, we identified spelling or formatting errors in 9 to 14 percent of the Pew open-ended responses and corrected them. For the Kaiser surveys, the comparable error rates were 1 to 2 percent. We then conduct standard preprocessing, including stemming words (Porter 1980), removing stop words, and removing words of one and two letters. There are 3,715 unique word stems in the corpus as a whole; we remove all but the 225 word stems that appear in at least 0.25 percent of the documents. We again experiment with various numbers of clusters, from four to twelve, before choosing six as a maximally coherent representation that distinguishes the major frames.

92. For the technical details, see Hopkins 2018a.

93. More technically, we begin by representing a given set of surveys or press releases as a probability distribution across the V words in the overall vocabulary. The distribution of interest is the share of the total words in a given corpus accounted for by each particular word w_v. We can then calculate the distance $p_{pr}(w_v)$ between the distribution of words in a group of press releases $p_{sur}(w_v)$ and the distribution of the same words among the public $p_{sur}(w_n)$, using any of several distance metrics.

94. To measure whether such differences are statistically meaningful, we use bootstrapping, randomly drawing ten thousand new data sets of press releases and open-ended responses and repeating the measurement procedure outlined earlier. The increase in the symmetrized KL divergence between Democratic press releases and citizens' language is in the unexpected direction but insignificant for the early period between July and November ($p = 0.95$, one-sided), as illustrated on the left-hand side of figure 7.6. We see the same insignificant result on the Republican side ($p = 0.925$).

95. As the center panel of figure 7.6 shows, we reach the same conclusion when estimating a more intuitive metric: the average absolute difference between the word frequencies in the open-ended responses and those in the press releases. For Democrats

that figure drops from 0.0102 to 0.0098 between November 2009 and May 2010, while for Republicans it drops from 0.0094 to 0.0088.

96. Fowler et al. 2017.

97. See Hopkins, Schwarz, and Chainani, forthcoming.

98. For example, Bail et al. 2018; Bhanot and Hopkins 2020; Druckman 2001; Gadarian, Goodman, and Pepinsky 2021b; Golos et al. 2022; Pacheco, Haselswerdt, and Michener 2020; Zaller 1992; but see Gadarian, Goodman, and Pepinsky 2021a.

99. See especially Lerman, Sadin, and Trachtman 2017; Sances and Clinton 2019; Trachtman 2018.

100. Shafer et al. 2020.

101. See also Gollust et al. 2018; Gollust, Fowler, and Niederdeppe 2019; Ogilvy 2018.

102. See also Yokum et al. 2022.

103. For a related field experiment, see Levine 2015.

104. *Time* 1965.

105. See also Noel 2014; Smith 2007.

106. False claims about "death panels" were a descendant of attacks on the 1993–1994 Clinton health care plan. The ACA's backers may have reacted with the failure of that earlier health reform effort in mind (Rutenberg and Calmes 2009).

107. This pattern of findings is consistent with the results of Lodge and Taber (2013), a study that emphasizes unconscious, often affective processes in shaping public opinion.

108. Pomerantsev 2015, 69.

109. Greene 2020, 5.

110. Berinsky and Kinder 2006; Heath and Heath 2007; Lakoff 1981; Shiller 2019; Tilly 2002.

111. Baumgartner, De Boef, and Boydstun 2008; Baumgartner et al. 2009; Noel 2014; Smith 2007.

Chapter 8: Conclusion

1. To an important extent, the debate focused on the role of racial issues in Democrats' messaging (Bacon 2021; English and Kalla 2021; Haney-López 2019; Klein 2021a).

2. See Hacker and Pierson 2019; Levendusky 2009; McCarty 2019; Pacheco, Haselswerdt, and Michener 2020.

3. Ambrose 1997, 22.

4. Internal Revenue Service, "Affordable Care Act Items," https://www.irs.gov/businesses/corporations/affordable-care-act-items.

5. Also, if enacting policies were a surefire way to build political support, why do researchers so consistently observe that politicians and parties tend to lose support during their time in office? (Green and Jennings 2017).

6. Fowler et al. 2020; Grossman et al. 2020.

7. Bhanot and Hopkins 2020; Golos et al. 2022; Kushner Gadarian, Goodman, and Pepinsky 2021. On the waning influence of elite-level rhetoric and policy during the pandemic, see Gupta, Simon, and Wing 2020; Herby 2021; Whaley et al. 2021; see also Guntermann and Lenz 2022.

8. Klein 2022; see also Jaroszewicz, Jachimowicz, and Hauser 2022.

9. Hopkins and Noel 2022.

10. Smith 2021.

11. Hopkins 2021; Hopkins and Washington 2020.

12. Hopkins 2018b; Hopkins, Schickler, and Azizi 2022; Iyengar et al. 2019; Lee 2016; McCarty 2019.

13. On mass-membership organizations, see Putnam 2000; Skocpol 2003; but see Schlozman 2015. On the fragmentation of the media landscape, see Bennett and Iyengar 2008.

14. Gurri 2018; Naím 2013; Pildes 2021.

15. Patashnik 2008.

16. Béland, Rocco, and Waddan 2016; Hertel-Fernandez, Skocpol, and Lynch 2016; Jones 2017; Patashnik and Zelizer 2013; Rocco and Haeder 2018.

17. Bawn et al. 2012; but see Canes-Wrone 2015.

18. Kaiser Family Foundation 2010.

19. Frean, Gruber, and Sommers 2017.

20. Caughey and Warshaw 2022.

21. *New York Times* 2010.

22. Wlezien 1995.

23. Lee 2009.

24. See Bawn et al. 2012; Mansbridge 1986.

25. Wlezien 1995.

26. Lee 2016; Trende 2012.

27. See Blum 2020; Han 2014; Parker and Barreto 2014; Skocpol and Williamson 2016.

28. Gerber and Green 2000, 2012; Morton and Williams 2010; Mutz 2011; Sniderman and Grob 1996.

29. Sen and Wasow 2016.

30. Hall 2003.

31. Bacon 2018.

32. Witters 2019.

33. Fording and Patton 2020; Kaiser Family Foundation 2021.

34. Jaffe 2021.

35. Bartels 2022.

Appendix C

1. These questions were asked in fourteen surveys between 2010 and early 2014 ($n \approx 18,000$).

2. Manning, Raghavan, and Schütze 2008.

3. We have twenty-nine respondents who were uninsured in both waves, twenty-three who were uninsured only in 2016, and seventeen who were uninsured only in 2018. When predicting changes in insurance status, we do find that Republicans were marginally less likely to become uninsured in this period.

REFERENCES

Abraham, Jean Marie. 2020. "Individual Market Volatility and Vulnerability, 2015 to 2019." *RSF: The Russell Sage Foundation Journal of the Social Sciences* 6(2): 206–22. DOI: https://doi.org/10.7758/RSF.2020.6.2.09.

Abramowitz, Alan. 2013. *The Polarized Public? Why American Government Is So Dysfunctional.* Boston: Pearson.

Acharya, Avidit, Matthew Blackwell, and Maya Sen. 2018. *Deep Roots: How Slavery Still Shapes Southern Politics.* Princeton, N.J.: Princeton University Press.

Achen, Christopher H., and Larry Bartels. 2016. *Democracy for Realists: Why Elections Do Not Produce Responsive Government.* Princeton, N.J.: Princeton University Press.

Achen, Christopher H., and W. Phillips Shively. 1995. *Cross-Level Inference.* Chicago: University of Chicago Press.

Ahler, Douglas J., and Gaurav Sood. 2018. "The Parties in Our Heads: Misperceptions about Party Composition and Their Consequences." *Journal of Politics* 80(3): 964–81.

Akesson, Jesper, Robert W. Hahn, Robert D. Metcalfe, and Itzhak Rasooly. 2022. "Race and Redistribution in the United States: An Experimental Analysis." Working Paper Series 30426. National Bureau of Economic Research, September.

Aklin, Michael, and Matto Mildenberger. 2020. "Prisoners of the Wrong Dilemma: Why Distributive Conflict, Not Collective Action, Characterizes the Politics of Climate Change." *Global Environmental Politics* 20(4): 4–27.

Ambrose, Stephen. 1997. *Undaunted Courage: Meriwether Lewis, Thomas Jefferson, and the Opening of the American West.* New York: Simon & Schuster.

Anderson, Soren, Ioana Elena Marinescu, and Boris Shor. 2019. "Can Pigou at the Polls Stop Us Melting the Poles?" Working Paper 26146. National Bureau of Economic Research, August. DOI: https://doi.org/10.3386/w26146.

Angrist, Joshua D., and Jörn-Steffen Pischke. 2010. "The Credibility Revolution in Empirical Economics: How Better Research Design Is Taking the Con Out of Econometrics." *Journal of Economic Perspectives* 24(2): 3–30.

Antonisse, Larisa, Rachel Garfield, Robin Rudowitz, and Samantha Artiga. 2016. "The Effects of Medicaid Expansion under the ACA: Updated Findings from a Literature Review." Kaiser Family Foundation, June. http://www.nationaldisabilitynavigator.org /wp-content/uploads/news-items/KFF_Effects-of-Medicaid-Expansion_June-2016.pdf.

Anzia, Sarah, Jake Alton Jares, and Neil Malhotra. 2021. "Does Receiving Government Assistance Shape Political Attitudes? Evidence from Agricultural Producers." *American Political Science Review* (April 19): 1–18. DOI: https://doi.org/10.1017/S0003055422000314.

Arceneaux, Kevin. 2012. "Cognitive Biases and the Strength of Political Arguments." *American Journal of Political Science* 56(2): 271–85.

Arceneaux, Kevin, and Martin Johnson. 2013. *Changing Minds or Changing Channels? Partisan News in an Age of Choice.* Chicago: University of Chicago Press.

Arceneaux, Kevin, Martin Johnson, and Chad Murphy. 2012. "Polarized Political Communication, Oppositional Media Hostility, and Selective Exposure." *Journal of Politics* 74(1): 174–86.

Arceneaux, Kevin, and Ryan J. Vander Wielen. 2017. *Taming Intuition: How Reflection Minimizes Partisan Reasoning and Promotes Democratic Accountability.* Cambridge: Cambridge University Press.

Arnold, R. Douglas. 1992. *The Logic of Congressional Action.* New Haven, Conn.: Yale University Press.

Ashok, Vivekinan and Gregory A. Huber. 2020. "Do Means of Program Delivery and Distributional Consequences Affect Policy Support? Experimental Evidence about the Sources of Citizens' Policy Opinions." *Political Behavior* 42(4): 1097–1118.

Ashworth, Scott. 2012. "Electoral Accountability: Recent Theoretical and Empirical Work." *Annual Review of Political Science* 15(1): 183–201.

Associated Press. 2013. "Policy Notifications and Current Status, by State." *Yahoo News,* December 26, 2013. https://finance.yahoo.com/news/policy-notifications-current -status-state-204701399.html.

Azari, Julia. 2018. "Forget Norms. Our Democracy Depends on Values." *FiveThirtyEight,* May 24, 2018. https://fivethirtyeight.com/features/forget-norms-our-democracy-depends -on-values/.

Bachrach, Peter, and Morton S. Baratz. 1962. "Two Faces of Power." *American Political Science Review* 56(4): 947–52.

Bacon, Perry, Jr. 2018. "Republicans Killed Much of Obamacare without Repealing It." *FiveThirtyEight,* December 18, 2018. https://fivethirtyeight.com/features/republicans -killed-much-of-obamacare-without-repealing-it/.

———. 2021. "The Problem with Our Election Obsession." *Washington Post,* October 7, 2021. https://www.washingtonpost.com/opinions/2021/10/07/perry-bacon-america -election-obsession/.

Bagley, Nicholas. 2017. "Trump's Ominous Threat to Withhold Payment from Health Insurers, Explained." *Vox,* March 29, 2017. https://www.vox.com/the-big-idea/2017/3/29/15107836 /lawsuit-aca-payments-reimbursement-unconstitutional.

Baicker, Katherine, and Amy Finkelstein. 2019. "The Impact of Medicaid Expansion on Voter Participation: Evidence from the Oregon Health Insurance Experiment." *Quarterly Journal of Political Science* 14(4): 383–400.

Baicker, Katherine, Sarah L. Taubman, Heidi L. Allen, Mira Bernstein, Jonathan H. Gruber, Joseph P. Newhouse, Eric C. Schneider, Bill J. Wright, Alan M. Zaslavsky, and Amy N. Finkelstein. 2013. "The Oregon Experiment—Effects of Medicaid on Clinical Outcomes." *New England Journal of Medicine* 368(18): 1713–22.

Bail, Christopher A. 2021. *Breaking the Social Media Prism: How to Make Our Platforms Less Polarizing.* Princeton, N.J.: Princeton University Press.

Bail, Christopher A., Lisa P. Argyle, Taylor W. Brown, John P. Bumpus, Haohan Chen, M. B. Fallin Hunzaker, Jaemin Lee, Marcus Mann, Friedolin Merhout, and Alexander Volfovsky. 2018. "Exposure to Opposing Views on Social Media Can Increase Political Polarization." *Proceedings of the National Academy of Sciences* 115(37): 9216–21.

Bailey, Michael A., Daniel J. Hopkins, and Todd Rogers. 2016. "Unresponsive and Unpersuaded: The Unintended Consequences of a Voter Persuasion Effort." *Political Behavior* 38(3): 713–46.

Baldwin, Laura-Mae, Eric H. Larson, Frederick A. Connell, D. Nordlund, K. C. Cain, M. L. Cawthon, P. Byrns, and R. A. Rosenblatt. 1998. "The Effect of Expanding Medicaid Prenatal Services on Birth Outcomes." *American Journal of Public Health* 88(11): 1623–29.

Banks, Antoine J. 2014a. *Anger and Racial Politics: The Emotional Foundation of Racial Attitudes in America.* New York: Cambridge University Press.

———. 2014b. "The Public's Anger: White Racial Attitudes and Opinions toward Health Care Reform." *Political Behavior* 36(3): 493–514.

Barabas, Jason, and Jennifer Jerit. 2010. "Are Survey Experiments Externally Valid?" *American Political Science Review* 104(2): 226–42.

Barberá, Pablo, Andreu Casas, Jonathan Nagler, Patrick J. Egan, Richard Bonneau, John T. Jost, and Joshua A. Tucker. 2019. "Who Leads? Who Follows? Measuring Issue Attention and Agenda Setting by Legislators and the Mass Public Using Social Media Data." *American Political Science Review* 113(4): 883–901.

Barnes, Robert. 2015. "Affordable Care Act Survives Supreme Court Challenge." *Washington Post*, June 25, 2015. https://www.washingtonpost.com/politics/courts_law/obamacare-survives-supreme-court-challenge/2015/06/25/af87608e-188a-11e5-93b7-5eddc056ad8a_story.html.

Barrilleaux, Charles, and Carlisle Rainey. 2014. "The Politics of Need: Examining Governors' Decisions to Oppose the 'Obamacare' Medicaid Expansion." *State Politics and Policy Quarterly* 14(4): 437–60.

Bartels, Larry M. 2002. "Beyond the Running Tally: Partisan Bias in Political Perceptions." *Political Behavior* 24(2): 117–50.

———. 2008. *Unequal Democracy: The Political Economy of the New Gilded Age.* New York: Russell Sage Foundation.

———. 2018. "Partisanship in the Trump Era." *Journal of Politics* 80(4): 1483–94.

———. 2022. "Public Opinion and the Crisis of Democracy in Europe." Unpublished book manuscript.

Baum, Matthew A. 2011. *Soft News Goes to War: Public Opinion and American Foreign Policy in the New Media Age.* Princeton, N.J.: Princeton University Press.

Baumgartner, Frank R., Jeffery M. Berry, Marie Hojnacki, Beth Leech, and David C. Kimball. 2009. *Lobbying and Policy Change: Who Wins, Who Loses, and Why.* Chicago: University of Chicago Press.

Baumgartner, Frank R., Suzanna De Boef, and Amber E. Boydstun. 2008. *The Decline of the Death Penalty and the Discovery of Innocence.* New York: Cambridge University Press.

Bawn, Kathleen, Martin Cohen, David Karol, Seth Masket, Hans Noel, and John Zaller. 2012. "A Theory of Political Parties: Groups, Policy Demands, and Nominations in American Politics." *Perspectives on Politics* 10(3): 571–97.

Beauregard, Kalimon Lisa, and Edward Alan Miller. 2020. "Why Do States Pursue Medicaid Home Care Opportunities? Explaining State Adoption of the Patient Protection and Affordable Care Act's Home and Community-Based Services Initiatives." *RSF: The Russell Sage Foundation Journal of the Social Sciences* 6(2): 154–78. DOI: https://doi.org/10.7758/RSF.2020.6.2.07.

Béland, Daniel, Andrea Louise Campbell, and R. Kent Weaver. 2022. *Policy Feedback: How Policies Shape Politics.* New York: Cambridge University Press.

Béland, Daniel, Philip Rocco, and Alex Waddan. 2016. *Obamacare Wars: Federalism, State Politics, and the Affordable Care Act.* Lawrence: University Press of Kansas.

———. 2019. "Policy Feedback and the Politics of the Affordable Care Act." *Policy Studies Journal* 47(2): 395–422.

———. 2020. "The Affordable Care Act in the States: Fragmented Politics, Unstable Policy." *Journal of Health Politics, Policy, and Law* 45(4): 647–60.

Benedictis-Kessner, Justin de, and Michael Hankinson. 2019. "Concentrated Burdens: How Self-Interest and Partisanship Shape Opinion on Opioid Treatment Policy." *American Political Science Review* 113(4): 1078–84.

Bennett, W. Lance, and Shanto Iyengar. 2008. "A New Era of Minimal Effects? The Changing Foundations of Political Communication." *Journal of Communication* 58(4): 707–31.

Berinsky, Adam J. 2007. "Assuming the Costs of War: Events, Elites, and American Public Support for Military Conflict." *Journal of Politics* 69(4): 975–97.

———. 2009. *In Time of War: Understanding American Public Opinion from World War II to Iraq.* Chicago: University of Chicago Press.

———. 2017. "Rumors and Health Care Reform: Experiments in Political Misinformation." *British Journal of Political Science* 47(2): 241–62.

Berinsky, Adam J., and Donald R. Kinder. 2006. "Making Sense of Issues through Media Frames: Understanding the Kosovo Crisis." *Journal of Politics* 68(3): 640–56.

Berman, Russell. 2017. "The Senate's Blind Vote on 'Skinny Repeal.'" *Atlantic*, July 27, 2017. https://www.theatlantic.com/politics/archive/2017/07/the-senates-blind-vote-on-skinny-repeal/535164/.

Berry, Christopher R., Barry C. Burden, and William G. Howell. 2010. "After Enactment: The Lives and Deaths of Federal Programs." *American Journal of Political Science* 54(1): 1–17.

Bertrand, Marianne, Esther Duflo, and Sendhil Mullainathan. 2004. "How Much Should We Trust Differences-in-Differences Estimates?" *Quarterly Journal of Economics* 119(1): 249–75.

Bhanot, Syon, and Daniel J. Hopkins. 2020. "Partisan Polarization and Resistance to Elite Messages: Results from Survey Experiments on Social Distancing." *Journal of Behavioral Public Administration* 3(2): 1–17.

Billings, Stephen, Eric Chyn, and Kareem Haggag. 2020. "The Long-Run Effects of School Racial Diversity on Political Identity." Working Paper 27302. National Bureau of Economic Research, June. DOI: https://doi.org/10.3386/w27302.

Biskupic, Joan. 2019. *The Chief: The Life and Turbulent Times of Chief Justice John Roberts.* New York: Basic Books.

Blei, David M., Andrew Y. Ng, and Michael I. Jordan. 2003. "Latent Dirichlet Allocation." *Journal of Machine Learning Research* 3: 999–1022.

Blendon, Robert J., and John M. Benson. 2014. "Voters and the Affordable Care Act in the 2014 Election." *New England Journal of Medicine* 371(20): e31.

———. 2017. "Public Opinion about the Future of the Affordable Care Act." *New England Journal of Medicine* 377(9): e12.

Blinder, Scott, Robert Ford, and Elisabeth Ivarsflaten. 2013. "The Better Angels of Our Nature: How the Antiprejudice Norm Affects Policy and Party Preferences in Great Britain and Germany." *American Journal of Political Science* 57(4): 841–57.

Blum, Rachel M. 2020. *How the Tea Party Captured the GOP: Insurgent Factions in American Politics.* Chicago: University of Chicago Press.

Bode, Leticia, Ceren Budak, Jonathan M. Ladd, Frank Newport, Josh Pasek, Lisa O. Singh, Stuart N. Soroka, and Michael W. Traugott. 2020. *Words That Matter: How the News and Social Media Shaped the 2016 Presidential Campaign.* Washington, D.C.: Brookings Institution Press.

Boudreau, Cheryl, and Scott A. MacKenzie. 2014. "Informing the Electorate? How Party Cues and Policy Information Affect Public Opinion about Initiatives." *American Journal of Political Science* 58(1): 48–62.

Bowler, Shaun, and Todd Andrew Donovan. 1998. *Demanding Choices: Opinion, Voting, and Direct Democracy.* Ann Arbor: University of Michigan Press.

Boyd-Graber, Jordan, Jonathan Chang, Sean Gerrish, Chong Wang, and David M. Blei. 2009. "Reading Tea Leaves: How Humans Interpret Topic Models." In *Advances in Neural Information Processing Systems* 22, edited by Yoshua Bengio, Dale Schuurmans, John D. Lafferty, Christopher K. I. Williams, and Aron Culotta, proceedings of the twenty-third Annual Conference on Neural Information Processing Systems, 288–96. Vancouver, B.C. (December 7–10).

Boydstun, Amber E., Rebecca A. Glazier, Matthew T. Pietryka, and Philip Resnik. 2014. "Real-Time Reactions to a 2012 Presidential Debate: A Method for Understanding Which Messages Matter." *Public Opinion Quarterly* 78(S1): 330–43.

Brill, Steven. 2015. *America's Bitter Pill: Money, Politics, Backroom Deals, and the Fight to Fix Our Broken Healthcare System.* New York: Random House.

Broder, David, and Haynes Johnson. 1996. *The System: The American Way of Politics at the Breaking Point.* New York: Hachette Book Group.

Brodie, Mollyann, Elizabeth Hamel, and Ashley Kirzinger. 2019. "Partisanship, Polling, and the Affordable Care Act." *Public Opinion Quarterly* 83(2): 423–49.

Broockman, David E., and Daniel M. Butler. 2017. "The Causal Effects of Elite Position-Taking on Voter Attitudes: Field Experiments with Elite Communication." *American Journal of Political Science* 61(1): 208–21.

Broockman, David E., and Joshua Kalla. 2016. "Durably Reducing Transphobia: A Field Experiment on Door-to-Door Canvassing." *Science* 352(6282): 220–24.

———. 2022. "The Manifold Effects of Partisan Media on Viewers' Beliefs and Attitudes: A Field Experiment with Fox News Viewers." OSF Preprints, April 1. https://osf.io/jrw26/.

———. Forthcoming. "When and Why Are Campaigns' Persuasive Effects Small? Evidence from the 2020 U.S. Presidential Election." *American Journal of Political Science*.

Broockman, David E., and Christopher Skovron. 2018. "Bias in Perceptions of Public Opinion among Political Elites." *American Political Science Review* 112(3): 542–63.

Brooke, Steven, Youssef Chouhoud, and Mike Hoffman. Forthcoming. "The Friday Effect: How Communal Religious Practice Heightens Exclusionary Attitudes." *British Journal of Political Science*.

Brunner, Eric, Stephen Ross, and Ebonya Washington. 2011. "Economics and Policy Preferences: Causal Evidence of the Impact of Economic Conditions on Support for Redistribution and Other Ballot Proposals." *Review of Economics and Statistics* 93(3): 888–906.

Bullock, John. 2011. "Elite Influence on Public Opinion in an Informed Electorate." *American Political Science Review* 105(3): 496–515.

Bullock, John, Alan Gerber, Seth Hill, and Gregory Huber. 2015. "Partisan Bias in Factual Beliefs about Politics." *Quarterly Journal of Political Science* 10(4): 519–78.

Bursztyn, Leonardo, Jonathan Kolstad, Aakaash Rao, Pietro Tebaldi, and Noam Yuchtman. 2022. "Political Adverse Selection." Working Paper 2022-87. Becker Friedman Institute, June. https://bfi.uchicago.edu/wp-content/uploads/2022/06/BFI_WP_2022-87.pdf.

Byers, Dylan. 2012. "CNN's Jeffrey Toobin: 'I Got It Wrong.'" *Politico*, June 28, 2012. https://www.politico.com/blogs/media/2012/06/cnns-jeffrey-toobin-i-got-it-wrong-127605.

Campbell, Andrea L. 2003. *How Policies Make Citizens: Senior Political Activism and the American Welfare State.* Princeton, N.J.: Princeton University Press.

———. 2011. "Policy Feedbacks and the Impact of Policy Designs on Public Opinion." *Journal of Health Politics, Policy, and Law* 36(6): 961–73.

———. 2012. "Policy Makes Mass Politics." *Annual Review of Political Science* 15(1): 333–51.

———. 2014. *Trapped in America's Safety Net: One Family's Struggle.* Chicago: University of Chicago Press.

Campbell, Andrea L., and Lara Shore-Sheppard. 2020. "The Social, Political, and Economic Effects of the Affordable Care Act: Introduction to the Issue." *RSF: The Russell Sage Foundation Journal of the Social Sciences* 6(2): 1–40. DOI: https://doi.org/10.7758/RSF.2020.6.2.01.

Canes-Wrone, Brandice. 2015. "From Mass Preferences to Policy." *Annual Review of Political Science* 18(1): 147–65.

Canes-Wrone, Brandice, David W. Brady, and John F. Cogan. 2002. "Out of Step, Out of Office: Electoral Accountability and House Members' Voting." *American Political Science Review* 96(1): 127–40.

Carmines, Edward G., Paul M. Sniderman, and Beth C. Easter. 2011. "On the Meaning, Measurement, and Implications of Racial Resentment." *Annals of the American Academy of Political and Social Science* 634(1): 98–116.

Carmines, Edward G., and James A. Stimson. 1989. *Issue Evolution: Race and the Transformation of American Politics.* Princeton, N.J.: Princeton University Press.

Cattaneo, Matias D., Nicolás Idrobo, and Rocío Titiunik. 2017. *A Practical Introduction to Regression Discontinuity Designs.* Cambridge: Cambridge University Press.

Caughey, Devin, and Christopher Warshaw. 2022. *Dynamic Democracy: Public Opinion, Elections, and Policy Making in the American States.* Chicago: University of Chicago Press.

Cebul, Brent. 2023. *Illusions of Progress: Business, Poverty, and Liberalism in the American Century.* Philadelphia: University of Pennsylvania Press.

Centers for Medicare & Medicaid Services. 2021. "NHE Fact Sheet." Last updated December 15, 2021. https://www.cms.gov/Research-Statistics-Data-and-Systems/Statistics-Trends-and -Reports/NationalHealthExpendData/NHE-Fact-Sheet.

Chan, Nathan Kar Ming, Jae Yeon Kim, and Vivien Leung. 2022. "COVID-19 and Asian Americans: How Elite Messaging and Social Exclusion Shape Partisan Attitudes." *Perspectives on Politics* 20(2): 618–34.

Chattopadhyay, Jacqueline. 2017. "Is the ACA's Dependent Coverage Provision Generating Positive Feedback Effects among Young Adults?" *Poverty and Public Policy* 9(1): 42–70.

———. 2018. "Is the Affordable Care Act Cultivating a Cross-Class Constituency?" *Journal of Health Politics, Policy, and Law* 43(1): 19–67. DOI: https://doi.org/10.1215/03616878-4249805.

Chong, Dennis, and James N. Druckman. 2007a. "Framing Public Opinion in Competitive Democracies." *American Political Science Review* 101(4): 637–55.

———. 2007b. "A Theory of Framing and Opinion Formation." *Journal of Communication* 57(1): 99–118.

———. 2010. "Dynamic Public Opinion: Communication Effects over Time." *American Political Science Review* 104(4): 663–80.

———. 2011. "Public-Elite Interactions: Puzzles in Search of Researchers." In *The Oxford Handbook of American Public Opinion and the Media*, edited by Robert Y. Shapiro and Lawrence R Jacobs. New York: Oxford University Press.

Cillizza, Chris. 2017. "How the 'Jimmy Kimmel Test' Became the Health Care Fight's Measuring Stick." *The Point*, CNN, September 20, 2017. https://www.cnn.com /2017/09/20/politics/health-care-kimmel/index.html.

Clemans-Cope, Lisa, and Nathaniel Anderson. 2015. "QuickTake: Health Insurance Policy Cancellations Were Uncommon in 2014." Urban Institute Health Policy Center, March 12. https://hrms.urban.org/quicktakes/Health-Insurance-Policy-Cancellations-Were -Uncommon-in-2014.html.

Clerk of the U.S. House of Representatives. 2003. "Final Vote Results for Roll Call 332." June 27. http://clerk.house.gov/evs/2003/roll332.xml.

Clinton, Joshua D., and Michael W. Sances. 2018. "The Politics of Policy: The Initial Mass Political Effects of Medicaid Expansion in the States." *American Political Science Review* 112(1): 167–85.

Cohen, Geoffrey L. 2003. "Party over Policy: The Dominating Impact of Group Influence on Political Beliefs." *Journal of Personality and Social Psychology* 85(5): 808.

Cohn, Jonathan. 2008. *Sick: The Untold Story of America's Health Care Crisis—and the People Who Pay the Price*. New York: Harper Perennial.

———. 2021. *The Ten Year War: Obamacare and the Unfinished Crusade for Universal Coverage*. New York: St. Martin's Press.

Cohn, Nate. 2016. "There Are More White Voters than People Think. That's Good News for Trump." *New York Times*, June 9, 2016. https://www.nytimes.com/2016/06/10/upshot/there-are-more-white-voters-than-people-think-thats-good-news-for-trump.html.

Cohodes, Sarah R., Daniel S. Grossman, Samuel A. Kleiner, and Michael F. Lovenheim. 2016. "The Effect of Child Health Insurance Access on Schooling: Evidence from Public Insurance Expansions." *Journal of Human Resources* 51(3): 727–59.

Collier, David, and Henry E. Brady. 2004. *Rethinking Social Inquiry: Diverse Tools, Shared Standards*. Lanham, Md.: Rowman & Littlefield Publishers.

Committee for a Responsible Federal Budget. 2018. "American Health Care: Health Spending and the Federal Budget." Committee for a Responsible Federal Budget, May 16. https://www.crfb.org/papers/american-health-care-health-spending-and-federal-budget.

Congressional Research Service. 2021. "U.S. Health Care Coverage and Spending." January 26. https://crsreports.congress.gov/product/pdf/IF/IF10830/9.

Conover, Pamela Johnston, and Stanley Feldman. 1984. "Group Identification, Values, and the Nature of Political Beliefs." *American Politics Quarterly* 12(2): 151–75.

Constant, Benjamin. 1988. *Constant: Political Writings*. New York: Cambridge University Press.

Converse, Phillip E. 1964. "The Nature of Belief Systems in Mass Publics." In *Ideology and Discontent*, edited by David Apter. New York: Free Press.

Conway, Madeline. 2017. "Ryan: 'Obamacare Is the Law of the Land' for Foreseeable Future." *Politico*, March 17, 2017. https://www.politico.com/story/2017/03/obamacare-repeal-failed-paul-ryan-reaction-236478.

Coppock, Alexander. 2017. "The Persistence of Survey Experimental Treatment Effects." February 21. https://alexandercoppock.com/coppock_2017b.pdf.

———. 2021. *Persuasion in Parallel: How Information Changes Minds about Politics*. Chicago: University of Chicago Press.

Coppock, Alexander, and Donald P. Green. 2022. "Do Belief Systems Exhibit Dynamic Constraint?" *Journal of Politics* 84(2): 725–38.

Courtemanche, Charles, James Marton, and Aaron Yelowitz. 2020. "The Full Impact of the Affordable Care Act on Political Participation." *RSF: The Russell Sage Foundation Journal of the Social Sciences* 6(2): 179–204. DOI: https://doi.org/10.7758/RSF.2020.6.2.08.

Cowley, Philip, and Robert Ford. 2019. *Sex, Lies and Politics: The Secret Influences That Drive Our Political Choices*. London: Biteback Publishing.

Cramer, Katherine J. 2016. *The Politics of Resentment: Rural Consciousness in Wisconsin and the Rise of Scott Walker*. Chicago: University of Chicago Press.

Cramer Walsh, Katherine. 2007. *Talking about Race: Community Dialogues and the Politics of Difference*. Chicago: University of Chicago Press.

Cuddy, Amy J. C., Susan T. Fiske, Virginia S. Y. Kwan, Peter Glick, Stéphanie Demoulin, Jacques-Philippe Leyens, Michael Harris Bond, et al. 2009. "Stereotype Content Model across Cultures: Towards Universal Similarities and Some Differences." *British Journal of Social Psychology* 48(1): 1–33.

Cunha, Darlena. 2019. "How Florida Republicans Are Talking about Impeachment." *New York Times*, October 21, 2019. https://www.nytimes.com/2019/10/21/opinion/florida-republicans-impeachment.html.

Currie, Janet, and Jonathan Gruber. 1996. "Saving Babies: The Efficacy and Cost of Recent Changes in the Medicaid Eligibility of Pregnant Women." *Journal of Political Economy* 104(6): 1263–96.

Dawes, Daniel. 2016. *150 Years of ObamaCare*. Baltimore: Johns Hopkins University Press.

Dawson, Michael C. 1994. *Behind the Mule: Race and Class in African-American Politics*. Princeton, N.J.: Princeton University Press.

DeBonis, Mike. 2019. "McCarthy Blames Republican Loss of House Majority on GOP Health Care Bill." *Washington Post*, February 12, 2019. https://www.washingtonpost.com/powerpost/mccarthy-blames-republican-loss-of-house-majority-on-gop-health-care-bill/2019/02/12/651e967a-2eed-11e9-813a-0ab2f17e305b_story.html.

Delli Carpini, Michael X., and Scott Keeter. 1996. *What Americans Know about Politics and Why It Matters*. New Haven, Conn.: Yale University Press.

DePillis, Lydia. 2022. "Pace of Climate Change Sends Economists Back to Drawing Board." *New York Times*, August 25, 2022.

de Vreese, Claes H. 2003. *Framing Europe: Television News and European Integration*. Amsterdam: Het Spinhuis.

Dorn, Stan, Bowen Garrett, and John Holahan. 2014. "Redistribution under the ACA Is Modest in Scope." Urban Institute, February. https://www.urban.org/sites/default/files/alfresco/publication-pdfs/413023-Redistribution-Under-the-ACA-is-Modest-in-Scope.PDF.

Druckman, James N. 2001. "On the Limits of Framing Effects: Who Can Frame?" *Journal of Politics* 63(4): 1041–66.

Druckman, James N., and Toby Bolsen. 2011. "Framing, Motivated Reasoning, and Opinions about Emergent Technologies." *Journal of Communication* 61(4): 659–88.

Druckman, James N., Jordan Fein, and Thomas J. Leeper. 2012. "A Source of Bias in Public Opinion Stability." *American Political Science Review* 106(2): 430–54.

Druckman, James N., and Lawrence R. Jacobs. 2015. *Who Governs? Presidents, Public Opinion, and Manipulation*. Chicago: University of Chicago Press.

Druckman, James N., and Thomas J. Leeper. 2012. "Learning More from Political Communication Experiments: Pretreatment and Its Effects." *American Journal of Political Science* 56(4): 875–96.

Druckman, James N., and Matthew S. Levendusky. 2019. "What Do We Measure When We Measure Affective Polarization?" *Public Opinion Quarterly* 83(1): 114–22.

Druckman, James N., Erik Peterson, and Rune Slothuus. 2013. "How Elite Partisan Polarization Affects Public Opinion Formation." *American Political Science Review* 107(1): 57–79.

Du Bois, W.E.B. 1903. *The Souls of Black Folk*. New York: Oxford University Press.

Duggan, Mark, Atul Gupta, and Emilie Jackson. 2019. "The Impact of the Affordable Care Act: Evidence from California's Hospital Sector." Working Paper 25488. National Bureau of Economic Research, January. DOI: https://doi.org/10.3386/w25488.

Eckles, David L., and Brian F. Schaffner. 2010. "Loss Aversion and the Framing of the Health Care Reform Debate." *Forum* 8(1): article 7.

Edsall, Thomas B. 1991. *Chain Reaction: The Impact of Race, Rights, and Taxes on American Politics.* New York: W. W. Norton & Co.

Edwards, George C. 2009. *The Strategic President: Persuasion and Opportunity in Presidential Leadership.* Princeton, N.J.: Princeton University Press.

———. 2012. *Overreach: Leadership in the Obama Presidency.* Princeton, N.J.: Princeton University Press.

Einhorn, Robin. 2006. *American Taxation, American Slavery.* Chicago: University of Chicago Press.

Eisenstein, Jacob, Brendan O'Connor, Noah A. Smith, and Eric P. Xing. 2010. "A Latent Variable Model for Geographic Lexical Variation." In *Proceedings of the 2010 Conference on Empirical Methods in Natural Language Processing*, 1277–87. Stroudsburg, Penn.: Association for Computational Linguistics.

Eissler, Rebecca, and Bryan D. Jones. 2019. "The US Policy Agendas Project." In *Comparative Policy Agendas: Theory, Tools, Data*, edited by Frank R. Baumgartner, Christian Breunig, and Emiliano Grossman. New York: Oxford University Press.

Ellis, Christopher, and Christopher Faricy. 2020. "Race, 'Deservingness,' and Social Spending Attitudes: The Role of Policy Delivery Mechanism." *Political Behavior* 42(3): 819–43.

Ellis, Christopher, and James A. Stimson. 2012. *Ideology in America.* Cambridge: Cambridge University Press.

Elmendorf, Douglas W. 2010. "Letter to Speaker Nancy Pelosi: Estimated Budgetary Impact of H.R. 3590." Congressional Budget Office, March 20. https://images.procon.org/wp-content/uploads/sites/49/cboestimateofhealthcarelawspendingrevenue.pdf.

Elster, Jon. 1989. "Social Norms and Economic Theory." *Journal of Economic Perspectives* 3(4): 99–117.

Emanuel, Ezekiel J. 2020. *Which Country Has the World's Best Health Care?* New York: Public Affairs.

Engelhardt, Andrew M. 2019. "Trumped by Race: Explanations for Race's Influence on Whites' Votes in 2016." *Quarterly Journal of Political Science* 14(3): 313–28.

———. 2020. "Racial Attitudes through a Partisan Lens." *British Journal of Political Science* 51(3): 1062–79.

English, Micah, and Joshua Kalla. 2021. "Racial Equality Frames and Public Policy Support: Survey Experimental Evidence." OSF Preprints, April 23. DOI: https://doi.org/10.31219/osf.io/tdkf3.

Enns, Peter K. 2018. "Clarifying the Role of Racism in the 2016 U.S. Presidential Election: Opinion Change, Anti–Immigrant Sentiment, and Vote Choice." Paper presented at the annual meeting of the American Political Science Association. Boston (August 30–September 2).

Enos, Ryan D. 2017. *The Space between Us: Social Geography and Politics.* Cambridge: Cambridge University Press.

Entman, Robert M. 2004. *Projections of Power: Framing News, Public Opinion, and U.S. Foreign Policy.* Chicago: University of Chicago Press.

Feldman, Stanley, and Leonie Huddy. 2005. "Racial Resentment and White Opposition to Race-Conscious Programs: Principles or Prejudice?" *American Journal of Political Science* 49(1): 168–83.

Fernandez, Raquel, and Dani Rodrik. 1991. "Resistance to Reform: Status Quo Bias in the Presence of Individual-Specific Uncertainty." *American Economic Review* 81(5): 1146–55.

Finkelstein, Amy, Sarah Taubman, Bill Wright, Mira Bernstein, Jonathan Gruber, Joseph P. Newhouse, Heidi Allen, Katherine Baicker, and Oregon Health Study Group. 2012. "The Oregon Health Insurance Experiment: Evidence from the First Year." *Quarterly Journal of Economics* 12(3): 1057–1106.

Fording, Richard C., and Dana Patton. 2020. "The Affordable Care Act and the Diffusion of Policy Feedback: The Case of Medicaid Work Requirements." *RSF: The Russell Sage Foundation Journal of the Social Sciences* 6(2): 131–53. DOI: https://doi.org/10.7758/RSF.2020.6.2.06.

Fowler, Anthony. 2020. "Partisan Intoxication or Policy Voting?" *Quarterly Journal of Political Science* 15(2): 141–79.

Fowler, Erika Franklin, Laura Baum, Colleen Barry, Jeff Niederdeppe, and Sarah Gollust. 2017. "Media Messages and Perceptions of the Affordable Care Act during the Early Phase of Implementation." *Journal of Health Politics, Policy, and Law* 42(1): 167–95.

Fowler, James H., Seth J. Hill, Remy Levin, and Nick Obradovich. 2020. "The Effect of Stay-at-Home Orders on Covid-19 Cases and Fatalities in the United States." arXiv:2004.06098v4 [stat.AP]. DOI: https://doi.org/10.48550/arXiv.2004.06098.

Fraga, Bernard L. 2018. *The Turnout Gap: Race, Ethnicity, and Political Inequality in a Diversifying America.* Cambridge: Cambridge University Press.

Frank, Thomas. 2016. *Listen, Liberal, or, What Ever Happened to the Party of the People?* New York: Metropolitan Books.

Frean, Molly, Jonathan Gruber, and Benjamin D. Sommers. 2017. "Premium Subsidies, the Mandate, and Medicaid Expansion: Coverage Effects of the Affordable Care Act." *Journal of Health Economics* 53(May): 72–86.

Fredrickson, George M. 1982. *White Supremacy: A Comparative Study of American and South African History.* Oxford: Oxford University Press.

Friend, Zach. 2013. *On Message: How a Compelling Narrative Will Make Your Organization Succeed.* New York: Turner Publishing.

Froelich, Jacqueline. 2019. "In Arkansas, Thousands of People Have Lost Medicaid Coverage over New Work Rule." *All Things Considered,* NPR, February 18, 2019. https://www.npr.org/sections/health-shots/2019/02/18/694504586/in-arkansas-thousands-of-people-have-lost-medicaid-coverage-over-new-work-rule.

Frontline. 2004. "Interview: Frank Luntz." *Frontline,* PBS, November 9, 2004. https://www.pbs.org/wgbh/pages/frontline/shows/persuaders/interviews/luntz.html.

———. 2009. "Transcript: Dreams of Obama." *Frontline,* PBS, January 11, 2009. https://www.pbs.org/wgbh/pages/frontline/dreamsofobama/etc/script.html.

Fry, Carrie E., Thomas G. McGuire, and Richard G. Frank. 2020. "Medicaid Expansion's Spillover to the Criminal Justice System: Evidence from Six Urban Counties." *RSF: The*

Russell Sage Foundation Journal of the Social Sciences 6(2): 244–63. DOI: https://doi.org/10.7758/RSF.2020.6.2.11.

Fukuyama, Francis. 2018a. "Against Identity Politics: The New Tribalism and the Crisis of Democracy." *Foreign Affairs* 97(5): 90–114.

———. 2018b. *Identity: The Demand for Dignity and the Politics of Resentment.* New York: Farrar, Straus and Giroux.

Gadarian, Shana Kushner, Sara Wallace Goodman, and Thomas B. Pepinsky. 2021a. "Partisan Endorsement Experiments Do Not Affect Mass Opinion on Covid-19." *Journal of Elections, Public Opinion, and Parties* 31(suppl.): 122–31.

———. 2021b. "Partisanship, Health Behavior, and Policy Attitudes in the Early Stages of the Covid-19 Pandemic." *PLoS ONE* 16(4): e0249596.

Galewitz, Phil. 2013. "48 Million Americans Remain Uninsured, Census Bureau Reports." *Kaiser Health News*, September 17, 2013. https://khn.org/news/census-numbers-uninsured-numbers-remain-nearly-unchanged/.

Galvin, Daniel, and Chloe Thurston. 2017. "The Democrats' Misplaced Faith in Policy Feedback." *Forum* 15(2): 333–43.

Garz, Marcel, and Gregory J. Martin. 2021. "Media Influence on Vote Choices: Unemployment News and Incumbents' Electoral Prospects." *American Journal of Political Science* 65(2): 278–93.

Gaventa, John. 1980. *Power and Powerlessness: Quiescence and Rebellion in an Appalachian Valley.* Urbana: University of Illinois Press.

Gerber, Alan S., James G. Gimpel, Donald P. Green, and Daron R. Shaw. 2011. "How Large and Long-Lasting Are the Persuasive Effects of Televised Campaign Ads? Results from a Randomized Field Experiment." *American Political Science Review* 105(1): 135–50.

Gerber, Alan S., and Donald P. Green. 2000. "The Effects of Canvassing, Telephone Calls, and Direct Mail on Voter Turnout: A Field Experiment." *American Political Science Review* 94(3): 653–63.

———. 2012. *Field Experiments: Design, Analysis, and Interpretation.* New York: W. W. Norton & Co.

Gerstle, Gary. 2022. *The Rise and Fall of the Neoliberal Order: America and the World in the Free Market Era.* New York: Oxford University Press.

Gest, Justin. 2016. "The Untouchables: Who Can Appeal to the White Working Class?" In Justin Gest, *The New Minority: White Working Class Politics in an Age of Immigration and Inequality.* New York: Oxford University Press.

Gidron, Noam. 2020. "Many Ways to Be Right: Cross-Pressured Voters in Western Europe." *British Journal of Political Science* 52(1): 146–61. DOI: https://doi.org/10.1017/S0007123420000228.

Gilens, Martin. 1999. *Why Americans Hate Welfare: Race, Media, and the Politics of Anti-Poverty Policy.* Chicago: University of Chicago Press.

Gillion, Daniel Q. 2013. *The Political Power of Protest: Minority Activism and Shifts in Public Policy.* Cambridge: Cambridge University Press.

———. 2016. *Governing with Words: The Political Dialogue on Race, Public Policy, and Inequality in America.* Cambridge: Cambridge University Press.

————. 2020. *The Loud Minority: Why Protests Matter in American Democracy.* Princeton, N.J.: Princeton University Press.

Gingrich, Jane, and Sara Watson. 2016. "Privatizing Participation? The Impact of Private Welfare Provision on Democratic Accountability." *Politics and Society* 44(4): 573–613.

Ginsberg, Allen. 1986. *The Captive Public: How Mass Opinion Promotes State Power.* New York: Basic Books.

Glaser, James M., and Timothy J. Ryan. 2013. *Changing Minds, If Not Hearts: Political Remedies for Racial Conflict.* Philadelphia: University of Pennsylvania Press.

Gleckman, Howard. 2012. "The Rise and Fall of the CLASS Act: What Lessons Can We Learn?" In *Universal Coverage of Long-Term Care in the United States: Can We Get There from Here?*, edited by Douglas Wolf and Nancy Folbre. New York: Russell Sage Foundation.

Glied, Sherry, and Adlan Jackson. 2017. "The Future of the Affordable Care Act and Insurance Coverage." *American Journal of Public Health* 107(4): 538–40.

Goldman, Seth K., and Daniel J. Hopkins. 2019. "Past Place, Present Prejudice: The Impact of Adolescent Racial Context on White Racial Attitudes." *Journal of Politics* 82(2): 529–42.

Goldstein, Amy. 2016. "HHS Failed to Heed Many Warnings That HealthCare.Gov Was in Trouble." *Washington Post*, February 23, 2016. https://www.washingtonpost.com/national/health-science/hhs-failed-to-heed-many-warnings-that-healthcaregov-was-in-trouble/2016/02/22/dd344e7c-d67e-11e5-9823-02b905009f99_story.html.

Gollust, Sarah E., Colleen Barry, Jeff Niederdeppe, Laura Baum, and Erika Franklin Fowler. 2014. "First Impressions: Geographic Variation in Media Messages during the First Phase of ACA Implementation." *Journal of Health Politics, Policy, and Law* 39(6): 1253–62.

Gollust, Sarah E., Erika Franklin Fowler, and Jeff Niederdeppe. 2019. "Television News Coverage of Public Health Issues and Implications for Public Health Policy and Practice." *Annual Review of Public Health* 40(1): 167–85.

Gollust, Sarah E., Andrew Wilcock, Erika Franklin Fowler, Colleen L. Barry, Jeff Niederdeppe, Laura Baum, and Pinar Karaca-Mandic. 2018. "TV Advertising Volumes Were Associated with Insurance Marketplace Shopping and Enrollment in 2014." *Health Affairs (Project Hope)* 37(6): 956–63.

Golos, Aleksandra M., Daniel J. Hopkins, Syon P. Bhanot, and Alison M. Buttenheim. 2022. "Partisanship, Messaging, and the Covid-19 Vaccine: Evidence from Survey Experiments." *American Journal of Health Promotion* 36(4): 602–11. DOI: https://doi.org/10.1177/08901171211049241.

Goodman-Bacon, Andrew. 2021. "Difference-in-Differences with Variation in Treatment Timing." *Journal of Econometrics*, themed issue: "Treatment Effect 1," 225(2): 254–77.

Goodnough, Abby. 2017. "The Governor Blocked Medicaid Expansion. Now Maine Voters Could Overrule Him." *New York Times*, October 27, 2017. https://www.nytimes.com/2017/10/27/health/medicaid-maine-obamacare.html.

————. 2018. "As Some Got Free Health Care, Gwen Got Squeezed: An Obamacare Dilemma." *New York Times*, February 19, 2018. https://www.nytimes.com/2018/02/19/health/obamacare-premiums-medicaid.html.

Gordon, Sanford. 2011. "Politicizing Agency Spending Authority: Lessons from a Bush-Era Scandal." *American Political Science Review* 105(4): 717–34.

Goren, Paul. 2003. "Race, Sophistication, and White Opinion on Government Spending." *Political Behavior* 25(3): 201–20.

———. 2008. "The Two Faces of Government Spending." *Political Research Quarterly* 61(1): 147–57.

Gose, Leah E., and Theda Skocpol. 2019. "Resist, Persist, and Transform: The Emergence and Impact of Grassroots Resistance Groups Opposing the Trump Presidency." *Mobilization: An International Quarterly* 24(3): 293–317.

Grande, David, Sarah E. Gollust, and David A. Asch. 2011. "Polling Analysis: Public Support for Health Reform Was Broader than Reported and Depended on How Proposals Were Framed." *Health Affairs* 30(7): 1242–49.

Green, Donald P., Bradley Palmquist, and Eric Schickler. 2002. *Partisan Hearts and Minds: Political Parties and the Social Identities of Voters.* New Haven, Conn.: Yale University Press.

Green, Jane, and Will Jennings. 2017. *The Politics of Competence: Parties, Public Opinion, and Voters.* Cambridge: Cambridge University Press.

Greene, Brian. 2020. *Until the End of Time: Mind, Matter, and Our Search for Meaning in an Evolving Universe.* New York: Vintage Books.

Grimmer, Justin. 2010. "A Bayesian Hierarchical Topic Model for Political Texts: Measuring Expressed Agendas in Senate Press Releases." *Political Analysis* 18(1): 1–35.

Grimmer, Justin, and Gary King. 2011. "General Purpose Computer-Assisted Clustering and Conceptualization." *Proceedings of the National Academy of Sciences* 108(7): 2643–50.

Grimmer, Justin, and William Marble. 2019. "Who Put Trump in the White House? Explaining the Contribution of Voting Blocs to Trump's Victory." Working paper, December 12. https://williammarble.co/docs/vb.pdf.

Grimmer, Justin, Solomon Messing, and Sean J. Westwood. 2012. "How Words and Money Cultivate a Personal Vote: The Effect of Legislator Credit Claiming on Constituent Credit Allocation." *American Political Science Review* 106(4): 703–19.

———. 2014. *The Impression of Influence: Legislator Communication, Representation, and Democratic Accountability.* Princeton, N.J.: Princeton University Press.

Grimmer, Justin, and Brandon Stewart. 2013. "Text as Data: The Promise and Pitfalls of Automatic Content Analysis Methods for Political Texts." *Political Analysis* 21(3): 267–97.

Grogan, Colleen M., and Sunggeun (Ethan) Park. 2017. "The Racial Divide in State Medicaid Expansions." *Journal of Health Politics, Policy, and Law* 42(3): 539–72.

Grossman, Guy, Soojong Kim, Jonah M. Rexer, and Harsha Thirumurthy. 2020. "Political Partisanship Influences Behavioral Responses to Governors' Recommendations for Covid-19 Prevention in the United States." *Proceedings of the National Academy of Sciences* 117(39): 24144–53.

Grossmann, Matt, and Daniel Thaler. 2018. "Mass-Elite Divides in Aversion to Social Change and Support for Donald Trump." *American Politics Research* 46(5): 753–84.

Gruber, Jonathan, and Benjamin D. Sommers. 2019. "The Affordable Care Act's Effects on Patients, Providers, and the Economy: What We've Learned So Far." Working Paper 25932. National Bureau of Economic Research, June. DOI: https://doi.org/10.3386/w25932.

Grumbach, Jacob M. 2018. "From Backwaters to Major Policymakers: Policy Polarization in the States, 1970–2014." *Perspectives on Politics* 16(2): 416–35.

———. 2022. *Laboratories against Democracy: How National Parties Transformed State Politics*. Princeton, N.J.: Princeton University Press.

Guess, Andrew M. 2021. "(Almost) Everything in Moderation: New Evidence on Americans' Online Media Diets." *American Journal of Political Science* 65(4): 1007–22.

Guess, Andrew M., Pablo Barberá, Simon Munzert, and JungHwan Yang. 2021. "The Consequences of Online Partisan Media." *Proceedings of the National Academy of Sciences* 118(14). DOI: https://doi.org/10.1073/pnas.2013464118.

Guntermann, Eric, and Gabriel Lenz. 2022. "Still Not Important Enough? Covid-19 Policy Views and Vote Choice." *Perspectives on Politics* 20(2): 547–61.

Gupta, Sumedha, Kosali Simon, and Coady Wing. 2020. "Mandated and Voluntary Social Distancing during the Covid-19 Epidemic." *Brookings Papers on Economic Activity* (Summer): 269–326.

Gurri, Martin. 2018. *The Revolt of the Public and the Crisis of Authority in the New Millennium*. San Francisco: Stripe Press.

Gustafsson, Lovisa, and Sarah R. Collins. 2022. "The Inflation Reduction Act Is a Milestone Achievement in Lowering Americans' Health Care Costs." Commonwealth Fund blog. August 15. https://www.commonwealthfund.org/blog/2022/inflation-reduction-act -milestone-achievement-lowering-americans-health-care-costs (accessed September 11, 2022).

Guth, Madeline, Rachel Garfield, and Robin Rudowitz. 2020. "The Effects of Medicaid Expansion under the ACA: Studies from January 2014 to January 2020." Kaiser Family Foundation, March 17. https://www.kff.org/medicaid/report/the-effects-of-medicaid -expansion-under-the-aca-updated-findings-from-a-literature-review/.

Haberkorn, Jennifer, Burgess Everett, and Seung Min Kim. 2017. "Inside the Life and Death of Graham-Cassidy." *Politico*, September 27, 2017. https://politi.co/2GfmDur.

Hacker, Jacob. 1999. *The Road to Nowhere: The Genesis of President Clinton's Plan for Health Security*. Princeton, N.J.: Princeton University Press.

———. 2002. *The Divided Welfare State: The Battle over Public and Private Social Benefits in the United States*. Cambridge: Cambridge University Press.

———. 2004. "Privatizing Risk without Privatizing the Welfare State: The Hidden Politics of Social Policy Retrenchment in the United States." *American Political Science Review* 98(2): 243–60.

———. 2019. "Medicare Expansion as a Path as Well as a Destination: Achieving Universal Insurance through a New Politics of Medicare." *Annals of the American Academy of Political and Social Science* 685(1): 135–53.

Hacker, Jacob S., and Daniel J. Hopkins. 2010. "After Massachusetts, Why the Democrats Should Still Pass Health-Care Reform." *Washington Post*, January 19, 2010. http://www .washingtonpost.com/wp-dyn/content/article/2010/01/19/AR2010011902846.html.

Hacker, Jacob S., and Paul Pierson. 2018. "The Dog That Almost Barked: What the ACA Repeal Fight Says about the Resilience of the American Welfare State." *Journal of Health Politics, Policy, and Law* 43(4): 551–77. DOI: https://doi.org/10.1215/03616878-6527935.

————. 2019. "Policy Feedback in an Age of Polarization." *Annals of the American Academy of Political and Social Science* 685(1): 8–28.

————. 2020. *Let Them Eat Tweets: How the Right Rules in an Age of Extreme Inequality.* New York: Liveright Publishing.

Hafner-Burton, Emilie M., D. Alex Hughes, and David G. Victor. 2013. "The Cognitive Revolution and the Political Psychology of Elite Decision Making." *Perspectives on Politics* 11(2): 368–86.

Hagan, Elizabeth. 2016. "ACA Assisters Can Help Consumers Register to Vote." Families USA, July 4. https://familiesusa.org/resources/aca-assisters-can-help-consumers-register-to-vote/.

Hajnal, Zoltan L. 2020. *Dangerously Divided: How Race and Class Shape Winning and Losing in American Politics.* New York: Cambridge University Press.

Hajnal, Zoltan L., and Taeku Lee. 2011. *Why Americans Don't Join the Party: Race, Immigration, and the Failure (of Political Parties) to Engage the Electorate.* Princeton, N.J.: Princeton University Press.

Hall, Mark A. 2020. "The Effects of Political versus Actuarial Uncertainty on Insurance Market Stability." *RSF: The Russell Sage Foundation Journal of the Social Sciences* 6(2): 223–42. DOI: https://doi.org/10.7758/RSF.2020.6.2.10.

Hall, Peter A. 2003. "Aligning Ontology and Methodology in Comparative Politics." In *Comparative Historical Analysis in the Social Sciences*, edited by James Mahoney and Dietrich Rueschemeyer. New York: Cambridge University Press.

Hamel, Liz, Mira Norton, and Mollyann Brodie. 2015. "Survey of Kentucky Residents on State Health Policy." Kaiser Family Foundation, December 11. https://www.kff.org/health-reform/poll-finding/survey-of-kentucky-residents-on-state-health-policy/.

Hancock, Ange-Marie. 2004. *The Politics of Disgust: The Public Identity of the Welfare Queen.* New York: New York University Press.

Haney-López, Ian. 2019. *Merge Left: Fusing Race and Class, Winning Elections, and Saving America.* New York: New Press.

Han, Hahrie. 2014. *How Organizations Develop Activists: Civic Associations and Leadership in the 21st Century.* New York: Oxford University Press.

Hankinson, Michael. 2018. "When Do Renters Behave Like Homeowners? High Rent, Price Anxiety, and NIMBYism." *American Political Science Review* 112(3): 473–93.

Hargrove, Brantley. 2009. "How Rep. Jim Cooper Became a Fighter—and a Target—in the Health Care Wars." *Nashville Scene*, October 29, 2009. https://www.nashvillescene.com/news/how-rep-jim-cooper-became-a-fighter-and-a-target-in-the-health-care-wars/article_86ff2cde-201a-5e65-bb10-1e7f91e0fcf3.html.

Hartz, Louis. 1955. *The Liberal Tradition in America: An Interpretation of American Political Thought since the Revolution.* New York: Harcourt, Brace & Co.

Haselswerdt, Jake. 2017. "Expanding Medicaid, Expanding the Electorate." *Journal of Health Politics, Policy, and Law* 42(4): 667–95.

————. 2020. "Carving Out: Isolating the True Effect of Self-Interest on Policy Attitudes." *American Political Science Review* 114(4): 1103–16.

Haselswerdt, Jake, and Jamila D. Michener. 2019. "Disenrolled: Retrenchment and Voting in Health Policy." *Journal of Health Politics, Policy, and Law* 44(3): 423–54.

Hayes, Danny. 2008. "Does the Messenger Matter? Candidate-Media Agenda Convergence and Its Effects on Voter Issue Salience." *Political Research Quarterly* 61(1): 134–46.

Healy, Andrew, and Neil A. Malhotra. 2013. "Retrospective Voting Reconsidered." *Annual Review of Political Science* 16(May): 285–306.

Heath, Chip, and Dan Heath. 2007. *Made to Stick: Why Some Ideas Survive and Others Die.* New York: Random House.

Henderson, Michael, and D. Sunshine Hillygus. 2011. "The Dynamics of Health Care Opinion, 2008–2010: Partisanship, Self-Interest, and Racial Resentment." *Journal of Health Politics, Policy, and Law* 36(6): 945–60.

Herby, Jonas. 2021. "A First Literature Review: Lockdowns Only Had a Small Effect on Covid-19." SSRN Scholarly Paper 3764553, January 6. DOI: http://dx.doi.org/10.2139/ssrn.3764553.

Hersh, Eitan D. 2020. *Politics Is for Power: How to Move beyond Political Hobbyism, Take Action, and Make Real Change.* New York: Simon & Schuster.

Hersh, Eitan D., and Clayton Nall. 2016. "The Primacy of Race in the Geography of Income-Based Voting: New Evidence from Public Voting Records." *American Journal of Political Science* 60(2): 289–303.

Hertel-Fernandez, Alexander. 2019a. "Asymmetric Partisan Polarization, Labor Policy, and Cross-State Political Power-Building." *Annals of the American Academy of Political and Social Science* 685(1): 64–79.

———. 2019b. *State Capture: How Conservative Activists, Big Businesses, and Wealthy Donors Reshaped the American States—and the Nation.* New York: Oxford University Press.

Hertel-Fernandez, Alexander, Theda Skocpol, and Daniel Lynch. 2016. "Business Associations, Conservative Networks, and the Ongoing Republican War over Medicaid Expansion." *Journal of Health Politics, Policy, and Law* 41(2): 239–86.

Hetherington, Marc. 2005. *Why Trust Matters: Declining Political Trust and the Demise of American Liberalism.* Princeton, N.J.: Princeton University Press.

Hill, Seth J., James Lo, Lynn Vavreck, and John Zaller. 2013. "How Quickly We Forget: The Duration of Persuasion Effects from Mass Communication." *Political Communication* 30(4): 521–47.

Hiltzik, Michael. 2014. "Did Obamacare Destroy the Democratic Party? Another Look." *Los Angeles Times*, December 3, 2014. https://www.latimes.com/business/hiltzik/la-fi-mh-obamacare-destroy-the-democratic-20141203-column.html.

Hindman, Matthew. 2008. *The Myth of Digital Democracy.* Princeton, N.J.: Princeton University Press.

Hobbs, William R. 2019. "Text Scaling for Open-Ended Survey Responses and Social Media Posts." August 7. DOI: http://dx.doi.org/10.2139/ssrn.3044864.

Hobbs, William R., and Daniel J. Hopkins. 2021. "Offsetting Policy Feedback Effects: Evidence from the Affordable Care Act." *Journal of Politics* 83(4): 1800–1817. DOI: https://doi.org/10.1086/715063.

Hochschild, Jennifer L. 1981. *What's Fair? American Beliefs about Distributive Justice.* Cambridge, Mass.: Harvard University Press.

———. 1995. *Facing Up to the American Dream: Race, Class, and the Soul of the Nation.* Princeton, N.J.: Princeton University Press.

———. 2018. *Strangers in Their Own Land: Anger and Mourning on the American Right.* New York: New Press.

Hodge, Jamila. 2021. "Fifty Years Ago Today, President Nixon Declared the War on Drugs." Vera Institute of Justice, June 17. https://www.vera.org/news/fifty-years-ago-today-president-nixon-declared-the-war-on-drugs.

Holan, Angie Drobnic. 2009. "Obama Flip-Flops on Requiring People to Buy Health Care." *PolitiFact*, July 20, 2009. https://www.politifact.com/truth-o-meter/statements/2009/jul/20/barack-obama/obama-flip-flops-requiring-people-buy-health-care/.

Holl, Kristen, Jeff Niederdeppe, and Jonathon P. Schuldt. 2018. "Does Question Wording Predict Support for the Affordable Care Act? An Analysis of Polling during the Implementation Period, 2010–2016." *Health Communication* 33(7): 816–23.

Hollingsworth, Alex, Aparna Soni, Aaron E. Carroll, John Cawley, and Kosali Simon. 2019. "Gains in Health Insurance Coverage Explain Variation in Democratic Vote Share in the 2008–2016 Presidential Elections." *PLoS ONE* 14(4): e0214206.

Hopkins, Daniel J. 2012. "Whose Economy? Perceptions of National Economic Performance during Unequal Growth." *Public Opinion Quarterly* 76(1): 50–71.

———. 2017. "Trump's Election Doesn't Mean Americans Are More Opposed to Immigration." *FiveThirtyEight*, January 26, 2017. https://fivethirtyeight.com/features/while-trump-is-closing-the-borders-americans-are-warming-to-immigration/.

———. 2018a. "The Exaggerated Life of Death Panels?" *Political Behavior* 40(3): 681–709. DOI: https://doi.org/10.1007/s11109-017-9418-4.

———. 2018b. *The Increasingly United States: How and Why American Political Behavior Nationalized.* Chicago: University of Chicago Press.

———. 2021. "The Activation of Prejudice and Presidential Voting: Panel Evidence from the 2016 U.S. Election." *Political Behavior* 43(2): 663–86.

———. Forthcoming. "Stable Views in a Time of Tumult: Assessing Trends in American Public Opinion, 2007–2020." *British Journal of Political Science.*

Hopkins, Daniel J., and Anna Maria Barry-Jester. 2017. "Republicans' Obamacare Repeal Would Cut Taxes—But Mostly in Blue States." *FiveThirtyEight*, June 20, 2017. https://fivethirtyeight.com/features/republicans-obamacare-repeal-would-cut-taxes-but-mostly-in-blue-states/.

Hopkins, Daniel J., and Tori Gorton. 2022. "On the Internet, No One Knows You're an Activist: Patterns of Participation and Response in an Online, Opt-in Survey Panel." Paper presented at the Annual Meeting for the American Association for Public Opinion Research. Chicago, Ill., May.

Hopkins, Daniel J., Eunji Kim, and Soojong Kim. 2017. "Does Newspaper Coverage Influence or Reflect Public Perceptions of the Economy?" *Research and Politics* 4(4): 2053168017737900.

Hopkins, Daniel J., and Gary King. 2010. "A Method of Automated Nonparametric Content Analysis for Social Science." *American Journal of Political Science* 54(1): 229–47.

Hopkins, Daniel J., and Jonathan M. Ladd. 2014. "The Consequences of Broader Media Choice: Evidence from the Expansion of *Fox News*." *Quarterly Journal of Political Science* 9(1): 115–35.

Hopkins, Daniel J., and Jonathan Mummolo. 2017. "Assessing the Breadth of Framing Effects." *Quarterly Journal of Political Science* 12(May): 37–57.

Hopkins, Daniel J., and Diana C. Mutz. 2022. *Institute for the Study of Citizens and Politics Panel.* Harvard Dataverse, V1. DOI: https://doi.org/10.7910/DVN/CYISG1.

Hopkins, Daniel J., and Hans Noel. 2022. "Trump and the Shifting Meaning of 'Conservative': Using Activists' Pairwise Comparisons to Measure Politicians' Perceived Ideologies." *American Political Science Review* 116(3): 1133–40.

Hopkins, Daniel J., and Kalind Parish. 2019. "The Medicaid Expansion and Attitudes toward the Affordable Care Act." *Public Opinion Quarterly* 83(1): 123–34. DOI: https://doi.org /10.1093/poq/nfz004.

Hopkins, Daniel J., Susanne Schwarz, and Anjali Chainani. Forthcoming. "Officially Mobilizing: Repeated Reminders and Feedback from Local Officials Increase Turnout." *Journal of Politics.*

Hopkins, Daniel J., Eric Schickler, and David Azizi. 2022. "From Many Divides, One? The Polarization and Nationalization of American State Party Platforms, 1918–2017." *Studies in American Political Development* 36(1): 1–20.

Hopkins, Daniel J., John Sides, and Jack Citrin. 2019. "The Muted Consequences of Correct Information about Immigration." *Journal of Politics* 81(1): 315–20.

Hopkins, Daniel J., and Samantha Washington. 2020. "The Rise of Trump, the Fall of Prejudice? Tracking White Americans' Racial Attitudes via a Panel Survey, 2008–2018." *Public Opinion Quarterly* 84(1): 119–40.

Hosek, Adrienne. 2019. "Ensuring the Future of the Affordable Care Act on the Health Insurance Marketplaces." *Journal of Health Politics, Policy, and Law* 44(4): 589–630.

Howard, Christopher. 1999. *The Hidden Welfare State: Tax Expenditures and Social Policy in the United States.* Princeton, N.J.: Princeton University Press.

Howell, William G., and Terry M. Moe. 2020. *Presidents, Populism, and the Crisis of Democracy.* Chicago: University of Chicago Press.

Huber, Gregory A., Seth J. Hill, and Gabriel S. Lenz. 2012. "Sources of Bias in Retrospective Decision Making: Experimental Evidence on Voters' Limitations in Controlling Incumbents." *American Political Science Review* 106(4): 720–41.

Huber, Gregory A., and John S. Lapinski. 2006. "The Race Card Revisited: Assessing Racial Priming in Policy Contests." *American Journal of Political Science* 50(2): 421–40.

Huber, Gregory A., and Celia Paris. 2013. "Assessing the Programmatic Equivalence Assumption in Question Wording Experiments: Understanding Why Americans Like Assistance to the Poor More than Welfare." *Public Opinion Quarterly* 77(1): 385–97.

Huddy, Leonie. 2018. "The Group Foundations of Democratic Political Behavior." *Critical Review* 30(1/2): 71–86.

Huddy, Leonie, Lilliana Mason, and Lene Aarøe. 2015. "Expressive Partisanship: Campaign Involvement, Political Emotion, and Partisan Identity." *American Political Science Review* 109(1): 1–17.

Hundt, Reed. 2019. *A Crisis Wasted: Barack Obama's Defining Decisions.* New York: Rosetta Books.

Hurwitz, Jon, and Mark Peffley. 2005. "Playing the Race Card in the Post–Willie Horton Era: The Impact of Racialized Code Words on Support for Punitive Crime Policy." *Public Opinion Quarterly* 69(1): 99–112.

Hutchings, Vincent L. 2009. "Change or More of the Same? Evaluating Racial Attitudes in the Obama Era." *Public Opinion Quarterly* 73(5): 917–42.

Hutchings, Vincent L., and Ashley E. Jardina. 2009. "Experiments on Racial Priming in Political Campaigns." *Annual Review of Political Science* 12(1): 397–402.

Hutchings, Vincent L., and Nicholas A. Valentino. 2004. "The Centrality of Race in American Politics." *Annual Review of Political Science* 7: 383–408.

Hutchings, Vincent L., Hanes Walton, and Andrea Benjamin. 2010. "The Impact of Explicit Racial Cues on Gender Differences in Support for Confederate Symbols and Partisanship." *Journal of Politics* 72(4): 1175–88.

Imbens, Guido W., and Karthik Kalyanaraman. 2012. "Optimal Bandwidth Choice for the Regression Discontinuity Estimator." *Review of Economic Studies* 79(3): 933–59.

Imbens, Guido W., and Donald B. Rubin. 2015. *Causal Inference for Statistics, Social, and Biomedical Sciences: An Introduction.* Cambridge: Cambridge University Press.

Internal Revenue Service. 2015. "SOI Tax Statistics—Historic Table 2." https://www.irs.gov/statistics/soi-tax-stats-historic-table-2.

———. 2019. "Affordable Care Act Items." https://www.irs.gov/businesses/corporations/affordable-care-act-items.

Ivarsflaten, Elisabeth, Scott Blinder, and Robert Ford. 2010. "The Anti-Racism Norm in Western European Immigration Politics: Why We Need to Consider It and How to Measure It." *Journal of Elections, Public Opinion, and Parties* 20(4): 421–45. DOI: https://doi.org/10.1080/17457289.2010.511805.

Iyengar, Shanto, and Donald R. Kinder. 1987. *News That Matters: Television and American Public Opinion.* Chicago: University of Chicago Press.

Iyengar, Shanto, Yphtach Lelkes, Matthew Levendusky, Neil Malhotra, and Sean J. Westwood. 2019. "The Origins and Consequences of Affective Polarization in the United States." *Annual Review of Political Science* 22(1): 129–46. DOI: https://doi.org/10.1146/annurev-polisci-051117-073034.

Jacobs, Alan M., and R. Kent Weaver. 2015. "When Policies Undo Themselves: Self-Undermining Feedback as a Source of Policy Change." *Governance* 28(4): 441–57.

Jacobs, Lawrence R., and Melanie Burns. 2004. "The Second Face of the Public Presidency: Presidential Polling and the Shift from Policy to Personality Polling." *Presidential Studies Quarterly* 34(3): 536–56.

Jacobs, Lawrence R., and Timothy Callaghan. 2013. "Why States Expand Medicaid: Party, Resources, and History." *Journal of Health Politics, Policy, and Law* 38(5): 1023–50. DOI: https://doi.org/10.1215/03616878-2334889.

Jacobs, Lawrence R., and Suzanne Mettler. 2011. "Why Public Opinion Changes: The Implications for Health and Health Policy." *Journal of Health Politics, Policy, and Law* 36(6): 917–33. DOI: https://doi.org/10.1215/03616878-1460515.

———. 2016. "Liking Health Reform but Turned Off by Toxic Politics." *Health Affairs* 35(5): 915–22.

———. 2018. "When and How New Policy Creates New Politics." *Perspectives on Politics* 16(2): 345–63.

———. 2020. "What Health Reform Tells Us about American Politics." *Journal of Health Politics, Policy, and Law* 4 (4): 581–93. DOI: https://doi.org/10.1215/03616878-8255505.

Jacobs, Lawrence R., Suzanne Mettler, and Ling Zhu. 2019. "Affordable Care Act Moving to New Stage of Public Acceptance." *Journal of Health Politics, Policy, and Law* 44(6): 911–17. DOI: https://doi.org/10.1215/03616878-7785811.

Jacobs, Lawrence R., Benjamin I. Page, Melanie Burns, Gregory McAvoy, and Eric Ostermeier. 2003. "What Presidents Talk About: The Nixon Case." *Presidential Studies Quarterly* 33(4): 751–71.

Jacobs, Lawrence R., and Robert Y. Shapiro. 2000. *Politicians Don't Pander: Political Manipulation and the Loss of Democratic Responsiveness.* Chicago: University of Chicago Press.

Jacobs, Lawrence R., and Theda Skocpol. 2015. *Health Care Reform and American Politics: What Everyone Needs to Know.* New York: Oxford University Press.

Jaffe, Alexandra. 2021. "Biden Administration to Undo Medicaid Work Requirements." *AP News*, February 12, 2021. https://apnews.com/article/politics-medicaid-coronavirus-pandemic-16f7d6600ee9f240b63e8a5bdfa90276.

Jardina, Ashley. 2019. *White Identity Politics.* Cambridge: Cambridge University Press.

Jaroszewicz, Ania, Jon Jachimowicz, and Oliver Hauser. 2022. "How Effective Is (More) Money? Randomizing Unconditional Cash Transfer Amounts in the U.S." July 5. DOI: http://dx.doi.org/10.2139/ssrn.4154000.

Johnson, Haynes, and David Broder. 1997. *The System: The American Way of Politics at the Breaking Point.* Boston: Back Bay Books.

Johnston, Richard, Michael G. Hagen, and Kathleen Hall Jamieson. 2004. *The 2000 Presidential Election and the Foundations of Party Politics.* Hackensack, N.J.: Cambridge University Press.

Jones, David K. 2017. *Exchange Politics: Opposing Obamacare in Battleground States.* New York: Oxford University Press.

Jones-Correa, Michael. 1998. *Between Two Nations: The Political Predicament of Latinos in New York City.* Ithaca, N.Y.: Cornell University Press.

Jost, Timothy. 2017. "The Senate's Health Care Freedom Act." *Health Affairs*, July 28. https://www.healthaffairs.org/do/10.1377/hblog20170728.061295/full/.

Judis, John B. 2000. *The Paradox of American Democracy: Elites, Special Interests, and the Betrayal of Public Trust.* New York: Pantheon.

Kahneman, Daniel, Jack L. Knetsch, and Richard H. Thaler. 1991. "Anomalies: The Endowment Effect, Loss Aversion, and Status Quo Bias." *Journal of Economic Perspectives* 5(1): 193–206. DOI: https://doi.org/10.1257/jep.5.1.193.

Kahneman, Daniel, and Amos Tversky. 1979. "Prospect Theory: An Analysis of Decision under Risk." *Econometrica* 47(2): 263–92.

Kaiser Family Foundation. 2010. "Kaiser Health Tracking Poll—January 2010." January 1. https://www.kff.org/health-reform/poll-finding/kaiser-health-tracking-poll-january-2010/.

———. 2017. "Medicaid Spending per Enrollee (Full or Partial Benefit)." June 9. https://www.kff.org/medicaid/state-indicator/medicaid-spending-per-enrollee/.

———. 2019. "Medicaid in the United States." October. https://files.kff.org/attachment/fact-sheet-medicaid-state-US.

———. 2021. "Medicaid Waiver Tracker: Approved and Pending Section 1115 Waivers by State." July 26. https://www.kff.org/medicaid/issue-brief/medicaid-waiver-tracker-approved-and-pending-section-1115-waivers-by-state/.

———. 2022. "Kaiser Family Foundation Health Tracking Poll: The Public's Views on the ACA." March 31. https://www.kff.org/interactive/kff-health-tracking-poll-the-publics-views-on-the-aca/#?response=Favorable--Unfavorable&aRange=all.

Kalla, Joshua L., and David E. Broockman. 2018. "The Minimal Persuasive Effects of Campaign Contact in General Elections: Evidence from 49 Field Experiments." *American Political Science Review* 112(1): 148–66. DOI: https://doi.org/10.1017/S0003055417000363.

———. 2020. "Reducing Exclusionary Attitudes through Interpersonal Conversation: Evidence from Three Field Experiments." *American Political Science Review* 114(2): 410–25. DOI: https://doi.org/10.1017/S0003055419000923.

Kalla, Joshua L., Adam Seth Levine, and David E. Broockman. 2021. "Personalizing Moral Reframing in Interpersonal Conversation: A Field Experiment." *Journal of Politics* 84(2): 1239–43. DOI: https://doi.org/10.1086/716944.

Kam, Cindy D. 2012. "The Psychological Veracity of Zaller's Model." *Critical Review* 24(4): 545–67. DOI: https://doi.org/10.1080/08913811.2012.788281.

Kaplan, Thomas, and Robert Pear. 2017. "House Passes Measure to Repeal and Replace the Affordable Care Act." *New York Times*, May 4, 2017. https://www.nytimes.com/2017/05/04/us/politics/health-care-bill-vote.html.

Karaca-Mandic, Pinar, Andrew Wilcock, Laura Baum, Colleen Barry, Erika Franklin Fowler, Jeff Niederdeppe, and Sarah Gollust. 2017. "The Volume of TV Advertisements during the ACA's First Enrollment Period Was Associated with Increased Insurance Coverage." *Health Affairs* 36(4): 747–54.

Keech, William R., and Kyoungsan Pak. 1989. "Electoral Cycles and Budgetary Growth in Veterans' Benefit Programs." *American Journal of Political Science* 33(4): 901–11. DOI: https://doi.org/10.2307/2111114.

Keith, Katie. 2019. "More Insurers Win Lawsuits Seeking Cost-Sharing Reduction Payments." *Health Affairs*, February 17. https://www.healthaffairs.org/do/10.1377/hblog20190217.755658/full/.

———. 2021. "American Rescue Plan Increases ACA Enrollment." *Health Affairs* 40(7): 1026–27. https://doi.org/10.1377/hlthaff.2021.00983.

Kellstedt, Paul M. 2003. *The Mass Media and the Dynamics of American Racial Attitudes.* New York: Cambridge University Press.

Kendi, Ibram X. 2019. *How to Be an Antiracist.* New York: One World.

Kersey, Lori. 2014. "Medicaid and the Affordable Care Act; Expansion Helps Former Inmates." *Charleston Gazette-Mail*, June 2, 2014. https://www.wvgazettemail.com/news/medicaid-expansion-may-help-former-inmates-get-treatment/article_c8315a0e-bfa2-51f5-b615-82fee26bde9c.html.

Kiefer, Francine. 2016. "Obamacare's Ups and Downs, as Seen by a Republican Doctor." *Christian Science Monitor*, October 25, 2016. https://www.csmonitor.com/USA/Politics /2016/1025/Obamacare-s-ups-and-downs-as-seen-by-a-Republican-doctor.

Kilgore, Ed. 2017. "LePage Insists Medicaid Is Welfare." *New York*, August 30, 2017. https:// nymag.com/intelligencer/2017/08/lepage-insists-medicaid-is-welfare.html.

Kim, Eunji. 2022. "Entertaining Beliefs in Economic Mobility." *American Journal of Political Science* (March 12): 1–16. DOI: https://doi.org/10.1111/ajps.12702.

Kimmel, Jimmy. 2013. "Six of One—Obamacare vs. the Affordable Care Act." *Jimmy Kimmel Live*. https://www.youtube.com/watch?v=sx2scvIFGjE.

Kinder, Donald R., and Allison Dale-Riddle. 2012. *End of Race? Obama, 2008, and Racial Politics in America*. New Haven, Conn.: Yale University Press.

Kinder, Donald R., and Nathan P. Kalmoe. 2017. *Neither Liberal nor Conservative: Ideological Innocence in the American Public*. Chicago: University of Chicago Press.

Kinder, Donald R., and Cindy D. Kam. 2009. *Us against Them: Ethnocentric Foundations of American Opinion*. Chicago: University of Chicago Press.

Kinder, Donald R., and Lynn M. Sanders. 1996. *Divided by Color: Racial Politics and Democratic Ideals*. Chicago: University of Chicago Press.

Kinder, Donald, and Nicholas Winter. 2001. "Exploring the Racial Divide: Blacks, Whites, and Opinion on National Policy." *American Journal of Political Science* 45(2): 439–56.

King, Gary. 1997. *A Solution to the Ecological Inference Problem: Reconstructing Individual Behavior from Aggregate Data*. Princeton, N.J.: Princeton University Press.

King, Gary, Michael Tomz, and Jason Wittenberg. 2000. "Making the Most of Statistical Analyses: Improving Interpretation and Presentation." *American Journal of Political Science* 44(2): 347–61. DOI: https://doi.org/10.2307/2669316.

Kirzinger, Ashley, Bianca DiJulio, Elizabeth Hamel, Elise Sugarman, and Mollyann Brodie. 2017. "Kaiser Health Tracking Poll—May 2017: The AHCA's Proposed Changes to Health Care." May 31. https://www.kff.org/health-costs/report/kaiser-health-tracking -poll-may-2017-the-ahcas-proposed-changes-to-health-care/.

Kirzinger, Ashley, Luna Lopes, Audrey Kearny, and Mollyann Brodie. 2020. "KFF Health Tracking Poll—October 2020: The Future of the ACA and Biden's Advantage on Health Care." Kaiser Family Foundation, October 16. https://www.kff.org/health-reform /report/kff-health-tracking-poll-october-2020/.

Klar, Samara, Yanna Krupnikov, and John Barry Ryan. 2018. "Affective Polarization or Partisan Disdain? Untangling a Dislike for the Opposing Party from a Dislike of Partisanship." *Public Opinion Quarterly* 82(2): 379–90. DOI: https://doi.org/10.1093/poq /nfy014.

Klein, Ezra. 2019. "The Republican Strategy to Pass Medicare-for-All Continues." *Vox*, July 9, 2019. https://www.vox.com/policy-and-politics/2018/12/14/18141670/obamacare-unconstitutional -texas-judge-strikes-down-reed-o-connor.

———. 2021a. "David Shor Is Telling Democrats What They Don't Want to Hear." *New York Times*, October 8, 2021, https://www.nytimes.com/2021/10/08/opinion/democrats-david -shor-education-polarization.html.

———. 2021b. "Obama Explains How America Went from 'Yes We Can' to 'MAGA.'" *New York Times*, June 1, 2021. https://www.nytimes.com/2021/06/01/opinion/ezra-klein -podcast-barack-obama.html.

———. 2022. "America Has Turned Its Back on Its Poorest Families." *New York Times*, April 17, 2022. https://www.nytimes.com/2022/04/17/opinion/biden-child-tax-credit.html.

Kliff, Sarah. 2013. "The White House's Obamacare Fix Is About to Create a Big Mess." *Washington Post*, November 14, 2013. https://www.washingtonpost.com/news/wonk /wp/2013/11/14/the-white-houses-obamacare-fix-is-about-to-create-a-big-mess/.

———. 2016. "Why Obamacare Enrollees Voted for Trump." *Vox*, December 13, 2016. https:// www.vox.com/science-and-health/2016/12/13/13848794/kentucky-obamacare-trump.

———. 2017a. "HHS Told Obamacare Workers Their Budget Was Safe — Then Slashed It 40 Percent." *Vox*, September 1, 2017. https://www.vox.com/health-care/2017/9/1 /16243232/voxcare-hhs-obamacare-budget.

———. 2017b. "Maine Will Decide Tuesday Whether to Give 80,000 People Health Coverage." *Vox*, November 6, 2017. https://www.vox.com/policy-and-politics/2017 /11/6/16614906/maine-medicaid-health-coverage.

———. 2017c. "The Obamacare Repeal Bill the House Just Passed, Explained." *Vox*, May 3, 2017. https://www.vox.com/policy-and-politics/2017/5/3/15531494/american-health-care -act-explained.

Kluegel, James R., and Eliot R. Smith. 1986. *Beliefs about Inequality: Americans' Views of What Is and What Ought to Be*. New York: Routledge.

Kluender, Raymond, Neale Mahoney, Francis Wong, and Wesley Yin. 2021. "Medical Debt in the U.S., 2009–2020." *JAMA* 326(3): 250–56. DOI: https://doi.org/10.1001/jama .2021.8694.

Knowles, Brian D., Brian Lowery, and Rebecca L. Schaumberg. 2010. "Racial Prejudice Predicts Opposition to Obama and His Health Care Reform Plan." *Journal of Experimental Social Psychology* 46(2): 420–23.

Kogan, Vladimir. 2020. "Do Welfare Benefits Pay Electoral Dividends? Evidence from the National Food Stamp Program Rollout." *Journal of Politics* 83(1): 58–70. DOI: https:// doi.org/10.1086/708914.

Kogan, Vladimir, and Thomas Wood. 2018. "Obamacare Implementation and the 2016 Election." February 6. DOI: http://dx.doi.org/10.2139/ssrn.3075406.

Kriesi, Hanspeter, and Alexander H. Trechsel. 2008. *The Politics of Switzerland: Continuity and Change in a Consensus Democracy*. Cambridge: Cambridge University Press.

Krimmel, Katherine, and Kelly Rader. 2017. "The Federal Spending Paradox: Economic Self-Interest and Symbolic Racism in Contemporary Fiscal Politics." *American Politics Research* 45(5): 727–54. DOI: https://doi.org/10.1177/1532673X17701222.

———. 2020. "Substantive Divergence: The Meaning of Public Opinion on Government Spending in Red and Blue." *Perspectives on Politics* 19(3): 824–37. DOI: https://doi.org /10.1017/S1537592720003588.

Kriner, Douglas L., and Andrew Reeves. 2012. "The Influence of Federal Spending on Presidential Elections." *American Political Science Review* 106(2): 348–66.

———. 2014. "Responsive Partisanship: Public Support for the Clinton and Obama Health Care Plans." *Journal of Health Politics, Policy, and Law* 39(4): 717–49.

———. 2015. "Presidential Particularism and Divide-the-Dollar Politics." *American Political Science Review* 109(1): 155–71.

Kristol, William. 1993. "William Kristol's 1993 Memo: Defeating President Clinton's Health Care Proposal." Project for the Republican Future, December 2. https://www.scribd .com/document/12926608/William-Kristol-s-1993-Memo-Defeating-President-Clinton -s-Health-Care-Proposal.

Krupnikov, Yanna, and John Barry Ryan. 2022. *The Other Divide: Polarization and Disengagement in American Politics*. Cambridge: Cambridge University Press.

Kumlin, Staffan. 2004. *The Personal and the Political: How Personal Welfare State Experiences Affect Political Trust and Ideology*. New York: Palgrave Macmillan.

Kushner Gadarian, Shana, Sara Wallace Goodman, and Thomas B. Pepinsky. 2021. "Partisanship, Trumpism, and Health Behavior in the Covid-19 Pandemic: Evidence from Panel Data." *PloS ONE* 16(4): e0249596. DOI: https://doi.org/10.1371 /journal.pone.0249596.

LaCasse, Alex. 2017. "After Five Vetoes from Gov. LePage, Maine Residents Will Vote on Medicaid Expansion." *Governing*, October 31, 2017. https://www.governing.com /archive/gov-maine-citizens-vote-medicaid-expansion.html.

Ladd, Jonathan M. 2012. *Why Americans Hate the Media and How It Matters*. Princeton, N.J.: Princeton University Press.

Lakoff, George. 1981. *Metaphors We Live By*. Chicago: University of Chicago Press.

———. 2004. *Don't Think of an Elephant! Know Your Values and Frame the Debate— The Essential Guide for Progressives*. White River Junction, Vt: Chelsea Green Publishing.

Lane, Robert E. 1962. *Political Ideology: Why the American Common Man Believes What He Does*. New York: Free Press of Glencoe.

Lanford, Daniel, and Jill Quadagno. 2016. "Implementing ObamaCare: The Politics of Medicaid Expansion under the Affordable Care Act of 2010." *Sociological Perspectives* 59(3): 619–39. DOI: https://doi.org/10.1177/0731121415587605.

Lantz, Paula M., and Sara Rosenbaum. 2020. "The Potential and Realized Impact of the Affordable Care Act on Health Equity." *Journal of Health Politics, Policy, and Law* 45(5): 831–45. DOI: https://doi.org/10.1215/03616878-8543298.

Lapinski, John S., and Gregory A. Huber. 2008. "Testing the Implicit-Explicit Model of Racialized Political Communication." *Perspectives on Politics* 6(1): 125–34.

Larsen, Erik Gahner. 2019. "Policy Feedback Effects on Mass Publics." *Policy Studies Journal* 47(2): 372–94.

Lassman, David, Micah Hartman, Benjamin Washington, Kimberly Andrews, and Aaron Catlin. 2014. "U.S. Health Spending Trends by Age and Gender: Selected Years 2002–10." *Health Affairs* 33(5): 815–22. DOI: https://doi.org/10.1377/hlthaff.2013.1224.

Lauderdale, Benjamin E., and Tom S. Clark. 2014. "Scaling Politically Meaningful Dimensions Using Texts and Votes." *American Journal of Political Science* 58(3): 754–71.

Lawrence, Regina G., and Matthew L. Schafer. 2012. "Debunking Sarah Palin: Mainstream News Coverage of 'Death Panels.'" *Journalism* 13(6): 766–82. DOI: https://doi.org /10.1177/1464884911431389.

Lecheler, Sophie, Claes H. de Vreese, and Rune Slothuus. 2009. "Issue Importance as a Moderator of Framing Effects." *Communication Research* 36(3): 400–425.

Lee, Frances E. 2009. *Beyond Ideology: Politics, Principles, and Partisanship in the U.S. Senate.* Chicago: University of Chicago Press.

———. 2016. *Insecure Majorities: Congress and the Perpetual Campaign.* Chicago: University of Chicago Press.

Lee, Peter V., Vishaal Pegany, James Scullary, and Colleen Stevens. 2017. "Marketing Matters: Lessons from California to Promote Stability and Lower Costs in National and State Individual Insurance Markets." Covered California, September. http://hbex .coveredca.com/data-research/library/CoveredCA_Marketing_Matters_9-17.pdf.

Lee, Taeku. 2002. *Mobilizing Public Opinion: Black Insurgency and Racial Attitudes in the Civil Rights Era.* Chicago: University of Chicago Press.

Leeper, Thomas J., and Rune Slothuus. 2018. "Can Citizens Be Framed? How Persuasive Information More than Emphasis Framing Changes Political Opinions." Working paper, June.

Lenz, Gabriel. 2012. *Follow the Leader? How Voters Respond to Politicians' Policies and Performance.* Chicago: University of Chicago Press.

Leonhardt, David. 2019. "The GOP Promotes Leftism." *New York Times*, April 17, 2019, https://www.nytimes.com/2019/04/17/opinion/progressive-democrats-republicans -2020.html.

Lerman, Amy E. 2019. *Good Enough for Government Work: The Public Reputation Crisis in America (and What We Can Do to Fix It).* Chicago: University of Chicago Press.

Lerman, Amy E., and Katherine T. McCabe. 2017. "Personal Experience and Public Opinion." *Journal of Politics* 79(2): 624–41.

Lerman, Amy E., Meredith Sadin, and Samuel Trachtman. 2017. "Policy Uptake as Political Behavior: Evidence from the Affordable Care Act." *American Political Science Review* 111(4): 755–70.

Lerman, Amy E., and Samuel Trachtman. 2021. "Where Policies and Politics Diverge: Awareness, Assessments, and Attribution in the ACA." *Public Opinion Quarterly* 84(2): 419–45. DOI: https://doi.org/10.1093/poq/nfaa028.

Lerman, Amy E., and Vesla Weaver. 2014. *Arresting Citizenship: The Democratic Consequences of American Crime Control.* Chicago: University of Chicago Press.

Levendusky, Matthew S. 2009. *The Partisan Sort: How Liberals Became Democrats and Conservatives Became Republicans.* Chicago: University of Chicago Press.

———. 2010. "Clearer Cues, More Consistent Voters: A Benefit of Elite Polarization." *Political Behavior* 32(1): 111–31. https://doi.org/10.1007/s11109-009-9094-0.

Levine, Adam Seth. 2015. *American Insecurity: Why Our Economic Fears Lead to Political Inaction.* Princeton, N.J.: Princeton University Press.

Levine, Phillip B., and Diane Schanzenbach. 2009. "The Impact of Children's Public Health Insurance Expansions on Educational Outcomes." *Forum for Health Economics and Policy* 12(1). DOI: https://doi.org/10.2202/1558-9544.1137.

Levitsky, Steven, and Daniel Ziblatt. 2018. *How Democracies Die.* New York: Crown.

Levy, Helen, Andrew Ying, and Nicholas Bagley. 2020. "What's Left of the Affordable Care Act? A Progress Report." *RSF: The Russell Sage Foundation Journal of the Social Sciences* 6(2): 42–66. DOI: https://doi.org/10.7758/RSF.2020.6.2.02.

Lieberman, Robert C. 1998. *Shifting the Color Line: Race and the American Welfare State.* Cambridge, Mass.: Harvard University Press.

Lieberman, Robert C., Suzanne Mettler, Thomas B. Pepinsky, Kenneth M. Roberts, and Richard Valelly. 2019. "The Trump Presidency and American Democracy: A Historical and Comparative Analysis." *Perspectives on Politics* 17(2): 470–79. DOI: https://doi.org/10.1017/S1537592718003286.

Lilla, Mark. 2018. *The Once and Future Liberal: After Identity Politics.* New York: Oxford University Press.

Lippmann, Walter. 1922. *Public Opinion.* New York: Harcourt, Brace & Co.

Liptak, Adam. 2021. "Affordable Care Act Survives Latest Supreme Court Challenge." *New York Times,* June 17, 2021. https://www.nytimes.com/2021/06/17/us/obamacare-supreme-court.html.

Lizza, Ryan. 2011. "Romney's Dilemma." *New Yorker,* May 30, 2011. https://www.newyorker.com/magazine/2011/06/06/romneys-dilemma.

Lodge, Milton, and Charles S. Taber. 2013. *The Rationalizing Voter.* New York: Cambridge University Press.

Lundberg, Kristjen B., B. Keith Payne, Josh Pasek, and Jon A. Krosnick. 2017. "Racial Attitudes Predicted Changes in Ostensibly Race-Neutral Political Attitudes under the Obama Administration." *Political Psychology* 38(2): 313–30. DOI: https://doi.org/10.1111/pops.12315.

Lupia, Arthur. 2016. *Uninformed: Why People Know So Little about Politics and What We Can Do about It.* New York: Oxford University Press.

Lynch, James Q. 2020. "Tom Harkin: 2020 Election about Health Care." *Gazette,* September 23, 2020. https://www.thegazette.com/government-politics/tom-harkin-2020-election-about-health-care/.

Lynch, Julia. 2020. *Regimes of Inequality: The Political Economy of Health and Wealth.* Cambridge: Cambridge University Press.

Lynch, Julia, and Sarah E. Gollust. 2010. "Playing Fair: Fairness Beliefs and Health Policy Preferences in the United States." *Journal of Health Politics, Policy, and Law* 35(6): 849–87.

MacGuill, Dan. 2017. "Did Nancy Pelosi Say Obamacare Must Be Passed to 'Find Out What Is in It'?" *Snopes,* June 22. https://www.snopes.com/fact-check/pelosi-healthcare-pass-the-bill-to-see-what-is-in-it/.

Malhotra, Neil, Yotam Margalit, and Cecilia Hyunjung Mo. 2013. "Economic Explanations for Opposition to Immigration: Distinguishing between Prevalence and Magnitude." *American Journal of Political Science* 57(2): 391–410. DOI: https://doi.org/10.1111/ajps.12012.

Manning, Christopher D., Prabhakar Raghavan, and Hinrich Schütze. 2008. *Introduction to Information Retrieval.* Cambridge: Cambridge University Press.

Mansbridge, Jane J. 1986. *Why We Lost the ERA.* Chicago: University of Chicago Press.

Mansfield, Edward D., and Diana C. Mutz. 2009. "Support for Free Trade: Self-Interest, Sociotropic Politics, and Out-Group Anxiety." *International Organization* 63(3): 425–57. DOI: https://doi.org/10.1017/S0020818309090158.

Marble, William, and Clayton Nall. 2018. "Where Interests Trump Ideology: The Persistent Influence of Homeownership in Local Development Politics." October 22. http://www .nallresearch.com/uploads/7/9/1/7/7917910/interest.3.3.pdf.

Margalit, Yotam. 2013. "Explaining Social Policy Preferences: Evidence from the Great Recession." *American Political Science Review* 107(1): 80–103.

Marmor, Theodore R. 1973. *The Politics of Medicare.* Chicago: Aldine Publishing Co.

Mason, Lilliana. 2018. *Uncivil Agreement: How Politics Became Our Identity.* Chicago: University of Chicago Press.

Mayer, Martin, Robert Kenter, and John C. Morris. 2015. "Partisan Politics or Public-Health Need? An Empirical Analysis of State Choice during Initial Implementation of the Affordable Care Act." *Politics and the Life Sciences: The Journal of the Association for Politics and the Life Sciences* 34(2): 44–51. DOI: https://doi.org/10.1017/pls.2015.15.

McCabe, Katherine T. 2016. "Attitude Responsiveness and Partisan Bias: Direct Experience with the Affordable Care Act." *Political Behavior* 38(4): 861–82.

———. 2019. "The Persistence of Racialized Health Care Attitudes: Racial Attitudes among White Adults and Identity Importance among Black Adults." *Journal of Race, Ethnicity, and Politics* 4(2): 378–98.

McCarty, Nolan. 2019. *Polarization: What Everyone Needs to Know.* New York: Oxford University Press.

McCarty, Nolan, Keith T. Poole, and Howard Rosenthal. 2006. *Polarized America: The Dance of Ideology and Unequal Riches.* Cambridge, Mass.: MIT Press.

McDonough, John E. 2015. "The Demise of Vermont's Single-Payer Plan." *New England Journal of Medicine* 372(17): 1584–85. DOI: https://doi.org/10.1056/NEJMp1501050.

McGhee, Heather C. 2021. *The Sum of Us: What Racism Costs Everyone and How We Can Prosper Together.* New York: One World.

McKean, Benjamin Laing. 2020. *Disorienting Neoliberalism: Global Justice and the Outer Limit of Freedom.* New York: Oxford University Press.

McKenna, Ryan M., Brent A. Langellier, Héctor E. Alcalá, Dylan H. Roby, David T. Grande, and Alexander N. Ortega. 2018. "The Affordable Care Act Attenuates Financial Strain According to Poverty Level." *INQUIRY: The Journal of Health Care Organization, Provision, and Financing* 55(January): 0046958018790164.

McWhorter, John. 2021. *Woke Racism: How a New Religion Has Betrayed Black America.* London: Swift Press.

Mendelberg, Tali. 2001. *The Race Card: Campaign Strategy, Implicit Messages, and the Norm of Equality.* Princeton, N.J.: Princeton University Press.

———. 2008. "Racial Priming Revived." *Perspectives on Politics* 6(1): 109–23.

Mettler, Suzanne. 2005. *Soldiers to Citizens: The GI Bill and the Making of the Greatest Generation.* New York: Oxford University Press.

———. 2011. *The Submerged State: How Invisible Government Policies Undermine American Democracy.* Chicago: University of Chicago Press.

————. 2018. *The Government-Citizen Disconnect.* New York: Russell Sage Foundation.

————. 2019. "Making What Government Does Apparent to Citizens: Policy Feedback Effects, Their Limitations, and How They Might Be Facilitated." *Annals of the American Academy of Political and Social Science* 685(1): 30–46.

Mettler, Suzanne, Lawrence R. Jacobs, and Ling Zhu. 2022. "Policy Threat, Partisanship, and the Case of the Affordable Care Act." *American Political Science Review.* DOI: https://doi.org/10.1017/S0003055422000612.

Metzl, Jonathan M. 2019. *Dying of Whiteness: How the Politics of Racial Resentment Is Killing America's Heartland.* New York: Basic Books.

Michener, Jamila D. 2017. "People, Places, Power: Medicaid Concentration and Local Political Participation." *Journal of Health Politics, Policy, and Law* 42(5): 865–900.

————. 2018. *Fragmented Democracy: Medicaid, Federalism, and Unequal Politics.* New York: Cambridge University Press.

————. 2019a. "Medicaid and the Policy Feedback Foundations for Universal Healthcare." *Annals of the American Academy of Political and Social Science* 685(1): 116–34.

————. 2019b. "Policy Feedback in a Racialized Polity." *Policy Studies Journal* 47(2): 423–50.

————. 2020. "Race, Politics, and the Affordable Care Act." *Journal of Health Politics, Policy, and Law* 45(4): 547–66.

Mildenberger, Matto. 2020. *Carbon Captured: How Business and Labor Control Climate Politics.* Cambridge, Mass.: MIT Press.

Miller, James. 2018. *Can Democracy Work? A Short History of a Radical Idea, from Ancient Athens to Our World.* New York: Farrar, Straus and Giroux.

Miller, Joanne M., and Jon A. Krosnick. 2000. "News Media Impact on the Ingredients of Presidential Evaluations: Politically Knowledgeable Citizens Are Guided by a Trusted Source." *American Journal of Political Science* 44(2): 301–15.

Morgan, Kimberly J., and Andrea L. Campbell. 2011. *The Delegated Welfare State: Medicare, Markets, and the Governance of Social Policy.* New York: Oxford University Press.

Morgan, Stephen L., and Christopher Winship. 2007. *Counterfactuals and Causal Inference.* New York: Cambridge University Press.

Morrisey, Michael. 2013. *Health Insurance,* 2nd ed. Chicago: Health Administration Press.

Morton, Rebecca B., and Kenneth C. Williams. 2010. *Experimental Political Science and the Study of Causality: From Nature to the Lab.* Cambridge: Cambridge University Press.

Munger, Kevin M. 2022. *Generation Gap: Why the Baby Boomers (Still!) Dominate American Politics and Culture.* New York: Columbia University Press.

Murray, John E. 2007. *Origins of American Health Insurance: A History of Industrial Sickness Funds.* New Haven, Conn.: Yale University Press.

Mutz, Diana C. 1992. "Mass Media and the Depoliticization of Personal Experience." *American Journal of Political Science* 36(2): 483–508.

————. 1994. "Contextualizing Personal Experience: The Role of Mass Media." *Journal of Politics* 56(3): 689–714.

————. 2011. *Population-Based Survey Experiments.* Princeton, N.J.: Princeton University Press.

————. 2015. *In-Your-Face Politics: The Consequences of Uncivil Media.* Princeton, N.J.: Princeton University Press.

————. 2018. "Status Threat, Not Economic Hardship, Explains the 2016 Presidential Vote." *Proceedings of the National Academy of Sciences* 115(19): E4330–39.

Nadash, Pamela, Edward Alan Miller, David K. Jones, Michael K. Gusmano, and Sara Rosenbaum. 2018. "A Series of Unfortunate Events: Implications of Republican Efforts to Repeal and Replace the Affordable Care Act for Older Adults." *Journal of Aging and Social Policy* 30(3/4): 259–81.

Naím, Moisés. 2013. *The End of Power: From Boardrooms to Battlefields and Churches to States, Why Being in Charge Isn't What It Used to Be*. New York: Basic Books.

Nall, Clayton. 2018. *The Road to Inequality: How the Federal Highway Program Polarized America and Undermined Cities*. Cambridge: Cambridge University Press.

National Public Radio. 2012. "Medicaid Expansion Hangs on Justices' Scale." *All Things Considered*, NPR, March 28, 2012. https://www.npr.org/2012/03/28/149556743/medicaid -expansion-hangs-on-justices-scale.

Nelson, Thomas. 2011. "Issue Framing." In *The Oxford Handbook of American Public Opinion and the Media*, edited by Robert Y. Shapiro and Lawrence R Jacobs. New York: Oxford University Press.

Nelson, Thomas E., Rosealee A. Clawson, and Zoe M. Oxley. 1997. "Media Framing of a Civil Liberties Conflict and Its Effect on Tolerance." *American Political Science Review* 91(3): 567–83.

New York Times. 2010. "Election 2010: House Exit Polls." *New York Times*. https://www .nytimes.com/elections/2010/results/house/exit-polls.html.

Noel, Hans. 2014. *Political Ideologies and Political Parties in America*. New York: Cambridge University Press.

Norris, Louise. 2021. "What Was the Goal of the ACA's Cadillac Tax and Why Was It Repealed?" Verywell Health, December 22. https://www.verywellhealth.com/what-is -the-aca-cadillac-tax-4092993.

Nyhan, Brendan. 2010. "Why the 'Death Panel' Myth Wouldn't Die: Misinformation in the Health Care Reform Debate." *Forum* 8(1): 1–24.

Nyhan, Brendan, Eric McGhee, John Sides, Seth Masket, and Steven Greene. 2012. "One Vote Out of Step? The Effects of Salient Roll Call Votes in the 2010 Election." *American Politics Research* 40(5): 844–79.

Oberlander, Jonathan. 2003. *The Political Life of Medicare*. Chicago: University of Chicago Press.

O'Donnell, Jayne. 2014. "The Doctor Won't See You Now; Some Obamacare Patients Are Finding Doors Shut to Them." *USA Today*, October 28, 2014.

Ogilvy. 2018. "Health Care Press Coverage 2017 Enrollment Period vs. 2018 Enrollment." Prepared for Covered California. January 18. https://board.coveredca.com/meetings /2018/01-18/Ogilvy-Enrollment_Coverage_Measurement-Final-01-18-18.pdf.

Ogorzalek, Thomas K. 2018. *The Cities on the Hill: How Urban Institutions Transformed National Politics*. Oxford: Oxford University Press.

O'Keefe, Ed. 2014. "The House Has Voted 54 Times in Four Years on Obamacare. Here's the Full List." *Washington Post*, March 21, 2014. https://www.washingtonpost.com/news /the-fix/wp/2014/03/21/the-house-has-voted-54-times-in-four-years-on-obamacare-heres -the-full-list/.

Orr, Lilla V., and Gregory A. Huber. 2020. "The Policy Basis of Measured Partisan Animosity in the United States." *American Journal of Political Science* 64(3): 569–86.

Pacheco, Julianna, Jake Haselswerdt, and Jamila Michener. 2020. "The Affordable Care Act and Polarization in the United States." *RSF: The Russell Sage Foundation Journal of the Social Sciences* 6(2): 114–30. DOI: https://doi.org/10.7758/RSF.2020.6.2.05.

Pacheco, Julianna, and Elizabeth Maltby. 2017. "The Role of Public Opinion—Does It Influence the Diffusion of ACA Decisions?" *Journal of Health Politics, Policy, and Law* 42(2): 309–40.

———. 2019. "Trends in State-Level Opinions toward the Affordable Care Act." *Journal of Health Politics, Policy, and Law* 44(5): 737–64.

Page, Benjamin I., and Robert Y. Shapiro. 1992. *The Rational Public: Fifty Years of Trends in Americans' Policy Preferences.* Chicago: University of Chicago Press.

Parker, Christopher S., and Matt A. Barreto. 2014. *Change They Can't Believe In: The Tea Party and Reactionary Politics in America,* rev. ed. Princeton, N.J.: Princeton University Press.

Patashnik, Eric M. 2008. *Reforms at Risk: What Happens after Major Policy Changes Are Enacted.* Princeton, N.J.: Princeton University Press.

———. 2019. "Limiting Policy Backlash: Strategies for Taming Countercoalitions in an Era of Polarization." *Annals of the American Academy of Political and Social Science* 685(1): 47–63.

Patashnik, Eric, and Jonathan Oberlander. 2018. "After Defeat: Conservative Postenactment Opposition to the ACA in Historical-Institutional Perspective." *Journal of Health Politics, Policy, and Law* 43(4): 651–82.

Patashnik, Eric M., and Julian E. Zelizer. 2013. "The Struggle to Remake Politics: Liberal Reform and the Limits of Policy Feedback in the Contemporary American State." *Perspectives on Politics* 11(4): 1071–87.

Payne, Stanley L. 1951. *The Art of Asking Questions.* Princeton, N.J.: Princeton University Press.

Pear, Robert. 2015. "Marco Rubio Quietly Undermines Affordable Care Act." *New York Times,* December 9, 2015. https://www.nytimes.com/2015/12/10/us/politics/marco-rubio-obamacare-affordable-care-act.html.

Pearl, Judea. 2000. *Causality: Models, Reasoning, and Inference.* Cambridge: Cambridge University Press.

Peck, Reece. 2019. *Fox Populism: Branding Conservatism as Working Class.* Cambridge: Cambridge University Press.

Peffley, Mark, Jon Hurwitz, and Paul M. Sniderman. 1997. "Racial Stereotypes and Whites' Political Views of Blacks in the Context of Welfare and Crime." *American Journal of Political Science* 41(1): 30–60.

Perlstein, Rick. 2012. "Exclusive: Lee Atwater's Infamous 1981 Interview on the Southern Strategy." *Nation,* November 13, 2012. https://www.thenation.com/article/archive/exclusive-lee-atwaters-infamous-1981-interview-southern-strategy/.

Peterson, Robert. 2017. "Medicaid Expansion Critical to Uninsured and Viability of Rural Hospitals." Millinocket Regional Hospital. https://www.mrhme.org/medicaid-expansion-critical-to-uninsured-and-viability-of-rural-hospitals/.

Pew Research Center. 2010. "2010 U.S. Religious Knowledge Survey." Pew Forum on Religion and Public Life, September 28. https://www.pewresearch.org/religion/2010/09/28/u-s-religious-knowledge-survey/.

Peyton, Kyle. 2020. "Does Trust in Government Increase Support for Redistribution? Evidence from Randomized Survey Experiments." *American Political Science Review* 114(2): 596–602.

Peyton, Kyle, and Gregory Huber. 2020. "Racial Resentment, Prejudice, and Discrimination." *Journal of Politics* 83(4): 1829–36.

Pierson, Paul. 1993. "When Effect Becomes Cause: Policy Feedback and Political Change." *World Politics* 45(4): 595–628.

———. 1994. *Dismantling the Welfare State? Reagan, Thatcher, and the Politics of Retrenchment.* Cambridge: Cambridge University Press.

Pildes, Richard H. 2021. "The Age of Political Fragmentation." *Journal of Democracy* 32(4): 146–59.

Politifact. 2020. "Obama: 'If You Like Your Health Care Plan, You'll Be Able to Keep Your Health Care Plan.'" https://www.politifact.com/obama-like-health-care-keep/.

Pollitz, Karen, Jennifer Tolbert, and Maria Diaz. 2019. "Limited Navigator Funding for Federal Marketplace States." Kaiser Family Foundation, November 19. https://web.archive.org/web/20210301104442/https://www.kff.org/private-insurance/issue-brief/data-note-further-reductions-in-navigator-funding-for-federal-marketplace-states/.

Polsky, Daniel, and Janet Weiner. 2015. "The Skinny on Narrow Networks in Health Insurance Marketplace Plans." Robert Wood Johnson Foundation website, June 23. https://www.rwjf.org/en/library/research/2015/06/the-skinny-on-narrow-networks-in-health-insurance-marketplace-pl.html.

Pomerantsev, Peter. 2015. *Nothing Is True and Everything Is Possible: The Surreal Heart of the New Russia.* New York: PublicAffairs.

Popkin, Samuel. 1994. *The Reasoning Voter: Communication and Persuasion in Presidential Campaigns.* Chicago: University of Chicago Press.

Porter, Ethan, and Thomas J. Wood. 2019. *False Alarm: The Truth about Political Mistruths in the Trump Era.* Cambridge: Cambridge University Press.

Porter, M. F. 1980. "An Algorithm for Suffix Stripping." *Program: Electronic Library and Information Systems* 14(3): 130–37.

Pratto, Felicia, Jim Sidanius, Lisa M. Stallworth, and Bertram F. Malle. 1994. "Social Dominance Orientation: A Personality Variable Predicting Social and Political Attitudes." *Journal of Personality and Social Psychology* 67(4): 741–63.

Prior, Markus. 2007. *Post-Broadcast Democracy: How Media Choice Increases Inequality in Political Involvement and Polarizes Elections.* New York: Cambridge University Press.

Putnam, Robert D. 2000. *Bowling Alone: The Collapse and Revival of American Community.* New York: Simon & Schuster.

———. 2007. "E Pluribus Unum: Diversity and Community in the 21st Century: The 2006 Johan Skytte Prize Lecture." *Scandinavian Political Studies* 30(2): 137–74.

Putnam, Robert D., and Shaylyn R. Garrett. 2020. *The Upswing: How America Came Together a Century Ago and How We Can Do It Again.* New York: Simon & Schuster.

Quadagno, Jill. 1994. *The Color of Welfare: How Racism Undermined the War on Poverty*. New York: Oxford University Press.

Quinn, Kevin M., Burt L. Monroe, Michael Colaresi, Michael H. Crespin, and Dragomir R. Radev. 2010. "How to Analyze Political Attention with Minimal Assumptions and Costs." *American Journal of Political Science* 54(1): 209–28.

Rabe, Barry G. 2018. *Can We Price Carbon?* Cambridge, Mass.: MIT Press.

Rae, Matthew, Cynthia Cox, Gary Claxton, Daniel McDermott, and Anthony Damico. 2021. "How the American Rescue Plan Act Affects Subsidies for Marketplace Shoppers and People Who Are Uninsured." Kaiser Family Foundation, March 25. https://www.kff.org/health-reform/issue-brief/how-the-american-rescue-plan-act-affects-subsidies-for-marketplace-shoppers-and-people-who-are-uninsured/.

Reny, Tyler T., and David O. Sears. 2020. "Symbolic Politics and Self-Interest in Post–Affordable Care Act Health Insurance Coverage." *Research and Politics* 7(3). DOI: https://doi.org/10.1177/2053168020955108.

Richardson, Lilliard, and David M. Konisky. 2013. "Personal and Collective Evaluations of the 2010 Health Care Reform." *Journal of Health Politics, Policy, and Law* 38(5): 921–56.

Ridout, Travis N., and Michael M. Franz. 2011. *The Persuasive Power of Campaign Advertising*. Philadelphia: Temple University Press.

Riffkin, Rebecca. 2015. "Americans with Government Health Plans Most Satisfied." Gallup, November 6. https://news.gallup.com/poll/186527/americans-government-health-plans-satisfied.aspx.

Rigby, Elizabeth, and Jake Haselswerdt. 2013. "Hybrid Federalism, Partisan Politics, and Early Implementation of State Health Insurance Exchanges." *Publius: The Journal of Federalism* 43(3): 368–91.

Roberts, Margaret E., Brandon M. Stewart, Dustin Tingley, Christopher Lucas, Jetson Leder-Luis, Shana Kushner Gadarian, Bethany Albertson, and David G. Rand. 2014. "Structural Topic Models for Open-Ended Survey Responses." *American Journal of Political Science* 58(4): 1064–82.

Rocco, Philip, and Simon F. Haeder. 2018. "How Intense Policy Demanders Shape Post-reform Politics: Evidence from the Affordable Care Act." *Journal of Health Politics, Policy, and Law* 43(2): 271–304.

Rocco, Philip, and Andrew S. Kelly. 2020. "An Engine of Change? The Affordable Care Act and the Shifting Politics of Demonstration Projects." *RSF: The Russell Sage Foundation Journal of the Social Sciences* 6(2): 67–84. DOI: https://doi.org/10.7758/RSF.2020.6.2.03.

Rodden, Jonathan. 2022. "The Great Recession and the Public Sector in Rural America." Working paper. Stanford University.

Rose, Shanna. 2015. "Opting In, Opting Out: The Politics of State Medicaid Expansion." *Forum* 13(1): 63–82.

Rosen, Eva. 2020. *The Voucher Promise: "Section 8" and the Fate of an American Neighborhood*. Princeton, N.J.: Princeton University Press.

Rosenthal, Andrew. 2012. "Romney Blames Loss on Obama 'Gifts.'" *New York Times*, November 14, 2012. https://takingnote.blogs.nytimes.com/2012/11/14/romney-blames-loss-on-obama-gifts/.

Rosenthal, Elisabeth. 2022. "The End of the Covid Emergency Could Mean a Huge Loss of Health Insurance." *New York Times*, April 4, 2022. https://www.nytimes.com/2022/04/04/opinion/covid-medicaid-loss.html.

Roubein, Rachel. 2020. "Oklahoma Voters Approve Medicaid Expansion as Coronavirus Cases Climb." *Politico*, July 1, 2020. https://www.politico.com/news/2020/07/01/oklahoma-expand-medicaid-pandemic-346681.

Roy, Avik. 2014. "ACA Architect: 'The Stupidity of the American Voter' Led Us to Hide Obamacare's True Costs from the Public." *Forbes*, November 10, 2014. https://www.forbes.com/sites/theapothecary/2014/11/10/aca-architect-the-stupidity-of-the-american-voter-led-us-to-hide-obamacares-tax-hikes-and-subsidies-from-the-public/.

Ruffin, David C. 2003. "Getting Back the Black Vote." *Black Enterprise*, October 1, 2003. https://www.blackenterprise.com/getting-back-the-black-vote/.

Rutenberg, Jim, and Jackie Calmes. 2009. "False 'Death Panel' Rumor Has Some Familiar Roots." *New York Times*, August 14, 2009. https://www.nytimes.com/2009/08/14/health/policy/14panel.html.

Saldin, Robert P. 2017. *When Bad Policy Makes Good Politics: Running the Numbers on Health Reform.* New York: Oxford University Press.

Saltzman, Evan. 2019. "Demand for Health Insurance: Evidence from the California and Washington ACA Exchanges." *Journal of Health Economics* 63(January): 197–222.

Samuelson, William, and Richard Zeckhauser. 1988. "Status Quo Bias in Decision Making." *Journal of Risk and Uncertainty* 1(1): 7–59.

Sances, Michael, and Joshua Clinton. 2019. "Who Participated in the ACA?" *Journal of Health Politics, Policy, and Law* 44(3): 349–79. DOI: https://doi.org/10.1215/03616878-7366988.

———. 2020. "Policy Effects, Partisanship, and Elections: How Medicaid Expansion Affected Public Opinion toward the Affordable Care Act." *Journal of Politics* 83(2): 498–514.

Sayers, Freddie. 2021. "David Shor: College Liberals Have Hijacked the Democratic Party." *UnHerd*, August 13, 2021. https://unherd.com/thepost/david-shor-college-liberals-have-hijacked-the-democratic-party/.

Schaffner, Brian F., Matthew Macwilliams, and Tatishe Nteta. 2018. "Understanding White Polarization in the 2016 Vote for President: The Sobering Role of Racism and Sexism." *Political Science Quarterly* 133(1): 9–34.

Schattschneider, E. E. 1935. *Politics, Pressures, and the Tariff: A Study of Free Private Enterprise in Pressure Politics, as Shown in the 1929–1930 Revision of the Tariff.* New York: Prentice-Hall.

Scherer, Michael. 2010. "The White House Scrambles to Tame the News Cyclone." *Time*, March 4, 2010. https://content.time.com/time/subscriber/article/0,33009,1969723,00.html.

Scheufele, Dietram A., and Shanto Iyengar. 2012. "The State of Framing Research: A Call for New Directions." In *The Oxford Handbook of Political Communication Theories*, edited by Robert Y. Shapiro and Lawrence Jacobs. New York: Oxford University Press.

Schickler, Eric. 2016. *Racial Realignment: The Transformation of American Liberalism, 1932–1965.* Princeton, N.J.: Princeton University Press.

Schlozman, Daniel. 2015. *When Movements Anchor Parties: Electoral Alignments in American History.* Princeton, N.J.: Princeton University Press.

Schumpeter, Joseph A. 1943. *Capitalism, Socialism, and Democracy.* London: Routledge.

Schuyler, Michael. 2014. "A Short History of Government Taxing and Spending in the United States." Tax Foundation, February 19. https://taxfoundation.org/short-history -government-taxing-and-spending-united-states/.

Sears, David O., and Jack Citrin. 1982. *Tax Revolt: Something for Nothing in California.* Cambridge, Mass.: Harvard University Press.

Sears, David O., and Carolyn L. Funk. 1991. "The Role of Self-Interest in Social and Political Attitudes." *Advances in Experimental Social Psychology* 24(1): 1–91.

Segers, Grace. 2021. "McCarthy Says GOP Members Are Concerned Cheney Can't 'Carry Out the Message.'" *CBS News,* May 5, 2021. https://www.cbsnews.com/news/liz-cheney -kevin-mccarthy-republican-party-message/.

Sekhon, Jasjeet S. 2009. "Opiates for the Matches: Matching Methods for Causal Inference." *Annual Review of Political Science* 12(1): 487–508.

Sen, Maya, and Omar Wasow. 2016. "Race as a Bundle of Sticks: Designs That Estimate Effects of Seemingly Immutable Characteristics." *Annual Review of Political Science* 19(1): 499–522.

Shafer, Paul R., David M. Anderson, Seciah M. Aquino, Laura M. Baum, Erika Franklin Fowler, and Sarah E. Gollust. 2020. "Competing Public and Private Television Advertising Campaigns and Marketplace Enrollment for 2015 to 2018." *RSF: The Russell Sage Foundation Journal of the Social Sciences* 6(2): 85–112. DOI: https://doi.org/10.7758 /RSF.2020.6.2.04.

Shapiro, Robert Y., and Lawrence Jacobs. 2010. "Simulating Representation: Elite Mobilization and Political Power in Health Care Reform." *Forum* 8(1): 1–15.

Shiller, Robert J. 2019. *Narrative Economics.* Princeton, N.J.: Princeton University Press.

Sides, John, Michael Tesler, and Lynn Vavreck. 2019. *Identity Crisis: The 2016 Presidential Campaign and the Battle for the Meaning of America.* Princeton, N.J.: Princeton University Press.

Sides, John, Lynn Vavreck, and Christopher Warshaw. 2022. "The Effect of Television Advertising in United States Elections." *American Political Science Review* 116(2): 702–18.

Simmons-Duffin, Selena. 2021. "12 Holdout States Haven't Expanded Medicaid, Leaving 2 Million People in Limbo." *All Things Considered,* NPR, July 1, 2021. https://www.npr .org/sections/health-shots/2021/07/01/1011502538/12-holdout-states-havent-expanded -medicaid-leaving-2-million-people-in-limbo.

Skocpol, Theda. 1996. "The Rise and Resounding Demise of the Clinton Health Security Plan." In *The Problem That Won't Go Away: Reforming U.S. Health Care Financing,* edited by Henry J. Aaron. Washington, D.C.: Brookings Institution.

———. 1997. *Boomerang: Health Care Reform and the Turn against Government.* New York: W. W. Norton & Co.

———. 2003. *Diminished Democracy: From Membership to Management in American Civic Life.* Norman: University of Oklahoma Press.

———. 2013. "Naming the Problem: What It Will Take to Counter Extremism and Engage Americans in the Fight against Global Warming." Prepared for the symposium on "The Politics of America's Fight against Global Warming," Harvard University, February 14.

Skocpol, Theda, and Vanessa Williamson. 2016. *The Tea Party and the Remaking of Republican Conservatism*. New York: Oxford University Press.

Slothuus, Rune, and Claes H. de Vreese. 2010. "Political Parties, Motivated Reasoning, and Issue Framing Effects." *Journal of Politics* 72(3): 630–45.

Smith, Allan. 2021. "Trump Booed at Alabama Rally after Telling Supporters to Get Vaccinated." NBC, August 22, 2021. https://www.nbcnews.com/politics/donald-trump/trump-booed-alabama-rally-after-telling-supporters-get-vaccinated-n1277404.

Smith, Mark A. 2007. *The Right Talk: How Conservatives Transformed the Great Society into the Economic Society*. Princeton, N.J.: Princeton University Press.

Smith, Rogers M. 1997. *Civic Ideals: Conflicting Visions of Citizenship in U.S. History*. New Haven, Conn.: Yale University Press.

Sniderman, Paul M., and Edward Carmines. 1997. *Reaching beyond Race*. Cambridge, Mass.: Harvard University Press.

Sniderman, Paul M., and Douglas B. Grob. 1996. "Innovations in Experimental Design in Attitude Surveys." *Annual Review of Sociology* 22(August): 377–99.

Sniderman, Paul M., and Thomas Piazza. 1993. *The Scar of Race*. Cambridge, Mass.: Harvard University Press.

Sniderman, Paul M., and Sean M. Theriault. 2004. "The Structure of Political Argument and the Logic of Issue Framing." In *Studies in Public Opinion: Attitudes, Nonattitudes, Measurement Error, and Change*, edited by Willem E. Saris and Paul M. Sniderman. Princeton, N.J.: Princeton University Press.

Snowden, Lonnie, and Genevieve Graaf. 2019. "The 'Undeserving Poor,' Racial Bias, and Medicaid Coverage of African Americans." *Journal of Black Psychology* 45(3): 130–42.

Sommers, Benjamin D., Atul A. Gawande, and Katherine Baicker. 2017. "Health Insurance Coverage and Health—What the Recent Evidence Tells Us." *New England Journal of Medicine* 377(6): 586–93.

Sommers, Benjamin D., Bethany Maylone, Robert J. Blendon, E. John Orav, and Arnold M. Epstein. 2017. "Three-Year Impacts of the Affordable Care Act: Improved Medical Care and Health among Low-Income Adults." *Health Affairs* 36(6): 1119–28.

Soroka, Stuart N. 2006. "Good News and Bad News: Asymmetric Responses to Economic Information." *Journal of Politics* 68(2): 372–85.

Soss, Joe. 1999. "Lessons of Welfare: Policy Design, Political Learning, and Political Action." *American Political Science Review* 93(2): 363–80.

Soss, Joe, Richard C. Fording, and Sanford F. Schram. 2011. *Disciplining the Poor: Neoliberal Paternalism and the Persistent Power of Race*. Chicago: University of Chicago Press.

Soss, Joe, and Sanford F. Schram. 2007. "A Public Transformed? Welfare Reform as Policy Feedback." *American Political Science Review* 101(1): 111–27.

Soss, Joe, and Vesla Weaver. 2016. "Learning from Ferguson: Welfare, Criminal Justice, and the Political Science of Race and Class." In *The Double Bind: The Politics of Racial and Class Inequalities in the Americas: A Report of the Task Force on Racial and Social Class,* edited by Juliet Hooker and Alvin B. Tillery Jr. Washington, D.C.: American Political Science Association.

Stanek, Becca. 2017. "Lindsey Graham Insists His Health-Care Bill Is the Only Thing Standing between America and Socialism." *Week*, September 19, 2017. https://theweek .com/speedreads/725599/lindsey-graham-insists-healthcare-bill-only-thing-standing -between-america-socialism.

Starr, Paul. 1982. *The Social Transformation of American Medicine: The Rise of a Sovereign Profession and the Making of a Vast Industry.* New York: Basic Books.

———. 1995. "What Went Wrong with Health Reform." *American Prospect* 20: 20–31.

———. 1997. "The Clinton Presidency, Take Three." *American Prospect* 30: 7.

Steinhauer, Jennifer, and Robert Pear. 2011. "GOP Newcomers Set Out to Undo Obama Victories." *New York Times*, January 2, 2011. https://www.nytimes.com/2011/01/03/us /politics/03repubs.html.

Steinmo, Sven, and Jon Watts. 1995. "It's the Institutions, Stupid! Why Comprehensive National Health Insurance Always Fails in America." *Journal of Health Politics, Policy, and Law* 20(2): 329–72.

Stelter, Brian. 2012. "CNN and Fox Trip Up in Rush to Get the News on the Air." *New York Times*, June 29, 2012. https://www.nytimes.com/2012/06/29/us/cnn-and-foxs-supreme -court-mistake.html.

Stephens-Dougan, LaFleur. 2020. *Race to the Bottom: How Racial Appeals Work in American Politics.* Chicago: University of Chicago Press.

Stimson, James. 2004. *Tides of Consent: American Government, Politics, and Policy.* New York: Cambridge University Press.

Stokes, Leah Cardamore. 2020. *Short Circuiting Policy: Interest Groups and the Battle over Clean Energy and Climate Policy in the American States.* New York: Oxford University Press.

Stroud, Natalie Jomini. 2011. *Niche News: The Politics of News Choice.* New York: Oxford University Press.

Supreme Court of the United States. 2015. "King et al. v. Burwell, Secretary of Health and Human Services et al.: Certiorari to the United States Court of Appeals for the Fourth Circuit." No. 14-114. Argued March 4, 2015, decided June 25, 2015. https://www .supremecourt.gov/opinions/14pdf/14-114_qol1.pdf.

Svallfors, Stefan. 2007. *The Political Sociology of the Welfare State: Institutions, Social Cleavages, and Orientations.* Stanford, Calif.: Stanford University Press.

Taber, Charles S., and Milton Lodge. 2006. "Motivated Skepticism in the Evaluation of Political Beliefs." *American Journal of Political Science* 50(3): 755–69.

Tallevi, Ashley. 2018. "Out of Sight, Out of Mind? Measuring the Relationship between Privatization and Medicaid Self-Reporting." *Journal of Health Politics, Policy, and Law* 43(2): 137–83.

Tesler, Michael. 2012. "The Spillover of Racialization into Health Care: How President Obama Polarized Public Opinion by Racial Attitudes and Race." *American Journal of Political Science* 56(3): 690–704.

———. 2015. "Priming Predispositions and Changing Policy Positions: An Account of When Mass Opinion Is Primed or Changed." *American Journal of Political Science* 59(4): 806–24.

————. 2016. *Post-Racial or Most-Racial? Race and Politics in the Obama Era.* Chicago: University of Chicago Press.

Tesler, Michael, and David O. Sears. 2010. *Obama's Race: The 2008 Election and the Dream of a Post-Racial America.* Chicago: University of Chicago Press.

Tikkanen, Roosa, and Melinda K. Abrams. 2020. "U.S. Health Care from a Global Perspective, 2019." Commonwealth Fund, January 30. https://www.commonwealthfund.org /publications/issue-briefs/2020/jan/us-health-care-global-perspective-2019.

Tilly, Charles. 2002. *Stories, Identities, and Political Change.* Lanham, Md.: Rowman & Littlefield.

Time. 1965. "Nation: Dr. Ward's Last Words." May 21, 1965. http://content.time.com/time /subscriber/article/0,33009,901686,00.html.

Tocqueville, Alexis de. 1863. *Democracy in America.* Cambridge, Mass.: Sever and Francis.

Tolkien, J.R.R. 1991. *The Lord of the Rings.* London: HarperCollins.

Trachtman, Samuel. 2018. "Polarization, Participation, and Policy Performance: The Case of ACA Marketplaces." May 10. DOI: http://dx.doi.org/10.2139/ssrn.3081991.

Trende, Sean. 2012. *The Lost Majority: Why the Future of Government Is Up for Grabs—and Who Will Take It.* New York: St. Martin's Press.

Trussler, Marc, and Stuart Soroka. 2014. "Consumer Demand for Cynical and Negative News Frames." *International Journal of Press/Politics* 19(3): 360–79.

Tufte, Edward R. 1978. *Political Control of the Economy.* Princeton, N.J.: Princeton University Press.

Tversky, Amos, and Daniel Kahneman. 1991. "Loss Aversion in Riskless Choice: A Reference-Dependent Model." *Quarterly Journal of Economics* 106(4): 1039–61.

U.S. Census Bureau. 2020. *American Community Survey, 2013–2017.* Washington: U.S. Department of Commerce. https://www.census.gov/programs-surveys/acs.

Valentino, Nicholas A. 1999. "Crime News and the Priming of Racial Attitudes during Evaluations of the President." *Public Opinion Quarterly* 63(3): 293–320.

Valentino, Nicholas A., Vincent L. Hutchings, and Ismail K. White. 2002. "Cues That Matter: How Political Ads Prime Racial Attitudes during Campaigns." *American Political Science Review* 96(1): 75–90.

Valentino, Nicholas A., Fabian G. Neuner, and L. Matthew Vandenbroek. 2017. "The Changing Norms of Racial Political Rhetoric and the End of Racial Priming." *Journal of Politics* 80(3): 757–71.

Vavreck, Lynn. 2009. *The Message Matters: The Economy and Presidential Campaigns.* Princeton, N.J.: Princeton University Press.

Verba, Sidney, Kay Lehman Schlozman, and Henry E. Brady. 1995. *Voice and Equality: Civic Volunteerism in American Politics.* Cambridge, Mass.: Harvard University Press.

Volden, Craig. 2006. "States as Policy Laboratories: Emulating Success in the Children's Health Insurance Program." *American Journal of Political Science* 50(2): 294–312.

Weaver, Vesla M., and Amy E. Lerman. 2010. "Political Consequences of the Carceral State." *American Political Science Review* 104(4): 817–33.

Weisman, Jonathan, and Robert Pear. 2013. "Cancellation of Health Care Plans Replaces Website Problems as Prime Target." *New York Times*, October 30, 2013. https://www.nytimes.com/2013/10/30/us/politics/cancellation-of-health-care-plans-replaces-website-problems-as-prime-target.html.

Wesleyan Media Project. 2018. "2018: The Health Care Election." October 18. http://mediaproject.wesleyan.edu/releases/101818-tv/.

Westwood, Sean J., and Erik Peterson. 2020. "The Inseparability of Race and Partisanship in the United States." *Political Behavior* (October 8).

Wetts, Rachel, and Robb Willer. 2018. "Privilege on the Precipice: Perceived Racial Status Threats Lead White Americans to Oppose Welfare Programs." *Social Forces* 97(2): 793–822.

Whaley, Christopher M., Jonathan Cantor, Megan Pera, and Anupam B. Jena. 2021. "Assessing the Association between Social Gatherings and Covid-19 Risk Using Birthdays." *JAMA Internal Medicine* 181(8): 1090–99.

Wherry, Laura R., and Sarah Miller. 2016. "Early Coverage, Access, Utilization, and Health Effects Associated with the Affordable Care Act Medicaid Expansions." *Annals of Internal Medicine* 164(12): 795–803.

White, Ismail K. 2007. "When Race Matters and When It Doesn't: Racial Group Differences in Response to Racial Cues." *American Political Science Review* 101(2): 339–54.

White House. 2021. "Executive Order on Strengthening Medicaid and the Affordable Care Act." The White House. January 28. https://www.whitehouse.gov/briefing-room/presidential-actions/2021/01/28/executive-order-on-strengthening-medicaid-and-the-affordable-care-act/.

Wilkerson, Isabel. 2020. *Caste: The Origins of Our Discontents*. New York: Random House.

Winter, Nicholas J. G. 2006. "Beyond Welfare: Framing and the Racialization of White Opinion on Social Security." *American Journal of Political Science* 50(2): 400–420.

———. 2008. *Dangerous Frames: How Ideas about Race and Gender Shape Public Opinion*. Chicago: University of Chicago Press.

Witters, Dan. 2019. "U.S. Uninsured Rate Rises to Four-Year High." Gallup, January 23. https://news.gallup.com/poll/246134/uninsured-rate-rises-four-year-high.aspx.

Wlezien, Christopher. 1995. "The Public as Thermostat: Dynamics of Preferences for Spending." *American Journal of Political Science* 39(4): 981–1000.

Yokum, David, Daniel J. Hopkins, Andrew Feher, Elana Safran, and Joshua Peck. 2022. "Effectiveness of Behaviorally Informed Letters on Health Insurance Marketplace Enrollment: A Randomized Clinical Trial." *JAMA Health Forum* 3(3): e220034.

Zaller, John R. 1992. *The Nature and Origins of Mass Opinion*. New York: Cambridge University Press.

———. 2012. "What Nature and Origins Leaves Out." *Critical Review* 24(4): 569–642.

Zelizer, Julian E. 2000. *Taxing America: Wilbur D. Mills, Congress, and the State, 1945–1975*. Cambridge: Cambridge University Press.

Zingher, Joshua N. 2022. *Political Choice in a Polarized Era: How Elite Polarization Shapes Mass Behavior*. New York: Oxford University Press.

INDEX

Tables and figures are listed in **boldface**.

Achen, Christopher, 44
Advance Premium Tax Credit subsidies, 2, 30, 93
Affordable Care Act (ACA). *See* Patient Protection and Affordable Care Act
Alabama, exit polls on racial attitudes, 135–37, **136**, 252*n*76
Ambrose, Stephen, 178
American Community Survey (ACS), 70, 238–39*n*23, 241*n*35
American Health Care Act (AHCA, 2017), 38
American Rescue Plan (ARP), 40, 112, 180
America's Bitter Pill (Brill), 85
Atwater, Lee, 117

Banks, Antoine, 121
Bartels, Larry, 44
Baucus, Max, 31
Bevin, Matt, 82, 98
Biden, Joe: on ACA, 65; Covid-19 pandemic policies and, 180; reversing Trump administration decisions on ACA, 40
Brill, Steven, 85
Broockman, David, 151
Brown, Scott, 32
Bush, George W., 91–92

California v. Texas (2021), 41
Campbell, Andrea L., 9, 91, 93, 245*n*41
Carmines, Edward, 120
Cassidy, Bill, 38, 39
Caughey, Devin, 184
Children's Health Insurance Program (CHIP), 26
Child Tax Credit, 180
Chong, Dennis, 231–32*n*14
climate change legislation, 16–17
Clinton, Bill: health insurance reform attempts, 1–2, 25–26, 28, 154; welfare reform, 117–18
Clinton, Hillary, 25, 26–27
Clinton, Joshua, 246*n*57
Collins, Susan, 22, 39
Community Living Assistance Services and Supports (CLASS) Plan, 33
Congress. *See specific legislation*
Converse, Philip, 19
Cooper, Jim, 28
Covid-19 pandemic: American Rescue Plan, 40, 112, 180; government overreach and, 56; health care access and, 9; Medicaid use increase during, 65; policy feedbacks, effects on public opinion, 180; political polarization and, 180
Cruz, Ted, 35
Cunha, Darlena, 130

Democratic Party: 2008 election and, 27; 2014 midterm elections and, 4; 2016 election and, 4–5; 2018 midterm elections and, 5; ACA as political liability, 2–3; ACA expansion possibilities, 177–78; ACA political saga and, 31–33; Covid-19 pandemic policies and, 180; framing effects and, 159–64, **161**, 257*n*83, 257*n*85; health care reform proposals, 15–16, 25; political messaging of, 2, 145–46, 252*n*2; racial attitudes and, 118–19, 128–29; socioeconomic status of voters and, 68; welfare reform, 117–18. *See also* Obama, Barack; political elites

discrimination: in insurance premium rates by sex, 2, 124; pre-existing conditions and, 2, 90

distrust of government and support for ACA, 151–57, **156**

Don't Think of an Elephant (Lakoff), 145

Druckman, James N., 147, 231–32*n*14

Dying of Whiteness (Metzl), 114

Edwards, George, 3

Ehrlichman, John, 250*n*20

election data, 66–73, 240*n*17

Emanuel, Rahm, 32

employer mandate of ACA, 235*n*1

exchanges. *See* health insurance exchanges

Fein, Jordan, 147

framing effects. *See* political messaging/ framing

Frean, Molly, 184

Gollust, Sarah, 162

Goren, Paul, 117

government overreach, 2–3, 55–56

Graham, Lindsey, 22, 39

Greene, Brian, 176

Gregory, Emily, 137

Grimmer, Justin, 159

Gruber, Jonathan, 8, 184

Harbin, Brielle, 137

Harkin, Tom, 55

Haselswerdt, Jake, 250*n*23

health care costs, 23–24

healthcare.gov, 35, 91

health insurance: benefits of, 9–10; cancellations of ACA noncompliant plans, 10, 35, 87, 89, 97; discrimination and, 2, 90, 124; employer-provided, 24, 235*n*1; lifetime caps on insurance payments, 2, 32; population gaps in coverage, 24, 28–29, 117; pre-existing conditions and, 2, 5, 9, 29, 38, 59, 90; price increases resulting from ACA, 102–4, **103**; private, 15–16; risk corridor payments for, 36. *See also* Medicaid; Medicare

health insurance exchanges, 19, 85–113; ACA attitudes by insurance type, 99–102, **100**, 207–10, **208–10**; complexity of ACA and, 92–94; Covid-19 relief legislation and, 112; creation of, 29–30; discontinuity for older adults, 104–8, **106**, **108**, 217, **217–18**; government messaging on, 172–74, **174**; implementation of, 33; Kentucky, ACA attitudes in, 98–99; overview, 91–92; policy feedbacks and, 89, 90–92; political partisanship and usage of, 92, 246*n*57; price increases and, 102–4, **103**, **215–16**; public opinion on, 4, 59; research design and data sets on, 94–97, **95**, **96**, 246*n*55; risk corridor payments for participation in, 36; tax credits and, 30; website issues, 35, 91; young adults remaining on parents' insurance, 109–10, **110**

health insurance reform, 18, 22–42; Clinton administration and, 1–2, 25–26, 28, 154; history of, 23–24; lead-up to ACA, 26–28. *See also* Patient Protection and Affordable Care Act

health insurance sources, data on, 96, **96**, **205**, 246*n*57

Health Tracking Poll (HTP): on ACA favorability and price changes, 102–3, **103**, **215–16**, 247–48*nn*76–77; on ACA favorability by insurance status, 96, **96**; on ACA favorability of dependent children, 109–10, **110**; on ACA favorability of older adults, 105–8, **106**, **108**; on attitudes toward ACA after Trump election, 79–80; on attitudes toward ACA in 2015, 4–5; on attitudes toward ACA in Medicaid expansion states, 75–77, **76**; on attitudes toward ACA over time, **50**, 50–51, 239*n*28; on benefits or harm of ACA, **96**, 205–7, **206**; distribution of respondents by insurance type, 95, **95**; on insurance sources of older adults, 105; overview, 50

Hetherington, Marc, 154

Hiltzik, Michael, 3

Hobbs, William R., 85, 88, 245*n*29, 247*n*65, 249*n*96, 252*n*73

Hopkins, Daniel, 238*n*23, 245*n*29, 247*n*65, 249*n*96

Imbens, Guido W., 249*n*94

individual mandate of ACA: adverse selection, limiting, 29–30, 91, 183, 245*n*42; creation of, 29–30, 91; election data on, 240*n*17; elimination of, 40, 91, 183–84; fines resulting from, 10, 12, 19, 87, 91; negativity biases, 94; politicians' changed positions on, 41–42; public opinion on, 56, 59–60, 183–84; Supreme Court decision on, 33–35, 86

Inflation Reduction Act (IRA, 2022), 16–17, 112, 181

Institute for the Study of Citizens and Politics (ISCAP) survey: dates and sample sizes, 191, **192**; demographics of respondents, 191, **193**; overview, 48, 238–39*n*23; repealing ACA, data on support for, 48–49, **48**, 99–101, **100**, 183; on who benefits from ACA, 122–26, **123**

Jacobs, John, 64

Jacobs, Lawrence, 74, 89

Johnson, Lyndon, 24

Jones, Doug, 135

Kagan, Elena, 34

Kaiser Family Foundation (KFF): on Kentucky's insurance exchange, 98, 246*n*61; on Medicaid expansion, 69, 118; open-ended questions on health care

reform, 149, 258*nn*90–91; on preexisting health conditions, 9; on public support for ACA, 59; on voter participation of Medicaid recipients, 82–83. *See also* Health Tracking Poll

Kalla, Joshua, 151

Kalyanaraman, Karthik, 249*n*94

Kamh, Cindy, 3

Kentucky: insurance exchanges, attitudes on, 98–99, 246*n*61; voter participation of Medicaid recipients in, 82–83

Kimmel, Jimmy, 38, 46

King v. Burwell (2015), 36

Klein, Ezra, 51–52, 235*n*96

Kliff, Sarah, 46–47

Knowledge Networks (KN), 154, **156**, 157, 255–56*n*64, 255*n*60

Kristol, Bill, 1–2, 113

Lakoff, George, 145

latent Dirichlet allocation (LDA), 158–62, **161**, 256*n*69, 256*n*71

Lee, Frances, 185

Leeper, Thomas, 147

Leonhardt, David, 16

LePage, Paul, 69

Lerman, Amy E., 246*n*57

Levy, Helen, 33

Lieberman, Joe, 31–32

Lippmann, Walter, 44–45

Lodge, Milton, 153

Luntz, Frank, 146, 164

Lupia, Arthur, 46

Lynch, Julia, 162

Magaziner, Ira, 25

Maine, Medicaid expansion in, 68–71, **71**, 118, **200**, 241–42*n*37

Manchin, Joe, 137

Margolis, Michele, 135, 137

Massachusetts, health insurance mandate in, 26, 41

McCabe, Katherine, 74

McCain, John, 22–23, 39

McCarthy, Kevin, 253*n*4

McConnell, Mitch, 38

McDonough, John, 232*n*17

media: control over political elites'
rhetoric, 148; coverage of health care
reform, 159, 257*n*75; coverage of political
battles over ACA, 92; increase in access
to, 238*n*9; political elites' framing effects
and, 158–64, **160–61**, **227**, 257*n*76,
258*n*86. *See also* political messaging/
framing
Medicaid: benefits to society, 64–65;
customer satisfaction with, 74; eligibility
for, 24; prescription drug program, 26;
race and ethnicity of enrollees, 13; work
requirements for, 40, 188
Medicaid expansion, 19, 64–84;
implementation of, 33; incentives for
states, 40; income cap for eligibility,
243*n*56; income of survey respondents,
77, 242–43*nn*55; in Maine, 68–71, **71**, 118,
200; in Oklahoma, 71–73, **73**, **201**;
policy feedbacks from, 65–66, 73–79,
76, 82–83, **202**; popularity of, 4, 12, 59,
67, 69, 115, 118, 179; racial attitudes and,
116–18, 144, 183; Republican attempts
to repeal, 38, 118; secondary limits on
feedback effects, 82–83; state ballot
measures on, 66, 69; states' responses to,
13, 66–67, 183, 240*n*16; Supreme Court
decision on, 33–35, 66, 86, 116; Trump's
election and attitudes toward, 79–82, **81**,
203; uninsured covered by, 2, 9, 29, 86
Medical Expenditure Panel Survey, 245*n*26
Medicare, 24, 105–8, 129–30, 162, 248*n*84
Medicare Modernization Act (MMA, 2003),
26, 91–92
The Message Matters (Vavreck), 147
Mettler, Suzanne, 74, 89
Metzl, Jonathan, 114
Michener, Jamila, 117
Mills, Wilbur, 24
Morgan, Kimberly, 91
Mummolo, Jonathan, 148, 158–59
Murkowski, Lisa, 22, 39

*National Federation of Independent Business
v. Sebelius* (2012), 34–35, 56, 66, 86, 116
The Nature and Origins of Mass Opinion
(Zaller), 3, 6, 148

negativity biases, 94, 246*n*54
Nelson, Ben, 31–32
neoliberalism, 244*n*21
Noel, Hans, 181

Obama, Barack: 2012 election and, 35;
ACA as signature policy achievement of,
2, 116–17; cancellations of ACA-
noncompliant plans and, 35;
congressional address on health care,
148; health insurance reform and, 2–3,
27–28, 32; on individual mandate, 27,
40, 41–42, 183; political messaging as
Senate candidate, 145; on popularity of
ACA, 51–52
Obamacare. *See* Patient Protection and
Affordable Care Act
Oklahoma, Medicaid expansion in, 71–73,
73, **201**
older adults and insurance exchanges, 90,
104–8, **106**, **108**, 217, **217–18**, 245*n*26,
248*nn*85–86
online surveys on racial attitudes, 137–39,
138, **140**

Palin, Sarah, 3, 28, 147, 167
Parish, Kalind, 137
Patient Protection and Affordable Care Act
(ACA, 2010): Advance Premium Tax
Credit subsidies of, 2, 30, 93; benefits
and features of, 2, 9–10, 28–31; employer
mandate, 235*n*1; expansion options for,
177–78; future policy battles over, 187–89;
implementation issues, 35, 87–88, 245*n*29;
lead-up to passage of, 26–28; legal
challenges to (*see* Supreme Court);
opposition to, 2–5, 13, 27–28, 33, 35–36,
129–30, 235*n*96; passage of, 2, 15; political
attitudes toward, 11–13; political saga of,
31–35; post-implementation issues, 36–41;
goal of study, 15–18; repeal attempts, 5,
22–23, 36–41, 60–61, 80, 118, 182–84,
188; states' responses to, 13, 36, 38, 116
(*see also specific states*). *See also* health
insurance exchanges; Medicaid expansion;
political messaging/framing; public
opinion; individual mandate of ACA

Pelosi, Nancy, 32, 59, 145
personal experiences: political attitudes and, 11–13, 75; salient social groups and, 57–59, **58**
Peterson, Robert, 241*n*37
Pew Research Center, 18, 52, 149, 258*nn*90–91
policy advocates, lessons for, 185–86
policy feedbacks: defined, 231*n*4; electoral gain and, 21; evaluating, 94–97, **95, 96**; heterogeneity of ACA's effects and, 112; indirect policies and, 87, 89–94, 108, 113, 244*n*12, 245*n*41; insurance exchanges and, 89, 90–92; from Medicaid expansion, 66–68, 73–79, **76**, 82–83, **202**; political actors' expectations of, 35; political science implications, 186–87; public opinion, effect on, 1–4, 6–7, 179–80, 231*n*4; research on, 2, 177–78
political elites: Covid-19 pandemic and rhetoric of, 180; defined, 231–32*n*14, 232*n*30; diffusion of language to public, 167–72, **169, 171**, 258–59*nn*93–95; framing effects and, 152–53, 158–64, **160–61**, 167, **227**, 254*n*47; partisanship and, 78, 181; public opinion, effect on, 3, 5–8, 12–13, 62–63, 148, 179–80, 259*n*7; racial attitudes, influence on, 14, 127–28; racialization and, 115; survey data on influence of, 55
political messaging/framing, 20, 145–76; defined, 151, 231–32*n*14, 254*n*40; diffusion of language from elites to public, 167–72, **169, 171**; effectiveness of, 3–4, 145–48, 178, 232*n*17, 253*n*26; electoral gain and, 21; government messaging on insurance exchanges, 172–74, **174**; observational data and results, 158–64, **160–61**; open-ended responses, analyzing, 164–67, **166, 229**; open-ended survey responses and, 158, **227**; political science implications, 186–87; prior research on, 151–53; public opinion, effect on, 6–7; racial attitudes and, 128–29, 250*n*20; trust in government and support for ACA, 151–57, **156, 226, 228–29**

political partisanship: ACA repeal attitudes, tracking over time, 47–49, **48**; attitudes toward ACA and, 11–13, 75, 85–86, 243*n*66; attitudes toward Medicaid expansion and, 72–73; climate change policy and, 16; Covid-19 pandemic and, 180; framing effects and, 152–53; insurance exchange usage and, 92, 246*n*57; political awareness and, 147–48; political elites and, 78, 181; public opinion, effect on, 7–8, 46–47; racial attitudes and, 118–20, 128–29, **220**
political science, implications for studying, 186–87
Pomerantsev, Peter, 146
poverty. *See* socioeconomic status
pre-existing conditions, insurance access based on: ACA guarantee of coverage, 5, 29, 38; discrimination and, 2, 90; public opinion on, 9, 59
prescription drug costs, 91–92, 124
priming effects: exit polls on racial attitudes, 135–37, **136**, 252*n*76; online surveys on racial attitudes, 137–39, **138, 140**; on political activists, 140–41, **141**; racial attitudes and attitudes on ACA, 125–29, **127**; results of, 143; on Trump supporters, 141–42, **142**
public opinion, 18–19, 43–63; on ACA, 4–5; complex issues and, 44–47, 144; HTP data on, 50–52, **50**; on Medicaid expansion (*see* Medicaid expansion); on Medicare Modernization Act, 92; personal experiences and political attitudes, 11–13, 75; personal experiences and salient social groups, 57–59, **58**; policy advocates, lessons for, 185–86; policy feedbacks, effect on, 1–4, 6–7, 179–80, 231*n*4; political elites' effect on, 3, 5–8, 12–13, 62–63, 148, 179–80, 259*n*7; pro-ACA public opinion shift after election of Trump, 5, 7, 18, **48**, 49, 51, 181; purpose of study, 15–18; research conclusions, 61–63, 182–84; status quo bias and, 60–61, **62**; survey data on, 52–57, **53–54**, 191, **192–93**, 192–97; tracking respondents over time, 47–49, **48**; on

public opinion (*cont*)
    whole vs. parts of ACA, 59–60. *See also*
    policy feedbacks; political messaging/
    framing; racial attitudes
Public Opinion (Lippmann), 44–45

Quayle, Dan, 1

racial attitudes, 19–20, 114–44; Medicaid
    expansion and, 116–18, 144, 183; other
    policies compared to ACA and, 129–34,
    221–23; perceptions of ACA beneficiaries,
    122–25, **123–24**; political elites' use of,
    14, 127–28; population-based panel
    evidence, 125–29, **127**, **220**; public
    opinion on ACA and, 13–14, 179–80;
    racialization and, 118–21; survey
    experiments with priming effects,
    134–43, **136**, **138**, **140–42**; testing
    concepts of racialization, 121–22
Reagan, Ronald, 117
Reid, Harry, 31
Republican Party: 2016 election and, 4–5;
    2018 midterm elections and, 5; ACA
    political saga and, 31–33; attempts to
    repeal or weaken ACA, 5, 22–23, 36–41,
    60–61, 80, 118, 182–84, 188; framing
    effects and, 159–64, **161**, 257n85; health
    insurance reform attitudes, 1, 26–28;
    individual mandate, elimination of, 91,
    183–84; Medicaid expansion and, 36,
    116; Medicare Modernization Act and,
    91–92; opposition to ACA, 2–5, 13,
    27–28, 33, 35–36, 129–30, 235n96;
    political messaging of, 146, 253n4; racial
    attitudes and, 117, 118–19, 128–29,
    250n20. *See also* political elites; Trump,
    Donald
Research Now, 130
Roberts, John, 34–35
Robert Wood Johnson Foundation, 247n75
Rodden, Jonathan, 241n27
Romney, Mitt, 9–10, 26–27, 35, 41–42
Rubio, Marco, 36
rural hospitals, 69, 71–72, 241–42n37,
    241n27, 241n33
Ryan, Paul, 38

Sadin, Meredith, 246n57
salient social groups, survey data on, 57–59,
    58
Sances, Michael, 246n57
Sanders, Bernie, 15
selection biases, 94, 97, 99–100, 246n57
self-purchased insurance. *See* health
    insurance exchanges
seniors: insurance exchanges and, 104–8,
    106, **108**; support for ACA on behalf of,
    57, 124
Shor, David, 68
Shore-Sheppard, Lara, 245n41
Skocpol, Theda, 25, 129
Snowe, Olympia, 31
social safety net: middle-class dependence
    on, 1; opposition to, 69, 114, 129–30;
    public perception and stigma of, 74;
    racial attitudes and, 117, 120, 122, 131–34,
    132–33, **221–23**; welfare reform bill,
    117–18; work requirements for
    qualification, 40, 188, 250n23. *See also*
    specific programs
socioeconomic status: public opinion on
    ACA and, 57, 67; support for ACA on
    behalf of poor, 57; voter turnout and,
    68, 82–83. *See also* Medicaid expansion
Sommers, Benjamin, 184
Specter, Arlen, 31
Starr, Paul, 25–26
states' responses: to ACA, 13, 36, 38, 116;
    to Medicaid expansion, 13, 66–67, 183,
    240n16. *See also specific states*
status quo bias, 60–61, **62**
Steinmo, Sven, 26
Stimson, James, 120
Stupak, Bart, 32
Supreme Court: on individual mandate,
    33–35, 86; legal challenges to ACA, 33–37,
    41, 56, 86; on Medicaid expansion, 33–35,
    66, 86, 116
Survey Sampling International (SSI),
    60–61, 130, 137–39, 154, **156**, 255n64

Taber, Charles, 153
taxes: Advance Premium Tax Credit
    subsidies, 2, 30, 93; Cadillac Tax on

high-end health plans, 33; Child Tax Credit, 180; individual mandate penalty fees, 10, 87, 91; to pay for ACA, 2, 10, 30, 56, 59, 130; penalties for income increases, 87–88

Trachtman, Samuel, 246*n*57

Trapped in America's Safety Net (Campbell), 9

Trump, Donald: 2020 election and, 150, 181; attempts to repeal or weaken ACA, 37–41, 80, 182–83, 188; Medicaid expansion, public opinion after election, 79–82, **81**, **203**; opposition to ACA, 4–5; pro-ACA public opinion shift after election of, 5, 7, 18, **48**, 49, 51, 181

trust in government and support for ACA, 151–57, **156**, **226**, **228–29**, 255–56*nn*60–66

Undaunted Courage (Ambrose), 178

undocumented immigrants, 123–24

uninsured persons: ACA benefiting, 29, 95, **95**; favorability of ACA, **96**, 97; increase under Trump administration, 40, 188; public opinion on ACA and, 57, 90, 245*n*29; support for ACA on behalf of,

53, 57, 239*n*33; survey data on harm from ACA, 207, **208**; survey data on support for ACA, 99–101, **100**, 210–15, **211–14**, 247*n*68, 260*n*3. *See also* Medicaid expansion

Vavreck, Lynn, 147

voters: exit polls on racial attitudes, 135–37, **136**, 252*n*76; participation rates, 11, 68, 82–83

Warnock, Raphael, 177

Warshaw, Christopher, 184

Washington, Samantha, 238*n*23

Watts, Jon, 26

welfare. *See* social safety net

West Virginia, exit polls on racial attitudes, 137

white Americans. *See* racial attitudes

Williamson, Vanessa, 129

Yokum, David, 148

young adults remaining on parents' insurance, 32, 109–10, **110**

Zaller, John, 3, 6, 148